Histories of Disability in Latin America

Histories of Disability in Latin America

Edited by Heather Vrana
and David Carey Jr.

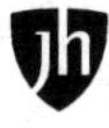

JOHNS HOPKINS UNIVERSITY PRESS   BALTIMORE

Johns Hopkins University Press
2715 North Charles Street
Baltimore, Maryland 21218
www.press.jhu.edu

Library of Congress Cataloging-in-Publication Data is available.
A catalog record for this book is available from the British Library.

ISBN 978-1-4214-5405-4 (paperback)
ISBN 978-1-4214-5406-1 (ebook)

Special discounts are available for bulk purchases of this book. For more information, please contact Special Sales at specialsales@jh.edu.

EU GPSR Authorized Representative
LOGOS EUROPE, 9 rue Nicolas Poussin, 17000, La Rochelle, France
E-mail: Contact@logoseurope.eu

For our teachers, *compas*, and students,
with hope for a more just world

Contents

Foreword

The Many Threads of Disability Woven Through Latin American History

Barbara Weinstein

To fully appreciate the moment in which this volume of essays is appearing with respect to the field of Latin American history, it might be useful to engage in a thought experiment and imagine how the category of disability or impairment would have been processed by historians and social scientists in the heyday of developmental nationalism (roughly, from the 1950s to the 1970s).[1] In the earlier stretch of that era, when scholars often regarded developmentalism as synonymous with modernization, disability would have been treated as a technical problem that could be solved or substantially mitigated with advances in hospital facilities or medical science. But even among Latin Americanists of a critical bent who emerged during the latter years of that era, the intense focus on social class as the principal category of resistance to capitalism and imperialism would have made disability, as an analytical category or subjectivity—much like race and gender—at best an "add-on" and at worst a distraction from class as the "true" basis for political consciousness.[2] Moreover, the analytical approach adopted by a historian studying disability at that time (if such a scholar had existed) would likely have started with the premise that Latin Americans, due to their neocolonial condition, would tend to have more numerous and more serious disabilities and suffer greater mistreatment or neglect because of insufficient public resources, government corruption, and a general *"atraso"* in developing new methods, treatments, and technologies.[3] And this lag, scholars would have been inclined to argue, would manifest itself both in the harsher experience of disability in Latin America and in the "belated" emergence of disability rights movements.

The point of this thought experiment is to highlight the degree to which it would have been difficult, if not impossible, to imagine a history of Latin America focused on disability back in the 1970s (when I began my training as a historian of Latin America); moreover, any such initiative, no matter how well intended, would likely have been freighted with certain Eurocentric assumptions about progress and development (despite the often fierce anti-imperialist rhetoric) that would have narrowed our historical perspective on disability. This is not to say that the developmentalist framework was entirely invalid. I can vividly recall, during my first stays in Brazil in the mid-to-late 1970s, being struck by the number of people I would routinely see with disabling conditions that would almost certainly have been surgically corrected soon after birth if that person had been born in the United States, as well as the many Brazilians with limited physical mobility who lacked access to wheelchairs and other assistive devices. And this was even more acutely the case when I went to live in Belém do Pará, then the largest urban center in the Amazon. The frequent sight of deformed bodies in public places became emblematic to me of the enduring inequalities—of caste, of class, of region—that had all worsened as a result of Brazil's long military dictatorship (1964–85) and that was indicative of the persistence of profound underdevelopment despite all the talk of a Brazilian economic miracle.[4] Even though today I no longer use the term "underdevelopment," and I understand aspects of the public visibility of disability differently (as I discuss below), I don't think those insights and reactions were completely off the mark.

Over the past half century, the field of history in general, and Latin American history in particular, has been reoriented in ways that have made us much more receptive to the types of approaches and interpretations offered in this volume. The intense focus on the categories of race and gender in recent decades (as well as, to a significant but lesser extent, sexual orientation), the questioning of stark binaries and a priori definitions, and the embrace of intersectionality have made it simultaneously more complex and more productive for historians to use "disability" as a category of analysis. And especially relevant for the Latin American historical context is the move toward decolonizing historical knowledge and decentering historical narratives, with the aim of recentering historical thinking so that Latin America is no longer relegated to the periphery of critical discussions about race, modernity, rights, and democracy.[5] And there has been a shift away from nation-centered research to more transnational and plurinational approaches that foreground Indigeneity and the African diaspora while also wrestling with questions of racialization and hybridity.

How do all of these new trends in historical thinking relative to Latin America create a more receptive academic environment for disability history? First, it means that the historical study of disability has broader implications than if it were just a move for recognition or inclusion in the pantheon of social movements. For example, the attention that several of the authors in this volume pay to degrees of "impairment" that might not initially register with many readers as equivalent to disability impels us to rethink boundaries between the able-bodied and the disabled previously treated as fixed and evident. And those kinds of impairments, which Julie Livingston and Jasbir K. Puar define as "debility,"[6] have impacted the minds and bodies of so many people—in some parts of the global south perhaps a majority—that "disability" becomes a category applicable to large swaths of the world's inhabitants. Indeed, considering the toxic and precarious working and living environments in which much of the earth's population finds employment and shelter, it is difficult to know how "able-bodied" would be defined beyond the wealthier nations.[7] The very same people performing the most physically taxing labor are the ones who are most likely to have damaged bodies, weakened lungs, and an assortment of chronic illnesses that, in a different context, would exempt them from heavy toil.

Given Latin America's unusually long history of "industrial" production—that is, large-scale colonial and neocolonial enterprises involving massive numbers of vulnerable or unprotected bodies engaged in often hazardous work under coercive conditions—the region's past offers mountains of evidence of work-related disabilities and debility. As early as the first century of Iberian imperial rule, we can point to the hundreds of thousands of Andean *mitayos* working in the fabled silver mines of Potosí in hair-raising circumstances, and even today, silicosis is a debilitating condition among those who continue to mine silver on the Cerro Rico. Early visitors to the New World's first major sugar economy, in the Brazilian Northeast, routinely noted the extreme hazards of work in the *engenhos*, where enslaved African and Indigenous workers could easily lose a limb while feeding cane into the crushing mechanisms or succumb to the extreme heat of the boiling houses. Every student of forced labor in the early modern Atlantic World is familiar with these accounts, but typically (and understandably) they are principally deployed to illustrate the horrors of human bondage in the context of a globalizing economy in the age of imperialism. Far less attention has been paid to what it meant for the Indigenous sending communities to care for the returning injured mine workers, and to what extent their injuries re-shaped broader attitudes about bodily difference; or to how maimed enslaved workers on sugar estates, no longer able to perform the primary tasks valued by their enslavers, managed to survive (or not).[8] To be sure, such questions might seem difficult or even impossible to answer given the nature of the archival evidence, but Adam Warren's article in this volume provides us with one path to illuminating how enslaved people claimed and portrayed their disabled status.

Similarly, the extended periods of continual, often low-intensity warfare that has characterized life in much of Latin America since the Conquest enables us to explore the relationship between disability, both physical and mental, and colonial and postcolonial violence. Moreover, the nature of "warfare" in Latin America—the vast majority of "wars" being internecine, not international, conflicts—has meant that those wounded and incapacitated, mentally or physically, rarely enjoy recognition as national heroes worthy of special care or state services. For the incapacitated former guerilla fighter there are few Latin American equivalents of the signs that for many years adorned the Paris Metro indicating certain seats as reserved for "*mutilés de guerre*"—a rather small token of national gratitude but a constant reminder of the veterans' heroic sacrifice. And some civilian casualties of Latin America's low-intensity conflicts, especially those who have been targets of sexual assaults, far from being consoled by public gratitude, struggle with physical and mental disabilities exacerbated by a deep sense of shame. Literary and cinematic works have focused in particular on sexual violence, typically portraying it as leading to degrees of madness among women victimized by men with guns. A recurring theme in the first segment of the classic Cuban film *Lucía* (1968), set during the war for independence, is a woman driven mad by the horrors of war and sexual violation. Some forty years later, the main character in the Peruvian film *La Teta Asustada* (*The Milk of Sorrow*) (2009) is portrayed as so disturbed by her mother's experience of repeated rape by soldiers during the campaign against Sendero Luminoso that her anxiety manifests as both mental and physical illness. Again, once we adopt a more capacious definition of disability or impairment and take into consideration the precarious circumstances of the regional populations, it becomes difficult to think of the disabled as a minority. And, as we can see in several of the chapters in this volume, even as medical conceptions of mental and physical impairment have radically changed over time, race and gender have continued to inform "expert" opinion about who is susceptible to what disease or disability.

But I want to avoid the implication that Latin America is of special interest to the historian of disability because its population has somehow been peculiarly damaged. As anyone who teaches Latin American history in the global north knows, it is easy to fall into the trap of making arguments that amount to a recitation of the region's social problems and to end up reinforcing negative stereotypes about Latin American society and culture. This tendency is particularly likely when we are discussing the hypervisible impact of violence, exploitation, and inequality. In effect, we run the risk of reinforcing pejorative stereotypes even as we seek to critique injustice and express sympathy and solidarity. Textual and visual examples abound, but for me the perfect illustration can be found in an inexpensive paperback published in São Paulo in 1984, *O que é Nordeste brasileiro?* (What is the Brazilian Northeast?). The image of the *nordestino* that accompanied the brief text was a drawing of a barefoot, stooped figure, bereft of any marker of modernity, over the caption "There are today, in the Northeast, more than 24 million Zecas-Tatu, the symbol of malnutrition, of laziness, of obstruction, of physical and mental incapacity."[9] In the guise of a compassionate portrayal of the long-suffering *nordestino*, the author offered a "diagnosis" that ended up placing the blame for regional atraso on the physical and mental deficiencies of the northeastern population. With this reiterative tendency in mind, it seems incumbent on historians of the global south who write about disability to avoid reproducing (unintentionally) such disparaging metaimages and to use with caution capacious categories like "debility."

To put it bluntly, might we consider whether there is a more "positive" perspective that can inform the study of Latin American history through the lens of disability? Going back to my discomfort with the sight of numerous disabled and divergent bodies in public spaces during my time in Belém do Pará, and my assumption that this reflected limited access to corrective surgeries in Brazilian Amazonia compared to the US (or even the Brazilian South), I would now suggest some other ways to reflect on my observations. One would be the possibility that this visibility indicated a higher degree of integration of disabled individuals into family life and social interaction, and a lesser inclination to warehouse or conceal disabled family members than was true at the time in the United States. Of course, poverty might limit recourse to institutional options, but historically, in the US, even low-income families have been known to resort to charity-financed institutionalization, either because of an inability to care for the disabled individual or for fear that the whole family would somehow be stigmatized or seen as "defective" for having a congenitally disabled family member. The purpose was often more to conceal divergent individuals from public scrutiny than to secure better care for them. So perhaps my observations, instead of being attributable to "atraso," were to some degree a reflection of cultural difference that we might assign a positive valence, as well as my own discomfort at the unaccustomed public display of disability.

To be sure, it is always risky to speak of "culture," or in this case, to overgeneralize or essentialize when speaking of "cultural" attitudes about mental and physical disabilities, and especially the acceptance (or not) of divergent bodies. Even as I was contemplating, back in the 1970s, the persistence of "correctible" physical disabilities in Belém, a phenomenon then easily interpreted as emblematic of atraso, countries like Brazil and Colombia were becoming ground zero for affordable (and cutting-edge) cosmetic surgery, thus demonstrating how problematic it would be to adopt a one-dimensional view of Latin American society.[10] The Brazilian plastic surgeon Ivo Pitanguy became a celebrated public figure not only for his skill at correcting perceived aesthetic defects but also for operating free of charge on burn and accident victims. How does an increasing obsession with the perfect face and body (including among women and men from relatively modest backgrounds), and the normalization of cosmetic-surgical "upgrades," impact perceptions of physical difference and reshape cultural attitudes about disability? Could it normalize potentially excessive surgical interventions to render disability less visible? How do we understand the simultaneous preoccupation with enforcing mainstream beauty standards and the growing rate of obesity in Brazil and other Latin American societies as processed foods have become an ever greater portion of the daily diet? And at what point does obesity transition from being seen as an undesirable physical trait to being categorized as a public health problem or even as a disabling condition?[11] Indeed, the signs in the Rio de Janeiro subway cars that indicate seating priority for, besides the usual cast of characters (the elderly, the physically disabled, pregnant women), the obese and people with autism strike me as raising uncomfortable questions about both visibility and sensitivity. It is perfectly possible that organized groups agitated for the inclusion of these two categories (which do not appear on the equivalent notices in any US context with which I am familiar) and that they reflect a broader Brazilian acceptance of accommodations for neurodivergent minds and nonstandardized bodies. But, to me, their inclusion inevitably begs certain awkward questions: How is the person giving up their seat expected to identify a passenger with autism, a disability that is often "invisible"? And who is responsible for identifying an individual as sufficiently overweight to deserve priority in seating? Ultimately, this inclusiveness—surely intended to signal sensitivity to the needs of the "incapacitated" broadly defined—may end up demonstrating a profound insensitivity to the way such categories operate and stigmatize in the context of social interaction.

As for the intersection of disability history and labor history, which has been the focus of much recent research, here again we can discern tendencies—actual and potential—that might be described, with some simplification, as negative and positive. Shopfloor accidents and work-related illnesses may be more frequent and severe in Latin America, where both domestic and foreign firms are less likely to be monitored or penalized for violations of workplace safety. During the decades of rapid industrialization in Brazil (roughly the 1950s through the 1980s), the country's manufacturing sector had the dubious distinction of being regularly described as the world champion in industrial accidents.[12] But there may also be fewer barriers to disabled workers engaging in occupations that would be closed to them in the more regulated global north. I recently took a taxi to an airport in Colombia and noticed that the driver, who appeared utterly in control of the vehicle, had deformed hands. It seemed highly unlikely to me that someone with this particular disability or, perhaps more accurately, this sort of physical difference, would have been licensed to drive a taxi anywhere in North America. In other words, in some situations adaptive attitudes may be more transformative than adaptive technologies.

As several chapters in this volume exemplify, the Latin American historical context also enables us to consider the intersection of Indigeneity and disability, and how Indigenous perspectives have informed attitudes about treatment or correction of physical or mental impairments. The plurinational character (whether officially or informally) of numerous Latin American nations allows us to think critically about our stubborn faith in "Western" expertise and progress with regard to disability. Historical and anthropological studies of Latin America have created particularly rich spaces for innovative research on African and Indigenous medical practices.[13] For example, Sidney Chalhoub's rethinking of the 1904 Revolt Against the Vaccine in Rio de Janeiro, by foregrounding the persistence of alternative medical forms of immunization, possibly derived from African practices, provides a way of understanding popular rejection of the smallpox vaccine that focuses on the actual medical issue, rather than treating it as a stand-in for other social concerns.[14] By the same token, we might consider to what extent Indigenous and African cultural practices produced different attitudes about disabilities as well as different treatments, or whether such conditions needed to be "treated" in the first place. But as Heather Vrana's chapter on disability and the guerilla struggle in El Salvador indicates, we cannot assume that non-Western identities automatically imply a preference for more natural or traditional healing practices. Conversely, Indigenous cultures that have rejected treatments that mainstream medicine regards as best practices for physical or mental disabilities may pose legal and ethical dilemmas, both for the larger society and for the historian.[15] My point here is not to facilely celebrate alternative approaches to disability or glibly disparage "medicalization" but to recognize that there are multiple analytical threads we can productively follow for studying disability history in the Latin American context, and for thinking critically about normative and Eurocentric approaches. Some of these threads reveal a history of attitudes and identities regarding disability that have resisted incorporation into more mainstream practices, while others have become thoroughly entwined with what we regard as "Western" medicine, with the result being a considerable degree of cultural hybridity.

No matter which of these threads a historian chooses to tease out or trace, I would venture that the history of disability offers the Latin Americanist an acute vantage point from which to think critically about linear notions of progress and development and to probe how they have contributed to normative assumptions about our minds and our bodies. And knowledge of alternative conceptions of disability can enable us to question the tendency to privilege technological solutions over supportive social programs and community-based resources that can address a wide range of mental and physical conditions, whether of the self-identified disabled, their often overtaxed caregivers, or the broader "debilitated" population whose numbers might make us question the very concept of "special" needs.

NOTES

1. On Latin America's leading role in postwar developmentalist policies, see Margarita Fajardo, *The World That Latin America Created: The United Nations Economic Commission for Latin America in the Development Era* (Harvard University Press, 2022).

2. There are many examples of this exclusive focus on class, but among the most influential was the early work of Aníbal Quijano, including *Nationalism and Capitalism in Peru: A Study in Neo-Imperialism* (Monthly Review Press, 1971), and *Clase obrera en América Latina* (Editorial Universitaria Centroamericana, 1976).

3. I am using "atraso" here instead of the usual translation, "backwardness," because I think the latter has a range of deeply disparaging connotations that "atraso" does not. Perhaps a better translation would be "lag."

4. On the many shortcomings of the supposed miracle, see Andre Pagliarini, "Believing in (Economic) Miracles in Brazil and Chile," *Radical History Review* 151 (January 2025): 211–226, https://doi.org/10.1215/01636545-11506819.

5. The historiography in this vein is literally too voluminous to list, but a good starting point is James Sanders, *The Vanguard of the Atlantic World: Creating Modernity, Nation, and Democracy in Nineteenth-Century Latin America* (Durham, NC: Duke University Press, 2014).

6. See the introduction to this volume, pp 1–26.

7. And even in wealthier nations, of course, there are regions, such as the Rio Grande Valley (discussed by Emily Xiao and Elizabeth O'Brien in this volume), where polluted drinking water or other environmental hazards have produced high rates of birth defects and disabilities.

8. A notable exception is a petition submitted by Chinese "coolies" in Cuba to an 1870s commission established to investigate conditions for these indentured workers, most of them located on sugar plantations. According to the petitioners, "When the contract expires, almost half of us have died. For those who have not died, a lot of them either become disabled or have internal injury." Petition reproduced in Lisa Yun, *The Coolie Speaks: Chinese Indentured Laborers and African Slaves in Cuba* (Temple University Press, 2008), 252–55.

9. Carlos Garcia, *O que é Nordeste brasileiro?* (Editora Brasiliense, 1984), 65. "Zeca-Tatu" is an adaptation of the disparaging figure (Jeca Tatu) created in 1918 by Paulista writer and publisher Monteiro Lobato to contrast the illiterate, sickly, and lazy country bumpkin with the civilized and industrious city dweller. See Barbara Weinstein, *The Color of Modernity: São Paulo and the Making of Race and Nation in Brazil* (Duke University Press, 2015), 33, 335.

10. Alvaro Jarrín, *The Biopolitics of Beauty: Cosmetic Citizenship and Affective Capital in Brazil* (University of California Press, 2017).

11. On the impact of changing diets on body types in Brazil, see Seth Garfield, *Guaraná: How Brazil Embraced the World's Most Caffeine-Rich Plant* (University of North Carolina Press, 2022), 167–70.

12. Amélia Cohn, Sedi Hirano, Ursula S. Karsch, and Ademar K. Sato, *Acidentes do Trabalho: Uma Forma de Violência* (Brasiliense; CEDEC, 1985); Barbara Weinstein, "The

Discourse of Technical Competence: Strategies of Authority and Power in Industrializing Brazil," *Political Power and Social Theory* 12 (1998): 137–75. Many conversations with Sofie Williams have shaped my views of the relationship between workplace accidents and the definition of disability in Brazil.

13. For example, Edward Anthony Polanco, *Healing like Our Ancestors: The Nahua Tiçitl, Gender, and Settler Colonialism in Central Mexico, 1535–1660* (University of Arizona Press, 2024).

14. Sidney Chalhoub, *Cidade Febril: Cortiços e Epidemias na Corte Imperial* (Companhia das Letras, 1996).

15. A number of anthropologists have explored the tensions and conflicts between liberal notions of human rights and rights as defined by Indigenous cultures. See, for example, Jean E. Jackson, "Rights to Indigenous Culture in Colombia," in *The Practice of Human Rights: Tracking Law Between the Global and the Local*, ed. Mark Goodale and Sally Engle Merry (Cambridge University Press, 2011), 204–41.

Histories of Disability in Latin America

Introduction

Disability in Latin America's Past

An Opening

David Carey Jr. and Heather Vrana

In highland Guatemala, the two closest words to "disability" in Kaqchikel Maya are *rusipanik Ajaw* (gift from God) and *ruloq'ob'al Ajaw* (blessing from God). Both terms reflect the Kaqchikel idea that every life's distinct characteristics are sacred.[1] Informed by those meanings and conceptions, Kaqchikel speakers do not assume that those with physical, sensory, or mental impairments are deficient or diminished. Instead of regarding disability as an illness, Kaqchikels often consider it a divine specialness or chosenness. As a result, Kaqchikel people with those "gifts" or "blessings" generally assume important roles in families and businesses, art and artisan production, agriculture, or healing.[2] By focusing on contributions rather than limitations, Kaqchikel Mayas mitigate the stigma often associated with disability.

Perceptions of bodily and intellectual difference vary across cultures.[3] Many Indigenous peoples normalize disability.[4] In colonial Mexico, Nahuatl terms for disability tended to be specific to individual bodies. Like *huihuilaxpol* (*tivulaxpul*), which describes a person who walks heavily, drags their feet, or otherwise has difficulty walking, *aoccan niyehuati* means "to get up with difficulty because one is thin and debilitated." Further along a continuum from mobility to immobility, *cecepoac* means "numb" or "paralyzed." The previously mentioned *aoccan niyehuati* can also describe someone who is unable to convalesce, as it is the negation (*aoc*) of the verb *ehua*, meaning "to get up, depart."[5] Although reading Nahuatl terms through a scientific medical lens might infer deficit-based diagnoses, Nahuatl worldviews encourage us to think of them as descriptions of physical difference rather than one's ability to contribute to society or wield power.[6]

Like Kaqchikel and Nahuatl conceptions of disability, this book centers the experiences, worldviews, and lives of disabled people and rejects deficit-based understandings of disability.[7] It considers what is unique about disability in Latin America, shaped by the region's distinct histories of race, class, gender, colonialism, development, and war. Very little has been written about disability in Latin America. Even as the burgeoning field of disability history expands from focusing on the United States and Europe to research in Africa, Asia, and the Middle East, Latin America remains obscure. What can research and scholarship on disability histories in Latin America teach us about the region and its people? How can Latin America expand our understanding of disability and its historical contingencies and significance?

Globally, people living with some form of disability number 1.6 billion (15 to 20 percent of the world's population).[8] With 80 percent of this group living in the global south (including at least 66 million disabled people living in Latin America), a history of disability in Latin America is long overdue.[9] But disability data should be considered critically. The experience of living with a disability in the global south has differed—still differs—in significant ways from that in the global north. While extant statistical counts can be useful for underscoring the importance of understanding disabilities, they are ill-equipped to recognize, much less explain and communicate, such distinctions.

Since the complex relationships of race and the persistent power of racism are integral components of Latin American historiography, examining disability histories in Latin America reveals new ways to conceptualize how race and disability shaped each other. As the modern Kaqchikel and colonial Nahuatl notions of disability suggest, Latin America has large Indigenous populations with distinct and overlapping conceptions of what disability is and is not, which have been dynamic through the pre-Hispanic, colonial, and postcolonial periods. The institution of slavery and the African diaspora shaped not only how disabled bodies came to be but also how they came to be understood. The fluidity of racial identities since slavery and the slave trade speaks to the malleable portrayals of disability in Latin America. Racialized forced labor systems (slavery, *encomienda*, *repartimiento*, debt peonage), colonialism, capitalism, imperialism, war, as well as decolonization, popular protests, and other manifestations of resistance have all produced disability.[10] Those forces also profoundly shaped how people with and without physical and mental impairments have identified, represented, and influenced the lives of those considered disabled.

Latin American disability histories can contribute to important interventions made by disability studies scholars. For instance, Nirmala Erevelles and Jasbir Puar have illustrated how imperialism actively constructs certain populations as disabled *and* creates disabling conditions of life, such as environmental pollution and malnutrition.[11] The long arc of Latin America's history of colonialism and neocolonialism points to institutions like slavery and military dictatorship that directly disabled enslaved people and political dissidents, respectively, and perhaps less directly disabled people by perpetuating poor public health and crushing poverty.[12] Whereas Central America, Mexico, and the Caribbean experienced intense postcolonial imperialism, with independence most South American nations enjoyed increased autonomy because of their distance from the United States. Compare, for example, the 1952 Bolivian Revolution with the 1954 coup in Guatemala, and Mexico's history of US intervention with that of Ecuador. In Guatemala and Mexico, US intrusions overdetermined historical fates, whereas Bolivia and Ecuador largely enjoyed the autonomy to shape their own realities. Such varied histories underscore the diversity of experiences within Latin America, something this volume also emphasizes.

If, as historian Pete Sigal asserts, Latin America had the "originating moment of colonialism," the region is crucial for understanding the intersections of disability and colonial power—particularly in light of the varied experiences of coloniality in Latin America—as Adam Warren and Martha Few demonstrate in this volume.[13] Likewise, Latin America's postcolonial disability histories offer insight into nation building, resource exploitation, and the costs of war, as the chapters by Bianca Premo, Paulo Drinot, David Carey Jr., and Heather Vrana explain. More recent histories of obstetric violence in the late twentieth and early twenty-first centuries, like those offered in the chapters by Elizabeth O'Brien and Emily Xiao and by Eliza Williamson, remind us that the disabling effects of racism and misogyny are ongoing.

This book centers disability—with all its nuances—in Latin American history. Largely ignored by historians and other scholars, disabled people have been important historical actors in Latin America. Disability history is not just rescue work or contributory scholarship that adds disabled people to the historical record.[14] Nor is it synonymous with the history of medicine, though histories of medicine and disability form "overlapping communities of thought."[15] Rather, productive tensions regularly characterize the complicated relationship between the fields of disability history and the history of medicine and public health.[16] Many scholars critique the medical model of disability for having ignored historical, cultural, social, political, and economic forces that have contributed to disability by locating disability in the individual and, often, their pathology.[17] Under the medical model, disability became synonymous with diagnosis, and its treatment or cure became the medical provider's, if not the patient's, primary goal. By contrast, much disability history explores processes by which people are categorized as disabled and the effects of this categorization, often by focusing on disabled people's experiences and perspectives. Disability history also addresses how these processes of categorization have been intertwined with broader political, economic, social, racial, and cultural projects and debates about how to understand, react to, and manage difference individually and collectively. With its diverse peoples and cultures, Latin America offers an ideal context in which to study how disability—as a concept and experience—has been a dynamic and malleable social and cultural construction.

Since Latin American governments seldom prioritized or could afford services for people with disabilities, those living with disabled bodies and minds experienced a range of reactions, from social stigmatization to social integration. Those experiences could change instantaneously as an Indigenous person left their highland community for the capital, for instance, or as an Afro-Latin American migrated to the highlands. As scholars focused on a region frequently defined by outsiders (and some insiders) as "backward" or "developing," Latin American historians can find the specter of disability in social reforms ranging from eugenics and carceral rehabilitation to public health and sanitation. Few have concentrated on disability in their pursuit of these themes. Disability histories can reorient scholarly focus away from medical authority, law, and knowledge systems toward disability's influence on everyday life and disabled people's agency.

A volume on Latin American disability history is vital not solely to the study of Latin America and the historiography of disability but also to debates within disability studies regarding the field's emphasis on white and US-centric or Eurocentric scholarship, regarding the role of religion and belief in disability cultures, and regarding approaches to care and therapy. Take, for instance, how some explanations for disabilities operated outside the etiologies defined by scientific medicine. Indigenous midwives insisted that lunar eclipses could cause birth defects, public health officials prescribed protections against *mal de ojo* (evil eye), and mestizos (people of mixed Spanish and Indigenous descent) and *indígenas* (Indigenous people) insisted *susto* (fright or spirit attack) could be debilitating.[18] Mal de ojo and susto both recognized that anger, jealousy, and rage in one person could disable another, even if that was not the intention. As these examples suggest, Indigenous approaches to disability could be guided by understandings rooted in deficit, even if translations of disability terminology from Kaqchikel and Nahuatl suggest alternative possibilities. Disability studies has, in recent years, responded to charges of "scholarship colonialism."[19] Focusing a critical disability lens on Latin America not only counteracts the bias toward North American and European perspectives that historian Sara Scalenghe decries as "disability imperialism" and the Achilles' heel of the field, but it also has the potential to change the terms of some important debates.[20]

In sum, Latin American disability histories expand existing disability scholarship in several ways: first, by centering the power of colonialism, neocolonialism, and imperialism in disabling people and places; second, by emphasizing the colonial and imperial components of scientific medicine that shaped disability; third, by revealing crucial fissures and contradictions in often celebrated national projects of democratic restoration and revolutionary uplift; fourth, by tracing the linkages between racial capitalism and disability; and, finally, by connecting resource extraction and labor to disability. Like other disability historians, the contributors to this volume come from the fields of the history of medicine, social history, and cultural anthropology. We have all been struck by US disability historian Douglas Baynton's axiom "Disability is everywhere in history, once you begin looking for it, but conspicuously absent in the histories we write."[21]

What does it mean to see disability everywhere in Latin America's past?

Disability Terminologies

One place to start is with language. Some scholars consider "disability" and "disabled" discrete categories that originated in Western Europe and the United States around the eighteenth century, or as early as the sixteenth century, largely depending on whether the author studies slavery, citizenship, suffrage, medicine, industrial labor, or social welfare.[22] There is little consensus around origins. By and large, this volume does not wade into those discussions. Instead, we and the other contributors to this volume understand disability as a historical construction, an analytical lens akin to gender, class, race, ethnicity, age, and sexuality whose terminologies have changed over time.[23] By exploring how these lenses combine, the chapters herein underscore how the meanings, conceptualizations, and experiences of embodied and intellectual difference have changed over time and across place. Take, for example, the discussion of modern Kaqchikel and colonial Nahuatl terms that begin this introduction. Several contributors' chapters raise other historical terms that denoted disabilities, like *lisiado* in eighteenth- and early-nineteenth-century Peru, late-nineteenth- and early-twentieth-century Ecuador, and civil war–era El Salvador.

Engaging the concept of impairment is crucial to our work. Like disability, this term has a history. Its roots lay in the changing structure of US life insurance after the abolition of slavery. After decades of fine-tuning their protocols for assessing the value of slaves, actuaries and underwriters began to use the term "impairment" to differentiate the values of human lives. By the 1880s, insurers shifted to using "impairment" as a shorthand for people with "weaker vital statistics."[24] Given this history and the term's easy medicalization, many disability scholars are keen to dismiss it. But others have argued for impairment's utility in pointing to aspects of disability that are not easily addressed by social factors.[25] Michael Rembis deftly argues that the social model, too, can be problematic as it risks erasing the body to the detriment of our understanding of "how disabled people in the past used, rather than denied, the biological realities and imperatives of their bodies to demand rights and much needed supports." He proposes—and we agree— that when understood as "socially created and historically contingent," impairment may be a more labile category than disability in contexts where people did not use notions of disability resonant with the term's later legal, medical, and social meanings.[26] Allowing impairment to challenge the social model also allows historians to consider pain and other experiences of embodiment.

A "revised social model" of disability could accommodate and even expand our understanding of impairment, as Carey demonstrates in his essay in this volume. After all, impairment is also historically contingent, subject to the social, cultural, and economic structures that produced it and in which it was experienced. "Rather than assuming impairment as either negative, a deficit, or at best neutral," Rembis suggests, "this approach [the revised social model] in turn enables impairment to assume a more generative role in shaping people's social interactions and their own identities." Importantly, this approach allows us to consider pain and suffering without viewing disability as pathology. Rembis continues: "Once historians acknowledge that impairment is socially created and that the biological, social, environmental and cultural work together not only to shape bodies, but also to shape the uses, meanings and values ascribed to those bodies, they can begin to think more critically about the important role that the body has played in disability history."[27] The payoff of this approach can benefit historians beyond the field of disability history.

Another term, "debility," has emerged in the work of scholars of disability outside the United States and Europe as a useful way to signal the effects of time, labor, racism, "active abandonment by the state," and other wearing factors on bodies.[28] Whereas "disability" is a term that can connote diagnosis, an injurious event, rights recognition, or an impaired or able-bodied binary; can gloss over more culturally specific definitions and meanings; and is readily coopted by states, debility is not freighted by such associations.[29] For historian Julie Livingston, "disability is a biosocial identity that is at once both biologically grounded and socially parsed, an umbrella term that denotes different things in different places and at different times." By contrast, "debility" signals "functional differences or losses in the body," especially those considered "normal" or even "expected" among Tswana in Botswana.[30] For Livingston, "debility" also acts as an umbrella term, including "experiences of chronic illness and senescence, as well as disability per se."[31] Puar, in turn, takes Livingston's concept of debility to explicate the violence of the liberal state's logic of what constitutes normal and expected impairments.[32] The essays gathered here (particularly those by Xiao and O'Brien, Warren, Williamson, and Carey) build on this important conversation as they show how "functional differences" and normal or expected impairments become endemic rather than exceptional in Black, Indigenous, working-class, and poor communities while still centering pain and other experiences of embodiment.

We recall Catherine Kudlick's exhortation "to refine our definition of disability so that it can hold a number of counterintuitive notions simultaneously" and call on Rembis's "socio-cultural-historical model."[33] Working from this foundation not only complicates our understanding of the myriad ways people have deployed and experienced disability but also suggests new approaches to researching, writing, and conceptualizing history.[34] Each author in this collection approaches disability terminology with attention to the historical context in which they are writing *and* about which they are writing. The chapters are empirically grounded and also written with awareness of the limitations of analytical categories that risk becoming overtheoretical or failing to "offer much in the way of practical help in understanding the lives of disabled people, let alone changing them for the better," to call on a third foundational thinker, Tom Shakespeare.[35] Indeed, the diversity of disability in Latin America and the complex ways people have experienced it over time sometimes diminish or obviate the usefulness, importance, and relevance of fine-grained theoretical interventions. At the same time, this diversity can open new theorizations of disability.

The authors herein pursue varied approaches. While some have embraced disability studies scholarship such as crip of color critique,[36] others have hewed more closely to traditional approaches articulated by disability history scholars who are now canonized in the field. This multiplicity of approaches both showcases a range of theoretical positions in the fields of disability studies and disability history and allows authors to explore theoretical interventions that map onto existing frameworks in Latin American history and their empirical evidence. Those choices and revelations also highlight contributors' varying expertise in disability studies and disability history. Since none of the contributors have been trained formally in disability history or studies, we approach our subjects as scholars who enter into the field from different locations, backstories, and (often interdisciplinary) areas of expertise. Most of us are historians, but some are also ethnographers, and one is trained as an anthropologist.

Regardless of their expertise, the authors herein approach the rich and long history of disability studies with respect and humility as they seek to center disability in Latin American history. Ableism and sanism are systems of power and ideologies that privilege people based on different notions of fitness (ability and sanity), such as their potential productivity, capacity, physical appearance, competitive success, and efficiency. Ableist and sanist ideologies are mutually constituting practices that systematically oppress and discriminate against people with physical or mental impairments, or both. Ableism and sanism have shaped and been shaped by other systems of power such as racism, sexism, colonialism, imperialism, and capitalism. Even as we recognize that focusing on Latin America decenters North American and European perspectives and content that have long dominated disability studies, our primary goal is not to make an internal intervention in disability studies but rather to deploy and incorporate disability studies in Latin American history. Taken as a whole, this volume extends, challenges, and aligns with earlier work in the field of disability studies. As readers encounter a range of entry points for thinking about disability in Latin America, our hope is that this volume not only starts new conversations but also offers solid bearings on which to continue ongoing debates.

Distinguishing Latin American from US and European Disability Histories

Latin American disability histories can be distinguished from European and US scholarship by chronology and terminology. These two factors are shaped by Indigenous knowledges, tensions between science and religion, colonialism, racial slavery, African diasporization, and imperialism, among other phenomena. As Latin American histories of disability expand, examining other regions similarly shaped by these phenomena is helpful.

In her study of debility (especially chronic illness and senescence) in Botswana, Livingston found it difficult to align her conceptions and questions with those of European and US historiography. Whereas people in Botswana embraced "somatic aspects of impairment," the field of disability studies marginalized them. Like many Latin American indígenas' notions of the interconnectedness of individuals and communities, Tswana notions stressed "the social permeability of the body and the person," which differed from a European-US emphasis on individuality and independence. With such distinct social constructions of the body, disability connotations also differed dramatically. As a result, the closest term to disability in Setswana, *bogole*, does not translate well to English, which fails to capture its range of meanings. Livingston found that *bogole*'s meaning changed as "colonialism, industrialization, globalization, missionary activity, and other complex interactions" unfolded during the twentieth century.[37]

The terms *rusipanik Ajaw*, *ruloq'ob'al Ajaw*, *Huihuilaxpol*, *aoccan niyehuati*, *cecepoac*, and *bogole* suggest other ways to comprehend distinctly abled bodies and minds. Ideas of injury and impairment varied in the cultural and social contexts of Mexico, Guatemala, El Salvador, Ecuador, Peru, and Brazil. The essays in this volume attend to these variations and how and why they changed over time. Acknowledging that impairments have not necessarily defined individuals as disabled, distinguishing impairment from disability and debility becomes imperative. Doing so allows scholars to separate functionality from social constructions of disability and to discern cultural perceptions of rehabilitation from its capacity to improve people's functionality and lives.[38]

One powerful example illustrates how focusing attention on Latin America contributes to rethinking the temporality of disability history. For years, disability historians pointed to mid-nineteenth-century industrialization, particularly in Europe and the United States, as marking a period when impairment took on new meaning. As economic rationality intensified with factory work under industrial capitalism, people unable to contribute to the productive economy were considered disabled, relegated to institutions and defined in opposition to society's contours and norms.[39] But recent work by David M. Turner and Daniel Blackie has added much-needed nuance to the "industrialization thesis" by foregrounding labor sites beyond factories (in their case, mines and pit villages) and examining disabled people's "domestic, spiritual, and social lives" beyond the workplace.[40] With empirical evidence, they demonstrate that contemporaries were much more concerned about the impact of the Industrial Revolution on the bodies of workers than on disabled workers' employment prospects. Going further, they argue, "Bodily non-normativity *defined* workers in industrializing Britain."[41]

Histories of Disability in Latin America further nuances the industrialization debate. Latin America can suggest how bodily nonnormativity defined laborers even earlier. Predating those periods, sixteenth-century European enslavement of Africans reduced men, women, and children to *piezas* (pieces) to assess their worth. An impaired, ill, or deformed body was less than a full pieza, for it was deemed not as productive as an able-bodied man or woman. Stefanie Hunt-Kennedy and Melanie J. Newton argue that the colonial Caribbean (and, we would argue, Latin America more broadly) disrupts the chronology of disability history by situating notions of disability in racial slavery in the Americas beginning in the sixteenth century. Owners, masters, and foremen of enslaved people often intentionally disfigured and impaired African bodies as a form of punishment, to remind them of their inferior position, and to prevent flight (as by severing a foot). With legal systems that endorsed and sometimes ordered such sentences, disability became part of enslaved Africans' social condition. The brutal living and working conditions marked by malnutrition, disease, and workplace (particularly sugar production) accidents meant that enslaved Africans and their children often lived in perpetual states of injury and endured long-term physical, psychological, and emotional damage.[42] These harsh corporeal and intellectual realities suggest that disability has a longer history than historians of Europe and the United States have heretofore envisioned.

Latin American case studies also demonstrate that conditions for disabled people did not necessarily improve over time. An example from Brazil is illustrative. Mothers of neurologically diverse children formed an advocacy group in the 1950s called the Associações de Pais e Amigos de Pessoas Excepcionais in order to, among other causes, support private schools called Pestalozzi Societies designed for intellectually disabled, gifted, or eccentric children. Despite these efforts, Brazilian medical professionals resisted the demedicalization and deinstitutionalization of people given psychiatric diagnoses.[43] Some disabled groups have become increasingly marginalized, while others have benefited from new technology and educational and employment opportunities. Disabled people shaped how physical and intellectual impairments did (or did not) become disabilities and how they were reconstituted and recrafted over time. They also advocated for their well-being and interests.[44]

We believe Latin American disability histories help all historians understand race more clearly. The historical confluence of colonialism and racism suggests why 80 percent of the world's disabled population live in the "poorest countries of the global South enduring some of the harshest levels of poverty."[45] Scientific and social scientific research in Latin America facilitated the disabling of the region, both in terms of the disablement of Latin Americans' bodies and the discursive construction of the region as backward or underdeveloped. Scientific conquest and colonization attracted mapmakers, physicians, botanists, and other scientists who sought out difference. European racialization of African and Indigenous peoples in the Americas distinctly shaped colonial exploitation and notions of disability, as Few and Warren demonstrate in this volume with their studies of colonial Guatemala and Peru, respectively. Racialized labor subjected certain bodies to horrific working conditions and punishment for the benefit of others. Just as eugenics and other scientific racisms sought to justify these labor practices and shore up national sentiment, eugenic ideas helped some Latin Americans argue for their nation's or their region's progress and exceptionalism. Intersections of race and disability point to distinct social constructions and specificities of impairment that may be unique to Latin America.

Latin American and US relations also have a place in histories of disability. Late-nineteenth- and early-twentieth-century US officials and authorities deployed disability to portray certain races and nationalities as "undesirable immigrants." By the late nineteenth century, notions of defect and disability had become embedded in US immigration policy. Concerned with "degeneration" in the United States, immigration officials excluded immigrants they considered "defectives," characterized by physical conditions ranging from missing limbs to blindness and psychiatric disorders such as intellectual limitations, mental illness, effeminacy in men, intersexuality, and other nonbinary identities.[46] Such exclusions were systemic and foundational. In his study of immigration and eugenics, Douglas Baynton argues, "The menacing image of the defective was the principal catalyst for the rapid expansion of immigration law and the machinery of its enforcement."[47] Beginning in the early twentieth century, authorities along the Texas-Mexico border regularly disinfected Mexican immigrants who they feared were bringing lice, typhus, and other diseases into the United States. In response to claims that Mexicans were less able to fight off tuberculosis because of their biological makeup, the US Public Health Service medicalized the border by placing physicians at US-Mexican ports of entry.[48] In those ways, social constructions of disability and race informed immigration policies.

Prior to the 1924 Immigration Act, which set no limits on Latin American immigration, US officials and capitalists extolled Mexicans' unique corporeal characteristics and diligence at a time when physical fitness and able bodies were crucial to assessing the value of immigrants. As historian Natalia Molina points out, perceived physical abilities were inextricably linked to racial classifications of Mexican migrants. Mexican immigrants countered anti-immigrationists who peddled perceptions of disability, disease, and race that decried Mexicans as unfit for manual, let alone cerebral, labor. Anti-immigrationists warned that Mexicans' diseased "Indian stock" would catalyze national degeneration. Mexican immigrants who withstood the deprivations that accompanied their peripatetic working and living conditions disproved officials who perpetuated such racialized knowledge and insisted Mexicans were less able-bodied than other races and thus dangerous vectors of tuberculosis.[49]

Eugenicists also peddled spurious public health and medical information to curb the immigration of certain groups. Citing diseases like tuberculosis, typhus, and typhoid, some US officials depicted Mexicans as less than able-bodied even if they were not necessarily deemed disabled. Representations of a model subject (white, heterosexual, able-bodied male) could be deployed to deport immigrants and exclude marginalized ethnic, gendered, or class groups. Those who enjoyed political, economic, or social power entwined social constructions of disability and race to serve their own interests and to disenfranchise particular groups from the body politic. At times marginalized groups like women, African Americans, and immigrants perpetuated disparaging disabled discourse by distinguishing themselves from "real disabled people" to advance their agendas.[50] The intersections of race, gender, class, and disability could empower or disempower marginalized populations in ways that could unite or divide them.

Ableist Archives and Other Evidentiary Questions

In Latin America, the omnipresence of disabled people, disability, and disabling life conditions has not buoyed an interest in disability history or archives.[51] Most archives in Latin America neglect the study of disability in their catalogues and in their inaccessibility to researchers. Few Latin American archival buildings are accessible to users of wheelchairs or other mobility aids. Researchers who enter archives often confront staircases, uneven walkways, narrow corridors, heavy doors, tripping hazards, small bathrooms, labyrinthine archival catalogs and information systems, outdated alarm systems that use only audio or visual signals, few or no resources in Braille, and lack of awareness of adaptive technology among archive staff.[52] A lack of adapted public transportation prevents many disabled researchers from ever arriving at archives.[53] Archives are inaccessible for people with all kinds of disabilities.

Methods of document organization and data management also obscure disability in the archive. Other than epidemics or people incarcerated in asylums, few finding aids highlight disabled people, and those that do, are defined narrowly by diagnoses or, often, charity and financial dependency. These omissions are borne partly of assumptions that range from discounting disabled people's capacity to leave their mark, perspectives, or voices in archival or material sources to assuming able-bodied individuals would mediate, obscure, or destroy historical traces disabled people left behind.[54] These challenges notwithstanding, most contributors in this volume conducted archival research to inform their analysis. The efficacy of their research—not to mention their cogent arguments and compelling narratives—offers proof that once historians and other scholars begin looking for disability, evidence of it abounds.

Prior to the mid- to late nineteenth century when public institutions from asylums to charities and organized welfare programs and services were on the rise, few clerks recorded conditions, events, or issues related to disabled people, at least in terminology easily recognizable to contemporary audiences. Yet these records are indispensable to postcolonial historians even when working with them can be challenging.[55] The term *discapacidad* in Spanish was not commonly used until the 1990s in Latin America, so historians must search for other words and phrases that denote and describe disability, such as the aforementioned lisiado. The challenge is even more acute for colonial historians. In an additional dimension to the challenge of searching for disability histories, documents pertaining to them are seldom grouped together in archives. For instance, desperate pleas in hand-written letters from family members inquiring about loved ones who have been institutionalized are strewn throughout the Archival General de Centroamérica (AGCA) public health *bultos* (bundles) of documents in Guatemala City.

In already limited archives of disability, Indigenous and Afro-Latin Americans are often invisible. At the AGCA, for example, neither the electronic nor the physical catalogs offer ethnic affiliations or surnames, so it is nearly impossible to trace particular ethnic groups, let alone individuals. Akin to the failure of medical systems and societies to acknowledge how class, race, and gender-based violence have disabled marginalized individuals and communities, archives perpetuate violence by occluding access to (or not collecting) records pertaining to marginalized people and groups. Sometimes archives perpetuate violence by collecting records only in moments of duress, loss, surveillance, or violence.

Disability historians using medical records face certain ethical considerations. Archival, oral, material, and other sources can evoke trauma and otherwise harm some people even as they inspire and empower others. In some cases, when researchers access mental health and other medical records, the absence of privacy measures for medical records is apparent, thereby compelling researchers to struggle with ethical questions and consider pseudonyms and other strategies to protect the identities of patients and their descendants. Historians in Canada and the United States have met these ethical challenges by anonymizing historical subjects, just as they would any other vulnerable group, such as guerrilla combatants, survivors of sexual assault, or former gang members.[56] Other disability historians have intentionally named disabled people at the center of their work and framed disabled people's perspectives as authoritative. In some Latin American nations, "public access to information" laws prioritize protection of information considered confidential or secret (*reservada*) over rights to access. In contexts where these laws have facilitated widespread government impunity, it is hard to believe that they are intended to protect vulnerable citizens. Thus, access to the very records that would enable some types of disability history research are limited by law. Making matters more complicated, enforcement of these laws seems to be left largely up to individual archivists who may intermittently permit or restrict access to records. Prejudice and stigma related to disability often inform these restrictions. In this context, while medical and institutional records of disability can be hard to access, they may also present possibility and accountability.

As a methodology and source, oral history can overcome some of the aforementioned challenges of archives. Researchers can arrive at their collaborators' residence, workplace, or other accessible site, thereby eliminating the barriers of many archive spaces. Similarly, setting up telephone and videoconference interviews can overcome some barriers. Interviews with disabled historical subjects can work to center disabled people in historical research methods and narratives.[57] Underscoring storytelling's transformative potential, Michi Saagiig Nsihnaabeg scholar Leanne Betasoamosake Simpson contends, "Storytelling is like air. It's that important especially as a tool of decolonization and transformation."[58] Demonstrating that oral history methodologies are not confined to spoken languages, Martin Atherton reminds us that deaf speakers of sign languages produce and preserve oral histories.[59] Oral histories that counter negative depictions of disability in archival materials can shift popular perceptions and dominant discourses of disability rooted in pity, shame, and exclusion.[60] Indeed, such methodology and evidence are crucial to understanding how disability influences worldviews and how disabled people have shaped and have been shaped by the past. On the other hand, oral histories can also cause harm and perpetuate violence, compelling scholars like Adria Imada to practice an "ethics of restraint."[61]

Material artifacts can help researchers move beyond state archival sources. Hand-woven *huipiles* (blouses) contain stories about Indigenous pasts, toys reveal patterns of childrearing, prostheses indicate how people with impairments adapted to able-dominated societies. These and other objects convey empathy and hold symbolic meaning.[62] In one particularly important manner, historians of disability face the same conundrum as their counterparts in other fields: not all information, particularly among Indigenous and Afro-descendant groups, is intended to be shared publicly. Researchers should follow community-articulated guidelines to protect sacred and special community knowledge and artifacts. Some of our contributors have long been working closely with disability communities in their activism, research, and everyday lives, while others are just now building these connections.

When scholars transform research into scholarship, another important ethical consideration is with whom to publish. As editors, we inquired with accessible presses that follow ethical publication standards. With varying commitments to open-access publishing, University of North Carolina Press, University of Illinois Press, University of Michigan Press, Syracuse University Press, and John Hopkins University Press all offer formats for readers with visual impairments and other disabilities. The University of Michigan Press clearly articulates its policies regarding accessibility and equity.[63] Johns Hopkins University (JHU) Press offers alternative electronic formats by email request for readers with "documented disabilities," under "Specialty Requests" on the "For Educators" page of the press website. Its "Guidelines for Illustration and Art" include color blindness standards for data legibility and accessibility, though they do not address alt text or image description. John Hopkins University Press's rapidly growing open access book program, Hopkins Open Publishing, publishes new, in-print, and out-of-print titles on Project Muse. Muse is transparent about the accessibility of its products and offers an Accessibility Guide for publishers. Our hope is that by publishing a book about disability histories, the press will go even further to accommodate all readers and to make their books and journals more accessible. We also considered working with a press without a track record of accessible publishing or an explicit statement regarding accessibility and equity as a way of encouraging them to embrace not only the fields of disability history and disability studies but also best practices in those fields. In the end, JHU Press most aligned with our digital accessibility plans, which include an inclusively designed ebook and inexpensive paperback option. We hope that our decision has facilitated this book finding its way to readers in Latin American history and disability history and, beyond, to readers who are new to one or both fields. To those ends, to the best of our abilities, the authors have followed accessibility practices such as thick description of visual sources and plain language.

Outline of the Chapters

Considered in light of the size and diversity of Latin America and the complexity of disability, this book is not intended to be a definitive disability history of Latin America. It is an invitation to cultivate new comprehensions of Latin America's past that disability history offers. Each chapter offers insight into the meanings of disability through the lens of a unique case study, often employing interdisciplinary approaches from history, anthropology, ethnology, literary studies, and public health. Many chapters address some of the most pressing topics emerging in recent disability histories and studies, such as representations of disability, agency, care, and interdependence.

In the first two chapters, Premo and Drinot consider how visual representations of disability circulated in newspapers and memoirs. Premo discusses Lina Medina, who became the world's youngest mother on record and a newspaper sensation after the story broke in Lima newspapers in April 1939. While the medical explanation for her pregnancy seems to rest on the condition of "precocious puberty" and, tragically, her rape as a child, the focus of Premo's chapter is on how Lina's handlers attempted to frame the public's desire to look at her as a national call to action. Rather than making her unnatural or pitiable, looking at Lina created a "staring but caring" national spectatorship that was set against "consumptive, capitalist, foreign spectatorship." Drinot examines another famous Peruvian, social theorist José Carlos Mariátegui. Drinot argues that disability is both present and absent in Mariátegui's work. For biographers, the famous thinker's disablement as a child serves as something of an origin story in which his genius was spurred by his long stay at a charity hospital where he became fond of reading and languages. It allows biographers to write heroic life narratives in which Mariátegui's disability was an identity but also a challenge. Yet most scholarship on Mariátegui neglects his experiences of disability and how disability may have shaped his political thought. Drinot's chapter considers Mariátegui's disability from two angles: first, by focusing on how

Mariátegui's disability has been represented, both visually and textually; second, by using a variety of sources, and in particular his correspondence, to explore how Mariátegui experienced impairment and disability.

Similarly, in chapters 3 and 4, family members, politicians, and public health officials vie for control of the lives of disabled children and youth. Like Premo, these authors bring analyses from the history of childhood and youth to bear on disability studies, but they also bring borderlands studies, environmental studies, and ethnic and race studies. In Xiao and O'Brien's chapter, a cluster of infant deaths caused by anencephaly activate racist, xenophobic, and ethnonationalist attitudes as public health authorities, news media, and doctors inscribed anencephaly within an imagined geography of race, poverty, and pollution at the border. Authorities blamed Mexican-origin women and claimed that cultural factors caused their children's deaths. Local activists, arguing that the cases clustered along lines of pollution at the Rio Grande, pointed to toxic water and land pollution from US corporations that exploited local workers and took advantage of lax environmental regulations on the border. The crisis resulted in the establishment of a state "birth defect registry" and a federally sponsored folic acid distribution campaign, outcomes that bolstered state surveillance but also created access to desired resources. Williamson's chapter examines a similar set of relations by drawing on ethnographic research with mothers raising children diagnosed with congenital Zika syndrome (CZS) in Bahia, Brazil. Williamson situates the Zika virus pandemic and its aftermath in longer histories of systematic debilitation of marginalized Brazilians. Dialoguing with disability studies scholarship that theorizes debility as produced through geopolitical violence on the bodies of those in the global south, she proposes the term "interembodied debility" to identify how debility is distributed in bodyminds (a term denoting how body and mind are entwined) in these intensive relations of care. These two chapters convey how individuals exercised power over or in relation to other people and institutions while drawing on and reworking racist, misogynistic, classist, and xenophobic assumptions that maligned them in order to make demands on the state. Together, they open a conversation around agency and interdependence within what Puar has termed the "biopolitics of debilitation."[64] Finally, as the most contemporary studies in this book, these two chapters remind us that the historical impacts of debility are ongoing.

Warren and Carey, in chapters 5 and 6, respectively, focus on how disabled people, and their family members and neighbors, navigated the legal regimes that mobilized medical definitions of disability in late colonial Lima and early-twentieth-century Ecuador. Faced with colonial and postcolonial archives that erase, minimize, and distort the lived histories of people considered mad or disabled, Warren and Carey read against the grain of archival sources, engage with absent presence (and present absence), and generate different centers and perspectives that counter some of this archival and historical violence. Warren's analysis of court records of redhibitory cases helps us to understand how ordinary people, including enslaved Africans and their owners, understood, constructed, and navigated what we would call disability in slaveholding settings. In some cases, enslaved people took their owners to court to make accusations and press for demands, among them the provision of treatment for their injuries and ailments, protection from violence and abuse, removal from specific labor sites, transfer to different owners, and exercise of the right to self-purchase. In others, slave owners engaged each other in litigation to contest the value, health, and labor capacity of the enslaved men, women, and children they purchased and sold. Warren's analysis extends beyond labor to show how Limeños and others constructed understandings of ability and disability and deployed them strategically for specific ends. Similarly, Carey's chapter examines the intersections of race, ethnicity, and disability through the lens of madness in Ecuador. Madness and perceptions thereof regularly reified racial hierarchies. By revealing the ranges, alternatives, and pluralism with which cultures, societies, and nations approached racially pathologized disabilities, Carey points to the limitation of the binary framings—exclusion-inclusion, discrimination-accommodation, institutionalization–social acceptance—common in disability studies.

In chapters 7 and 8, Few and Vrana explore networks of care that emerged in the wake of disabling events and consider how medical professionals and disabled people shaped contemporary narratives around disability. In analysis that allows her to pinpoint the origin of a new source of disability, Few examines the outbreak of a disease new to colonial doctors in Guatemala that they called *epidémica de la constitución* (epidemic of bodily constitution). The disease disabled people with hysteria, headaches, delirium, and anxiety. Few uses this unique case to demonstrate how medical professionals and authorities gendered debilitating diseases. Through her innovative methodology, she demonstrates how disasters reveal individuals' disabilities.

Vrana's chapter works with Tobin Siebers's concept of "disability masquerade" to show how the Farabundo Martí National Liberation Front (FMLN) politicized disabled combatants (*lisiados de guerra*) during and after the Salvadoran civil war. Representations of lisiados and wartime medicine in *testimonio* literature and propaganda films managed disability stigma by claiming "disability as a version of itself."[65] In the FMLN's masquerade, lisiados were lauded for their special knowledge and experience, compelled to be heroes, and presented as embodied evidence of Salvadoran military cruelty. Centering disability masquerade in wartime, El Salvador underscores the importance of disabled combatants to the war effort and reveals how the masquerade itself shaped how lisiados experienced the war and the postwar period.

This volume is the first of its kind expressly focused on disability history in Latin America. Rather than revising old histories, it posits the field as something new. At the same time, we acknowledge the value of many earlier studies that may not have been understood as disability history by their authors or accepted as such by the field.[66] The chapters herein also mark new directions for some authors who only recently have turned to disability history, following their interrogations of medicine, class, race, gender, labor, childhood, and birth. In the end, we hope that this volume sparks inquiry and new lines of research among scholars *within* Latin America, Latin American history, and disability history.

As a region, Latin America has persistently been framed as disabled or underdeveloped. As subjects of enduring racial discourses defined along a spectrum of disability, the region's populations responded in ways that ranged from empowerment and collaboration to co-optation and submission. Factors like neoliberal structural inequality, medical neglect, ableist and sanist social attitudes, and even medical understandings of disability have concentrated much of the world's disabled population in Latin America (and elsewhere in what the World Health Organization calls the "developing world"). Focusing on Latin America calls attention to the geopolitical topographies that privilege North American and European studies of disability and highlights the importance of expanding research and scholarship of disability in the global south.[67] We also believe disability histories of Latin America deepen our understanding of the discourses and practices of disablement and the experiences of disabled Latin Americans. We hope, most of all, that this volume convinces readers to be in conversation with one another across fields and areas of study and thereby expand our understanding of Latin America's past and how it has shaped and has been shaped by notions, experiences, and practices of disability.

NOTES

1. Based on his fluency in Kaqchikel and more than three decades living and working in Kaqchikel communities in highland Guatemala, Carey translated and glossed these Kaqchikel phrases with an eye toward maintaining orthographic structure without obscuring meaning. He favored explanation over direct translation. In *Diccionario Kaqchikel* (Proyecto Lingüístico Francisco Marroquín, 1998), Narciso Cojti, Martín Chacach Cutzal, and Marcos Armando Cal gloss *loq'ob'al* as "viruela" (180) and "gracias, bendición de Dios" (181). Stephen Eyman and Christopher Wheatley, "A Comparative Discourse of Inclusion in Iximulew and Pa Jotöl," unpublished paper prepared in collaboration with Oxlajuj B'atz' Byron Socorec, Aq' ab'al Gonzalo Ticun, Mokchewan Marco Tulio Guaján, Lajuj B'atz' Edy René Guaján, Ixkamey Magda Silvia Sotz' Mux, and Ixnal Ambrocia Cuma Chávez for Oxlajuj Aj, July 2020. Many Indigenous peoples associate disability with spirituality. See Minerva Rivas Velarde, "Indigenous Perspectives of Disability," *Disability Studies Quarterly* 38, no. 4 (Fall 2018).

2. Eyman and Wheatley, "Comparative Discourse of Inclusion in Iximulew and Pa Jotöl."

3. George S. Gotto, "Persons and Nonpersons: Intellectual Disability, Personhood, and Social Capital Among the Mixe of Southern Mexico," *Disabilities: Insights from Across Fields and Around the World*, ed. Mariah S. Glover (Bloomsbury, 2009), 193–210; Bryan Turner, "Disability and the Sociology of the Body," in *Handbook of Disability Studies*, ed. Gary Albrecht, Katherine Seelman, and Michal Bury (Sage, 2001), 252–66.

4. Rivas Velarde, "Indigenous Perspectives of Disability"; Sophie Kasonde-Ng'andu, "Bio-Medical Versus Indigenous Approaches to Disability," in *Disability in Different Cultures: Reflections on Local Concepts*, ed. Brigitte Holzer, Arthur Vreede, and Gabriele Weigt (Transcript Verlag, 1999), 118.

5. Nahuatl Dictionary, *aoccan niyehuati*, last accessed June 11, 2025, https://nahuatl .wired-humanities.org/content/aoccan-niyehuati. A special thanks to Rebecca Dufendach for helping us to understand these terms. See also Bernardino de Sahagún, *Florentine Codex: General History of the Things of New Spain*, Book 6: *Rhetoric and Moral Philosophy*, trans. Arthur J. O. Anderson and Charles Dibble (School of American Research, University of Utah Press, 1969), 121; Alonso de Molina, *Vocabulario en lengua castellana y mexicana y mexicana y castellana* (1571), part 2, "Nahuatl to Spanish," f. 6v. col. 1; f. 15v. col. 1; f. 29r.

6. Rebecca Dufendach, "'As If His Heart Died': A Reinterpretation of Moteuczoma's Cowardice in the Conquest History of the Florentine Codex," *Ethnohistory* 66, no. 4 (October 2019): 623–45.

7. Catherine Kudlick, "Disability History: Why We Need Another 'Other,'" *American Historical Review* 108 (2003): 763–93; Rosemarie Garland Thomson, *Extraordinary Bodies: Figuring Physical Disability in American Culture and Literature* (Columbia University Press, 1997); Lennard J. Davis, *Enforcing Normalcy: Disability, Deafness, and the Body* (Verso,

1995); Simi Linton, *Claiming Disability: Knowledge and Identity* (New York University Press, 1998).

8. Roy Hanes, "Introduction," in *The Routledge History of Disability*, ed. Roy Hanes, Ivan Brown, and Nancy E. Hansen (Taylor and Francis, 2017), 2; Michael Rembis, Catherine Kudlick, and Kim E. Nielsen, "Introduction," in *The Oxford Handbook of Disability History*, ed. Michael Rembis, Catherine Kudlick, and Kim E. Nielsen (Oxford University Press, 2018), 1.

9. Sara Scalenghe, *Disability in the Ottoman Arab World, 1500–1800* (Cambridge University Press, 2014), 8; Economic Commission for Latin America and the Caribbean, "Disability in Latin America and the Caribbean—Public Policy Changes," *ECLAC Notes*, no. 74 (December 2012), https://www.cepal.org/notes/74/Titulares2.

10. Stefanie Hunt-Kennedy, *Between Fitness and Death: Disability and Slavery in the Caribbean* (University of Illinois Press, 2020); Esme Cleall, ed., *Global Histories of Disability, 1700–2015: Power, Place, and People* (Routledge, 2023); Esme Cleall, *Colonizing Disability: Impairment and Otherness Across Britain and Its Empire, c. 1800–1914* (Cambridge University Press, 2022); Caroline Lieffers, "Imperial Ableism: Disability and American Expansion, c. 1850–1930," PhD dissertation, Yale University, 2020; Mary Mendoza, "La Tierra Pica / The Soil Bites: Hazardous Environments and the Degeneration of Bracero Health, 1942–1964," in *Disability Studies and the Environmental Humanities: Toward an Eco-Crip Theory*, ed. Sarah Jaquette Ray and Jay Sibara (University of Nebraska Press, 2018); John Kinder, *Paying with Their Bodies: American War and the Problem of the Disabled Veteran* (University of Chicago Press, 2020); Gildas Brégain, "An Entangled Perspective on Disability History: The Disability Protests in Argentina, Brazil, and Spain, 1968–1982," in *The Imperfect Historian: Disability Histories in Europe*, ed. Sebastian Barsch, Anne Klein, and Peter Verstraeten (Peter Lang, 2013); Íris Morais Araújo, "Dangerous Representations: 'Indigenous Infanticide,' Disability, and Karitiana Relations in Brazil," *Disability Studies Quarterly*, 41, no. 4 (Fall 2021).

11. Nirmala Erevelles, "The Color of Violence: Reflecting on Gender, Race, and Disability in Wartime," in *Feminist Disability Studies*, ed. Kim Q. Hall (Indiana University Press, 2011), 117–35; Nirmala Erevelles, "Thinking with Disability Studies," *Disability Studies Quarterly* 34, no. 2 (2014); Jasbir K. Puar, "Crip Nationalism: From Narrative Prosthesis to Disaster Capitalism," chapter 2 in *The Right to Maim: Debility, Capacity, Disability* (Duke University Press, 2017).

12. We understand "neocolonialism" to mean the often (but not always) subtler forms of political, economic, and cultural domination of Latin America, Africa, and Asia that followed decolonization. Of course, decolonization unfolded at different times and in different ways in each of these regions. Imperialism, by contrast, refers to more direct political, economic, or military intervention.

13. Pete Sigal, "Latin America and the Challenges of Globalizing the History of Sexuality," *American Historical Review* 114, no. 5 (December 2009): 1353.

14. Susan Burch and Hannah Joyner, "The Disremembered Past," in *Civil Disabilities*, ed. Nancy J. Hirschmann and Beth Linker (University of Pennsylvania Press, 2015), 67.

15. Julie Livingston, "Comment: On the Borderland of Medical and Disability History," *Bulletin of the History of Medicine* 87, no. 4 (Winter 2013): 560. For exemplary

ethnography that centers disabled actors and integrates these histories into broader narratives, see, for example, Joao Biehl, *Vita: Life in a Zone of Social Abandonment* (University of California Press, 2013).

16. For an exploration of the debates between historians of medicine and disability historians, see Beth Linker, "On the Borderland of Medical and Disability History: A Survey of the Fields," and comments by Livingston, Daniel J. Wilson, and Catherine Kudlick, *Bulletin of the History of Medicine* 87, no. 4 (Winter 2013): 499–535.

17. Susan Burch and Michael Rembis "Re-Membering the Past: Reflections on Disability Histories," in *Disability Histories*, ed. Susan Burch and Michael Rembis (University of Illinois Press, 2014), 3; Scalenghe, *Disability in the Ottoman Arab World*, 10; Rembis, Kudlick, and Nielsen, "Introduction," 3–4.

18. Archivo General de Centroamérica (AGCA), Guatemala City, Guatemala, índice 116 (1915), leg 16c, ex 39; Museo de Medicina, Quito, Ecuador, A0692, memo de Reglas Higiénicas para el niño, Director General de Sanidad, 1935.

19. Chris Bell, "Introducing White Disability Studies: A Modest Proposal," *The Disability Studies Reader*, 2nd ed., ed. Lennard J. Davis (Routledge, 2006), 272–82; Shaun Grech, "Disability and Development: Critical Connections, Gaps, and Contradictions," in *Disability in the Global South: The Critical Handbook*, ed. Shaun Grech and Karen Soldatic (Springer, 2016), 3–19; Sami Schalk, *Bodyminds Reimagined: (Dis)ability, Race, and Gender in Black Women's Speculative Fiction* (Duke University Press, 2018), Julie Avril Minich, "Enabling Whom? Critical Disability Studies Now," *Lateral* 5, no. 1 (2016); Minich, *Accessible Citizenships: Disability, Nation, and the Cultural Politics of Greater Mexico* (Temple University Press, 2014); Helen Meekosha, "Decolonising Disability: Thinking and Acting Globally," *Disability and Society* 26, no. 6 (October 2011): 668.

20. Scalenghe, *Disability in the Ottoman Arab World*.

21. Douglas Baynton, "Disability and the Justification of Inequality in American History," in *The New Disability History: American Perspectives*, ed. Paul K. Longmore and Lauri Umansky (New York University Press 2001), 51.

22. See Kudlick, "Disability History"; Davis, *Enforcing Normalcy*, 74; Anne Borsay, *Disability and Social Policy in Britain Since 1750* (Palgrave Macmillan, 2005); Colin Barnes, *Cabbage Syndrome: The Social Construction of Dependence* (Falmer Press, 1990); Brendan Gleeson, *Geographies of Disability* (Routledge, 1999); Hunt-Kennedy, *Between Fitness and Death*.

23. Paul Higgins, *Making Disability: Exploring the Social Transformation of Human Variation* (C. C. Thomas, 1992); Susan Wendell, *The Rejected Body* (Routledge, 1996); Burch and Rembis, "Re-Membering the Past," 1; Anna Stubblefield, "'Beyond the Pale': Tainted Whiteness, Cognitive Disability, and Eugenic Sterilization," *Hypatia* 22, no. 2 (2007): 162, 179; Kudlick, "Disability History."

24. Michael Ralph, "'Life . . . in the Midst of Death': Notes on the Relationship Between Slave Insurance, Life Insurance, and Disability," *Disability Studies Quarterly* 32, no. 3 (2012).

25. Lennard J. Davis, *Bending Over Backwards: Disability, Dismodernism, and Other Difficult Positions* (New York University Press, 2002); Tom Shakespeare, "The Social Model of Disability," in *The Disability Studies Reader*, ed. Lennard J. Davis (Routledge, 2010), 266–73.

26. Michael Rembis, "Challenging the Impairment/Disability Divide: Disability History and the Social Model of Disability," in *Routledge Handbook of Disability Studies*, ed. Nick Watson and Simo Vehmas (Routledge, 2020), 383, 380, 387.

27. Rembis, "Challenging the Impairment/Disability Divide," 381, 383. See also David Serlin, *Replaceable You: Engineering the Body in Postwar America* (University of Chicago Press, 2004).

28. Liat Ben-Moshe, "Weaponizing Disability," *Social Text Online*, October 25, 2018 https://socialtextjournal.org/periscope_article/weaponizing-disability/.

29. Puar, *Right to Maim*, xvii.

30. Julie Livingston, *Debility and the Moral Imagination in Botswana* (Indiana University Press, 2005), 7.

31. Julie Livingston, "Insights from an African History of Disability," *Radical History Review* 94 (Winter 2006): 113.

32. Puar, *Right to Maim*, xvi.

33. Catherine Kudlick, "Smallpox, Disability, and Survival in Nineteenth-Century France: Rewriting Paradigms from a New Epidemic Script." in Burch and Rembis, *Disability Histories*, 185–200; Rembis, "Challenging the Impairment/Disability Divide," 388.

34. Kudlick, "Smallpox, Disability, and Survival in Nineteenth-Century France," 4, 5–6.

35. Tom Shakespeare, *Disability Rights and Wrongs*, 3.

36. Jina B. Kim, "Toward a Crip-of-Color Critique: Thinking with Minich's 'Enabling Whom?,'" *Journal of the Cultural Studies Association* 6, no. 1 (Spring 2017), doi.org/10 .25158/L6.1.14.

37. Livingston, "Insights from an African History of Disability," 115, 113, 116.

38. Livingston, "Insights from an African History of Disability," 118.

39. Scalenghe, *Disability in the Ottoman Arab World*, 1; Davis, *Enforcing Normalcy*, 74; Borsay, *Disability and Social Policy*; Barnes, *Cabbage Syndrome*; Gleeson, *Geographies of Disability*.

40. David M. Turner and Daniel Blackie, *Disability in the Industrial Revolution: Physical Impairment in British Coalmining, 1780–1880* (Manchester University Press, 2018), 4–8.

41. Turner and Blackie, *Disability in the Industrial Revolution*, 7.

42. Stefanie Hunt-Kennedy and Melanie J. Newton, "The Hauntings of Slavery: Colonialism and the Disabled Body in the Caribbean," in *Disability in the Global South*, 381, 385–86; Hunt-Kennedy, *Between Fitness and Death*.

43. Pamela Block and Fátima Gonçalves Cavalcante, "Historical Perceptions of Autism in Brazil," in Burch and Rembis, *Disability Histories*, 80–83.

44. Daniel A. Rodríguez, *The Right to Live in Health: Medical Politics in Postindependence Havana* (University of North Carolina Press, 2020), 189–90.

45. Shaun Grech, "Disability, Communities of Poverty and the Global South," in *Inclusive Communities: A Critical Reader*, ed. Andrew Azzopardi and Shaun Grech (Sense, 2012), 69–70; Shaun Grech, "Recolonising Debates or Perpetuated Coloniality? Decentering the Spaces of Disability, Development, and Community in the Global South," *International Journal of Inclusive Education* 15 (2011): 87–100; Livingston, "Insights from an African History of Disability," 125n16.

46. Douglas Baynton, *Defectives in the Land: Disability and Immigration in the Age of Eugenics* (University of California Press, 2016).

47. Baynton, *Defectives in the Land*, 1.

48. John Raymond Mckiernan-González, *Fevered Measures: Public Health and Race at the Texas-Mexico Border, 1848–1942* (Duke University Press, 2012); Alexandra Minna Stern, "Buildings, Boundaries, and Blood: Medicalization and Nation-Building on the U.S.-Mexico Border, 1910–1930," *Hispanic American Historical Review* 79, no. 1 (1999): 41–81; Natalia Molina, "Medicalizing the Mexican: Immigration, Race, and Disability in Early Twentieth-Century United States," *Radical History Review* 94 (Winter 2006): 22–37.

49. Molina, "Medicalizing the Mexican," 23–27, 29–32.

50. Baynton, "Disability and the Justification of Inequality in American History," 33–57; Molina, "Medicalizing the Mexican," 23–27, 29–32.

51. Heather Vrana, "Hall of Miracles: Central American Disability Archives," in *Cripping in the Archive*, ed. Stefanie Hunt-Kennedy and Jenifer Barclay (University of Illinois Press, 2025).

52. Society of American Archivists, "Guidelines for Accessible Archives for People with Disabilities," February 2019.

53. Gildas Brégain, "An Entangled Perspective on Disability History: The Disability Protests in Argentina, Brazil and Spain, 1968–1982," in Barsch et al., *The Imperfect Historian*, 133–54.

54. Rembis, Kudlick, and Nielsen, "Introduction," 2, 9–10.

55. Hanes, "Introduction," 4–5; Burch and Rembis, "Re-Membering the Past," 4–5.

56. See David Wright and Renée Saucier, "Madness in the Archives: Anonymity, Ethics, and Mental Health History Research," *Journal of the Canadian Historical Association* 23, no. 2 (2012): 65–90; Geoffrey Reaume, *Remembrance of Patients Past: Patient Life at the Toronto Hospital for the Insane, 1870–1940* (Oxford University Press, 2000); John Harley Warner, "The Uses of Patient Records by Historians—Patterns, Possibilities and Perplexities," *Health and History* 1, nos. 2–3 (1999): 101–11; Guenter Risse and John Harley Warner, "Reconstructing Clinical Activities: Patient Records in Medical History," *Social History of Medicine* 5 (1992): 183–205; Carole Berkenkotter, *Patient Tales: Case Histories and the Uses of Narrative in Psychiatry* (University of South Carolina Press, 2008); Jonathan Gillis, "The Uses of the Patient History Since 1850," *Bulletin of the History of Medicine* 80, no. 3 (2006): 290–512; Gerald L. Higgins, "The History of Confidentiality in Medicine: The Physician Patient Relationship," *Canadian Family Physician* 35 (1989): 921–26.

57. David Carey Jr., *Oral History in Latin America: Unlocking the Spoken Archive* (Routledge, 2017); Fred Pelka, *What We Have Done: An Oral History of the Disability Rights Movement* (University of Massachusetts Press, 2012); Livingston, "Insights from an African History of Disability," 111; Rembis, Kudlick, and Nielsen, "Introduction," 10.

58. Betasoamosake Simpson quoted in Susan Burch, *Committed: Remembering Native Kinship in and Beyond Institutions* (University of North Carolina Press, 2021), 2.

59. Martin Atherton, "From Their Own Hands: Collecting Oral Testimony in Signing Communities," in *The Routledge History of Disability*, 247–48.

60. Karen Yoshida, Susan Ferguson, and Fady Shanouda, "Breaking the Rules: Sum-

mer Camping Experiences and the Lives of Ontario Children Growing Up with Polio in the 1940s and 1950s," in *The Routledge History of Disability*, 455–56.

61. Adria Imada, *An Archive of Skin, An Archive of Kin* (University of California Press, 2022), 27–29.

62. Burch and Rembis, "Re-Membering the Past," 5; Burch, *Committed*, 13; Rembis, Kudlick, and Nielsen, "Introduction," 10.

63. See "About: Equity, Justice, and Inclusion," University of Michigan Press, accessed August 29, 2022, https://www.press.umich.edu/about#equity.

64. Puar, *Right to Maim*, xix.

65. Tobin Siebers, "Disability as Masquerade," *Literature and Medicine* 23, no. 1 (Spring 2004): 5, 8.

66. The following books and articles stand out as texts that fit this description: Ann Zulawski, *Unequal Cures: Public Health and Political Change in Bolivia, 1900–1950* (Duke University Press, 2007); Stern, "Buildings, Boundaries, and Blood"; Alexandra Minna Stern, "Sterilized in the Name of Public Health," *American Journal of Public Health* 95 (July 2005): 1128–38; Natalia Molina, *How Race is Made in America: Immigration, Citizenship, and the Historical Power of Racial Scripts* (University of California Press, 2014); Jennifer Lambe, "In the Shadow of the Double: Psychiatry and Spiritism in Cuba," *History of Psychology* 21, no. 3 (2018): 223–39; Rocio Gomez, *Silver Veins, Dusty Lungs: Mining, Water, and Public Health in Zacatecas, 1835–1946* (University of Nebraska Press, 2020); and many books and articles by Anne-Emanuelle Birn, but especially "Doctors on Record: Uruguay's Infant Mortality Stagnation and Its Remedies, 1895–1945," *Bulletin of the History of Medicine* 82, no. 2 (2008): 311–54.

67. For work by scholars challenging those global north priorities and privileges, see, for example, Eunjung Kim, *Curative Violence: Rehabilitating Disability, Gender, and Sexuality in Modern Korea* (Duke University Press, 2017), 18; Nirmala Erevelles, *Disability and Difference in Global Contexts: Enabling a Transformative Body Politic* (New York: Palgrave Macmillan, 2011); Scalenghe, *Disability in the Ottoman Arab World*; Hunt-Kennedy, *Between Fitness and Death*.

1

Looking at Looking

Staring at and Caring for Peru's
Youngest Mother in the World (1939)

Bianca Premo

In 1939, at the age of five, Lina Medina became the world's youngest mother on record. On May 15, newspaper readers throughout the world exhaled on learning that this marvel, who had been diagnosed as pregnant only weeks before, had delivered her baby boy, healthy, via planned cesarean section, the day before, on Mother's Day. The medical explanation for her stunning pregnancy seems to have rested on the condition of "precocious puberty" and, tragically, her rape as a child.[1] This chapter looks at Peruvians as they looked at newspaper images of Lina when the story broke in April and May 1939. And it looks at us, looking at them.

The physicians and statesmen who took control of Lina's pregnancy and shaped the press reporting about it attempted to frame the ethics of looking at her as a communal—indeed, national—call to action, instead of a longer imperial gawking at Latin American bodies deemed spectacular, pitiable, or unnatural. Drawing from two strains of disability studies, one grounded in critical approaches to temporality and the other focused on "staring," this chapter theoretically foregrounds how Lina's condition, transitory and exclusive to children, adds the complicating issue of time to considerations of the ethics of looking. With this understanding established, the chapter then tracks the first two weeks of press coverage of Lina's pregnancy before her son Gerardo was born, following exclusives in Lima's tabloid daily *La Crónica*

The author thanks the editors and contributors of this volume, Alfredo Escudero Villanueva, Okezi Otovo, and Jessica Adler, and the 2024 Mellon Affirming Multivocal Humanities Workshop at the Center for Women and Gender Studies, led by Alex Cornelius at Florida International University.

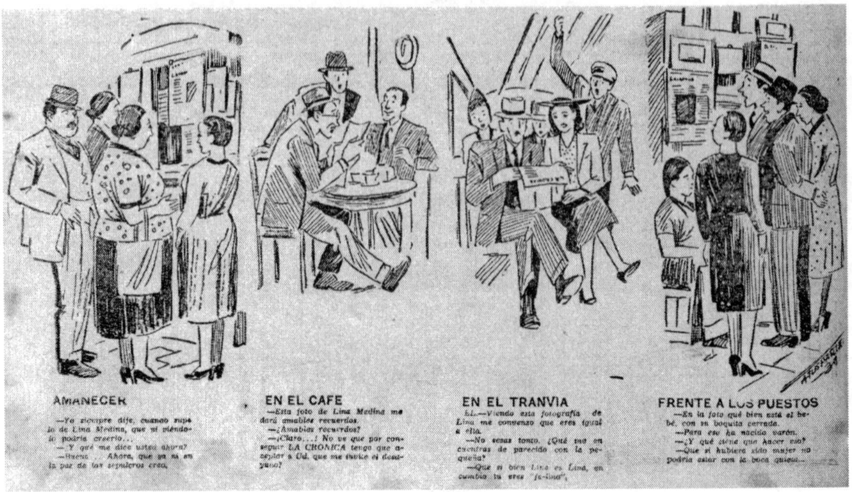

In this four-panel cartoon, slack-jawed readers of the tabloid daily, marveling at news of the birth of Gerardo Medina, gather throughout the day at the newsstand, in cafés, and on streetcars. The images feature bits of humorous or cartoonish dialogue; in the first image, a woman proclaims that, despite the photo of Lina, she would never believe the pregnancy was real as long as she lives and "even in the grave." "En el octavo día del nacimiento recibió ayer obsequios de diversas personas el bebecito de Lina Medina," *La Crónica*, May 22, 1939, 14.

as it published illustrations and photographs but held back on showing photos of Lina's actual body.[2]

As with the drawings shown in the adjacent figure, which appeared eight days after the birth in May 1939, the images Peruvians beheld as they sought news about the little mother as frequently focused on readers, professional spectators, and curious onlookers as they did on Lina herself. These images reveal the ongoing construction of a normate, or "able," staring public: an exclusive, national community of modern and active adult observers huddled around the paper. This construction of a staring but caring nation was explicitly contrasted with consumptive, capitalist, and foreign spectatorship. However, this was not the only way Peruvians regarded Lina. It is evident in *La Crónica*'s coverage that older legacies of looking, especially a fascination in imperial Western medicine with Latin American dwarfism, which rendered Lina a small adult rather than a growing child, endured and continued to frame her body.

Lina's pregnancy intersects with the history of disability at multiple points: It raises questions about how we define disability in terms of temporality or life course; it calls forth a tradition in disability studies focused on freakery and "extraordinary bodies"; and it resonates with more recent scholarly attention to the history of care, charity, and state welfare in Latin America's past. This chapter explores these themes theoretically first, before analyzing the visual coverage of the case in *La Crónica*. Each theoretical vector merges to create a sensitivity to the ways state agents and physicians used illustrations of Lina to create an abstracted, whitened, and "normal" child that could be a beneficiary of state care. Their intersection prepares us to see how the newspaper's images and photos primed readers to become active, emotive spectators and rally around a collective anti-imperial, nationalist, science-centered state regime of care. That effort would culminate in a presidential executive decree that removed both Lina and her son from her parents' guardianship. Two months after the birth, the children would be transferred to the custody and care of a consortium of state officials, representatives of private and public ministries of health and beneficence, and the Academy of Medicine. This meant Lina and her son were interned in a hospital in Lima for an entire year before the Supreme Court reversed the ruling in 1940 and returned them to her parents. Yet, even as this new, state-centered ethos of care developed, it competed with older, imperial ways of racialized gawking inherited from the nineteenth and early twentieth centuries, particularly that directed at disabled or extraordinary bodies.

Time, Childhood, and Extraordinary Bodies

Before delving into the unfolding visual representation of Lina's case during the first weeks of news coverage in April and May 1939, it is critical to lay out the problematics and promises of considering her record-shattering pregnancy within our own present concerns in disability histories in Latin America. This is especially important since, in contrast to more conventionally defined disabilities that occur in the life cycle of an otherwise non-disabled person, including old age, injury, or late-onset chronic illness, Lina would eventually shed the medical markers of precocious puberty as she grew. Her "disability" was, at least physiologically, neither permanent, progressive, nor irreversible.[3]

Today, Lina is an old woman. She is, as of this writing, presumably alive and residing in Lima, Peru. Her son, Gerardo, is gone, having died of a heart abnormality at age 40. For her entire adult life, she has refused invitations and insistence that she speak about what happened to her. But the intrusions have been near constant over the past eight decades. A Peruvian physician and erstwhile historian of Lina's case snapped a photo of her in 2018, seemingly without her knowledge, as she ambled home with plastic grocery bags over broken chunks of uneven concrete on a street in her neighborhood on the outskirts of the capital city. Her silver hair is pulled back in a ponytail, and she wears low-heeled shoes, a skirt, and the outdated pantyhose favored by grandmothers. A Spanish newspaper, which ran the photo beside an interview with the physician (who was seeking international publication of his book), commented on the irony that she looked young for her age.[4]

This unauthorized photo of an unsuspecting elderly Lina is an object lesson in how age conditions our sense of the ethics of looking. To see Lina as old is to see her as a historical actor, a person with a past, a person with agency. Yet the newspaper's remark on her youthful appearance subtly (re)places her in a timeless category, as a perpetual child. This temporal slippage in how we regard Lina, taken together with her refusals, complicates any simple attempt to fit her story within the political project of recovering voices and agency.

Children, arguably far more than disabled adults, remain a historical category of human actors whose full agency and ability to "speak" for themselves are still debated.[5] But Lina's refusal also exposes the conceit that we have reached a stage when historians must follow what might be called a recuperative imperative, a key foundational claim in disability history itself. "It is now time," write the editors of a sweeping handbook of the international history of disability, "to tell th[e] story and to provide a 'voice' to a population that has been traditionally silenced."[6] This seemingly straightforward ethics of recovering histories of disability becomes trickier when we consider the entanglements of circulating and consuming images of those who inhabited bodies deemed unnatural or unusual, especially images taken without consent in situations of direct violence and exploitation, often against a background of medical imperialism.[7]

And there's more. I also acknowledge my own tangled ethical relationship to Lina's advancing age and mortality. Any day now, Lina might pass away—she might have already. This would make it impossible for anyone to interview her. (To be clear, I have not sought to do so, to honor her past refusals to speak about her story, including to the physician who wrote a book about her.) Death will convert Lina from a living research subject into an archival object. She won't be able to stare back or turn away from an interested looker.[8] Alive and older, she can recoil from our gaze, berate us for our interest, or even stare back. These reactions help anchor us to the standard protocols of human subjects research.[9] That Lina is, or might still be, alive is an ethical rudder, a guilt maker that forces onlookers to be extremely cautious in viewing or exhibiting her if they do not avoid looking at her altogether.[10] It points to the thin line that distinguishes *Ripley's Believe It or Not* from academic disciplines such as history and anthropology and institutional practices such as museum culture.[11]

Starting with elderly Lina also reveals time to be an inescapable element in ethical questions about circulating historical images of the extraordinary, nonnormative, and disabled in Latin America. Time long has of course been a critical element especially in how we view photographic images.[12] But there is something more specific to be observed in the disorienting photograph of an old Lina. Child-mothers fundamentally disturb standardized notions of biological chronology and the natural order in multiple ways. As feminist scholar Carla Rice points out, precocious puberty, especially in girls, provokes a sense of crisis because of the perceived "mismatch" between possessing the body of an adult and the mind of a child, and this mismatch is simultaneously temporal and visual. Rice argues that a case like Lina's "enacts a new way of seeing that, through visual representations, medical measurements, and emotionally charged clinical descriptions, makes a spectacle of what are conceived as deviant, early-pubescent bodies, further entrenching notions of embodied normativity into the cultural and scientific imaginary."[13]

The crisis becomes particularly acute by attaching death to childhood, evincing what disability scholar Alison Kramer calls "curative time," which holds that disabled or extraordinary bodies must be subject to medical or sociopolitical intervention to force "normalcy" so that they bend to the arc of "standard" biological chronology.[14] We can see this at work in depictions of Lina in 1939 in which she was figured as a child whose life was jeopardized by giving life to her baby, making intervention necessary. It is perhaps not a surprise that studies of precocious puberty, including landmark research that included photographs of dozens of naked children's bodies from Denmark in 1952, rushed to postulate that many children would die early if they experienced what was classified as "true" precocious puberty—a medical classification that identified the early onset of hormonal processes that matured sex organs, processes distinct from others that might involve tumors on the reproductive organs or the manifestation of only one of multiple markers of this life stage.[15]

It is precisely by focusing on curative time that we may observe a different path than one plotted by the mere classification of Lina's pregnancy as some kind of impulsive "spectacle." When Lina is frozen in time as a child, onlookers today can imagine looking at her in a manner similar to the way Peruvians did in 1939: It is a looking that is life-affirming, even life-extending, rather than exploitive. If the imagined child, unable to either consent to or deny our gaze, might die or be harmed if she is not looked at, looking turns into saving or recovering. These impulses provide an ethical protocol for examining or studying historical subjects that changes depending on perceived chronological age and the extraordinary subject's embodied future.[16] By starting this section with the image of Lina as an elderly person who is said to resemble a child, we can see, however, that curative time offers only a twisted, narrow route to looking. Lina did not die in childbirth and her son, Gerardo, lived until his fortieth birthday. There is no urgency to look here and now.

Beyond the question of whether Lina's precocious puberty or her pregnancy can be usefully categorized as a disability or a state in urgent need of "cure," there are other ways her story and the public's reaction to it contribute to disability history. An interest in the early history and ethical implications of "staring" and "freakery" can enrich, and perhaps change, how we look at normate Latin American spectators in the past as they beheld what Rosemary Garland-Thompson has called the "spectacle of the extraordinary body."[17] While it might be easy to imagine that Peruvians simply gawked or were driven by some kind of automatic impulse to exploit the story's sensationalism, in fact both Lina's handlers and the public struggled, as we do, with the ethical murkiness of *wanting* to see.

Garland-Thompson theorizes about spectators' interior shame at their own curiosity about unusual or disabled bodies, and she presents this as a kind of censorship. She urges viewers to linger in the tension between the urge to, at once, look and look away from extraordinary bodies by promising us that "the contradiction between the desire to stare and the social prohibitions against it can be productive. . . . Who we think we are can shift into focus by staring at who we think we are not."[18] Theorist Jacques Rancière also promises productive looking by encouraging us, in a less self-, more community-oriented spirit, to take on the contradiction, to hesitate before sliding into consensus when approaching extraordinary bodies, unexpected images, and representations of human pain. Academically speaking, what he suggests involves resisting the scholarly impulse to make the history of disability—or photography, child abuse, or even freakery, for that matter— an "endless task of unmasking fetishes."[19]

Historians of disability might instead look at onlookers, seeing them as more than mere passive consumers in structured (capitalist) relations of power, inured to violence and instinctively bent on domination of unexpected bodies. Peruvians in the 1930s, at least at moments, attempted to distinguish their own looking from consumption or exploitation.[20] While never complete or universal, a method emerged in Peru as onlookers grappled to believe their eyes when looking at Lina. That method was rooted in nationalist notions of her "normality"—in whitewashing, quite literally, her appearance in illustrations to move her case from the realm of freakery into the domain of state-centered collective care, to fix her in time (as a white, normal, curable child) and to build faith in the masses' scientific capacities of scientific observation.

This method of looking derived in part from the evolving tenets of Peruvian "social medicine."[21] Social medicine—an approach focused on the environmental, political, and social origins of diseases and their cures—is best known for spawning nationalist medical imperialism throughout Latin America, and Peru was no exception. For example, physicians and statesman from Lima, some of European origin, were engaged in a literal "scientific colonization" of the Amazon precisely as Lina's case hit the news. Under the administrations of Peruvian presidents Oscar A. Benavides and Manuel Prado Ugarteche, the creation of academies of specialists, a ministry of health, and an institute for children's health meant that social medicine touched ordinary people. One signature effort was the establishment in the Amazon of colonies for lepers and children suffering parasitic infection. For social medicine advocates, active care involved not only internment and separation from others but also, critically, the creation of an internal community. As historian Marcos Cueto has argued concerning some of the very same doctors who became involved in Lina's case, social medicine in Peru wrapped Amazonians suffering from blindness, missing fingers, or swollen bellies in an ethos of care as it enacted its authoritarian medical paternalism.[22] That care, I contend, was more than a cover for medical conquest. Lina's case shows us that it could also be an effort, through the media, to foster an urgent collective enterprise that united the scientific expert and the "proletariat," state and society.

The stakes of attention to Lina's singular case can be instructive today. Closely following the sequence of images of press coverage in April and early May 1939 forces us to reflect on how twists in the story can impact, in turn, our own looking. After all, it is not only Lina's pregnancy and its ensuing press coverage in 1939 that were temporal. Reading this chapter itself is too. Acknowledging this fact might make visible something now invisible, something that can be revealed only over time as we examine in sequence the images readers beheld of Lina's extraordinary body: namely, our own consensus about how we should regard others as they looked at Lina Medina. Let's see, together.

La Crónica, April–May 1939

Peruvians were fascinated by Lina. And they were far from oblivious to their own fascination. Lina came from the heavily Indigenous district of Ticrapo, a tiny, isolated hamlet on the eastern edge of the Andes. She was diagnosed as seven months' pregnant by Dr. Gerardo Lozada in the provincial city of Pisco, where her family had taken her in mid-April when her abdomen began to swell visibly in her final month of pregnancy. Shortly after the diagnosis, when the story broke, newspaper reports in Lima built urgently toward two events: the birth of her baby and the presentation of her photographic image as proof to the paper's readers. As those two events drew closer, Peruvians began to fixate on the image of themselves straining to see her.

Limeños learned of Lina through increasingly breathless exclusives in *La Crónica*, an organ of Manuel Prado's financial empire with tight ties to the national elite and government. Almost no photographs of Lina, and none of her full body, were released through the press until the day before her son was delivered in a surgical feat on May 14, giving *La Crónica* four weeks' worth of near-daily coverage of the progress of the pregnancy without revealing a photo of the girl. After that date the paper was filled with carefully posed photographic portraits of child mother and son, surrounded by doctors and nurses. Perhaps this was the decision of the paper's editors, who worked in tight orchestration with President Benavides's administration. Perhaps it was the desire of Lina's medical handlers, including her diagnosing physician, Dr. Lozada, and Dr. Carlos Enrique Paz Soldán, founder of Peruvian social medicine and the powerful head of Peru's National Academy of Medicine. Probably both.

In the month leading up to the birth, the paper satisfied its readership's demand to see this marvelous case with illustrations rather than photos, often composed so as to build up suspense. The first account of Lina's pregnancy in the tabloid daily appeared on April 11, 1939, deep in the paper on page 14, near national and crime reports, with no accompanying image. This was followed by an article in which Pisco physician Lozada was featured and photographed. In the article's text, readers were treated to the story of an unnamed but intrepid reporter pushing his way past posted signs and hospital policies that kept the public away from Lina. The article draws the reader close by announcing Lina's name for the first time and claiming to have had the occasion to meet her (*"conocer a la menor"*) after making "multiple overtures before the public authorities for the concession to enter." He found her reticent and unresponsive to his questions, and the article ran no visual depiction of the girl.

The next day, readers got their first glimpse of Lina. This was in a drawing by the newspaper illustrator with the penname (or last name) Atusparia, who would compose most of the paper's illustrations of Lina over the coming weeks as the readership awaited the birth.[23] This article was again nestled alongside crime reports on page 14, and, in fact, this was where news of Lina would remain in *La Crónica*'s coverage almost every day of the coming months. Atusparia's drawing of Lina showed her lying on a table while being inspected by doctors and an unnamed man—possibly at this point standing in for a father—all wide-eyed. In a move the artist repeated multiple times as readers awaited the birth, in the drawing her belly was blocked from view.

Critically, the placement of the article among the crime reports positioned her prone body in parallel with a photograph of a corpse in the city's morgue. As we can see in the adjacent image, death was literally tracking Lina in the layouts of many stories, even as she was depicted with dolls and toys. Mortal threat would remain central to coverage of her pregnancy. For example, twelve days later, another article about the pregnancy, with no accompanying image, hovered above a photograph showing a close-up of the face of a dead three-year-old.[24] Lina and this birth were clearly surrounded by dangers to their very lives, a detail that would provide Peruvians permission to feel their attention to the case was at once virtuous, salvatory, and urgent.

Lina Medina debe ser traída a esta capital con intervención de las instituciones científicas

Ya está en poder de la policía José Peralta Gonzales, autor de la muerte de Justina Ramos

TAL ES EL CONCEPTO DE LA MAYORIA DE MEDICOS DE LIMA. — EL CASO SIGUE SUSCITANDO EXTRAORDINARIO INTERES. —SUCESOS PARECIDOS QUE REGISTRA LA LITERATURA MEDICA. — OPINAN DESTACADOS FACULTATIVOS. — LA ORIENTACION ASISTENCIAL SEGUIRA A CARGO DEL Dr. LOZADA.—EL ESTADO MENTAL DE LINA ACUSA RETARDO EN LA PERCEPCION. — EL SINDICATO NACIONAL DE OBSTETRICES CUIDARIA DE LA MENOR EN COLABORACION DE ENTIDADES FEMENINAS. — ¿EL HOGAR DE LA MADRE O LA CLINICA DE LA MATERNIDAD? — MEDICOS DE CHINCHA, ICA Y ALREDEDORES ACUDEN A CONOCER DE CERCA EL RARO FENOMENO QUE INTRIGA A LA CIENCIA

A medida que hemos dado a conocer detalles del extraordinario suceso de Lina Medina, la menor que teniendo cinco años y medio se halla en cinta de ocho meses, han brotado sugerencias y comentarios que revelan el apasionamiento con que se ha tomado un asunto de tanta importancia para los hombres de ciencia y para el público.

Apasionamiento e interés. Porque la diversidad de conceptos es un exponente de la trascendencia del caso.

Muchos, a través de nuestras informaciones, no obstante que ellas están trazadas en la más completa veracidad siguen poniendo en tela de juicio la exactitud de los datos. Es natural. El fenómeno ha producido revuelo no sólo en los profanos, sino hasta en los mismos hombres de estudio. Jamás, a estar por los datos que la investigación de gentes científicas ofrecen, se ha presentado un caso igual.

El de Lina Medina, merece toda dedicación. Se impone que las instituciones científicas del país, la Academia Nacional de Medicina, la Asociación de Médicos "Daniel A. Carrión", la Sociedad Peruana de Psiquiatría, etc., intervengan decididamente para que la menor sea traída a esta capital. Es aquí, como ya hemos dicho, donde se puede hacer de este caso un estudio notable, minucioso, profundo.

Hay entre nosotros, eminentes ginecólogo y psiquiatras que requieren ampliar sus conocimientos, ir desenvolviendo el proceso de Lina Medina, conforme se van sucediendo las diversas etapas de este desarrollo fisiológico. Un caso único en el mundo no puede pasar inadvertido por los estudiosos, médicos limeños. Sólo imperdonable negligencia podría poner al margen la oportunidad brillante que se ofrece para que nuestros hombres de ciencia investiguen nuevo, destellos en tan compleja y tan nutrido de sorpresas como es el de la medicina.

Recogemos, por otra parte, el clamor de la mayoría de los médicos de nuestra capital.

Y como sería injusto que al ser trasladada a Lima, la menor en referencia, fueran interrumpidas las investigaciones que está haciendo con admirable celo, el joven y notable médico doctor Lozada, es necesario que se le encomiende continúe bajo su dirección en esta Capital, la asistencia científica de Lina Medina.

DICE EL Dr. BAZUL, CATEDRATICO DE OBSTETRICIA

Tuvimos oportunidad, ayer, de entrevistar al doctor Bazul, catedrático de Obstetricia en la Facultad de Ciencias Médicas, y notable profesional. Como supiéramos que el doctor Bazul había estado en Pisco y conocido a la menor, en el hospital de aquella localidad, tuvimos interés en escuchar sus conceptos sobre el extraño caso.

—Considero que este asunto—está en muy buenas manos de mi distinguido colega, doctor Lozada, con lo cual yo prefiero inhibirme de opinar. Además, yo sólo fui a Pisco, porque al encontrarme en Ica, unos amigos me pedían con insistencia les explicara el fenómeno producido No tuve, pues, otro recurso que dirigirme a Pisco y ponerme al habla con mi colega, en cuya compañía, conocí a Lina Medina, tomando referencias, con toda atención de cuanto me dijera el doctor Lozada. He podido comprobar todo cuanto me dijo referente a las características exteriores.

UN CASO REALMENTE EXTRAORDINARIO

—En mi concepto—prosigue se trata de uno de esos grandes sucesos, que la ciencia ofrece como sorpresa. Un caso realmente extraordinario y digno de estudiarse hasta en sus menores detalles. He visto que la menor tiene sus órganos desarrollados. Pero no como los de una persona adulta, porque eso sería mucho decir, sino desarrollados en forma que guarda relación con la edad de la chica. También he observado los estudios radiográficos practicados por el doctor Lozada. He visto la situación del feto y lo considero que se trate de un embarazo normal.

ALGUNOS CASOS PARECIDOS

—Toda la literatura médica que conozco a través de mis estudios obstétricos, no menciona un caso igual, idéntico. Algo parecido sí hay algunos. Por ejemplo, el caso de Carus, citado por Auvard, en su obra, donde menciona que una menor de dos años había experimentado lo, síntomas periódicos de una mujer púber, habiendo quedado en cinta a los ocho años. Es lo más extraordinario en materia de precocidad maternal. Otro caso, el de Comar mout, que a los siete meses tuvo la regla mensual. Pero esto hecho, el de Lina Medina, es asombroso. Según los datos que proporcionó el doctor Lozada, esta chiquilla sufrió este fenómeno a los tres meses convirtiéndose en un período natural a los dos años.

INTERVENCION DE ENTIDADES CIENTIFICAS

Preguntamos al doctor Bazul si considera conveniente que debe traerse a Lima la menor:

—El Hospital de Pisco cuenta con los elementos necesario, como para la atención que ha de prestársele a la menor. Y el doctor Lozada no descuida en ningún momento la atención debida.

—Pero siendo un caso de tanta trascendencia para la Medicina, no cree, doctor, que es en esta ciudad donde debe estar la menor para que sea examinada por nuestros hombres de ciencia?

—Realmente, es un suceso, único. Considero que la chica debe estar en Lima. Pero debe hacerse de acuerdo y con intervención de las instituciones científicas. La Academia Nacional de Medicina por ejemplo; la Asociación de Médicos "Daniel A. Carrión" etc. tendrían que ser las que dirigieran la atención y protección de esta menor que, ya pertenece a la ciencia. Sin embargo, he de hacer presente, y estoy de acuerdo con una sugerencia de todos, en que al traerse a Lina Medina, debe también conseguirse que continúe la atención médica al doctor Lozada. No hay por qué poner al margen la investigación que con tanto esfuerzo viene practicando el médico-jefe del Hospital de Pisco.

HABRIA UNA SALA EN LA CLINICA DE LA MATERNIDAD

Conversamos ayer con un médico de una de las secciones, de la maternidad de Lima, cuyo nombre pidió que guardáramos en reserva.

—Yo conozco el caso sólo por las informaciones de LA CRONICA, que las considero notables porque conceptúo que revelan la realidad. Se trata de un fenómeno. No hay caso. Uno de esos, hechos que escapan a la imaginación de los mortales. Por algo en la medicina es la ciencia de las sorpresas. Al principio yo mismo hacía chirigota del suceso increíble. Hasta que LA CRONICA fue la misma pe-rio. Esa chica que viene a poner un jalón en capítulos interesantes de la obstetricia merece ser traída, no para que se haga de ella una exhibición vulgar ni se pregone a los cuatro vientos que sólo la ciencia puede decir, sino para que ella sea todo un laboratorio de estudio. Que los médicos, los muchacho estudiantes, en fin todos cuantos estamos en esta afán de conocer nuevos rumbos de la medicina, tengamos oportunidad de investigar el fenómeno. Que se la traiga. La medicina es una ciencia para todos, no exclusividad de uno de un grupo. Es para los estudiosos. Y así como no creo que el médico diga: 'mi enfermo' por que el enfermo, el paciente, es de todos; así también el extraordinario caso que ahora se opera en esa criatura, no debe ser privilegio de unos ano de todos, los que quieran ser algo más tarde. Lo cuerdo sería que se pusiera el hecho en conocimiento oficial a la Academia de Medicina para que interviniera inmediatamente.

EL Dr. ROBERTO ROMERO PACHECO

A poco de salir de la Maternidad, hablamos con el doctor Roberto Romero Pacheco, joven médico de la nueva hornada y cuyo, estudios científicos le han dado prestigio merecido. Sus conocimientos ginecológicos le han destacado en Lima, obteniendo renombre. Le interrogamos también acerca del caso de Lina Medina.

—LA CRONICA ha hecho recordar los casos que sobre el mismo tema conozco—nos dice—por libros y folletos que editan instituciones científicas; pero no hay parangón al caso de la menor que se encuentra en Pisco. Un caso expuesto en la obra científica, "Obstetricia", de Fabre, revela que Haller observó en Anna Mummen-thaler, que tuvo la regla periódica desde los dos años y que a los ocho fué madre, teniendo un parto normal dentro de los nueve meses.

El prestigioso facultativo nos siguió recordando otros casos, con gran acopio de datos que ponen de manifiesto su exquisita erudición científica. Nos habla de un suceso reciente, en Antioquía, Colombia, donde una menor fué madre a los siete años.

—Pero todo esto—agrega el doctor Romero Pacheco—nosotro, lo sabemos a través de esta bibliografía excelente, claro está, pero que muestra recursos extranjeros. Ahora que se presenta el caso de Lina Medina, considero que se haría una obra de beneficio oso para los médicos peruanos, trayéndola a esta capital.

—¿Considera posible un viaje prolongado sin hacer estrago, en el organismo de la menor?

—Hay medios de locomoción excelentes. La Asistencia Pública, por ejemplo, podría ceder uno de sus carros de ambulancia para que en él pudiera hacer viaje la chiquilla. Y reduciendo el inapreciable aporte que está realizando el doctor Lozada, muy competente y muy estudioso, creo que se a él, y sólo a él a quien se le debe seguir confiando la asistencia médica de la menor.

El joven médico a quien interrogamos, es como si se recogiera el clamor de los médicos nuevos de Lima. Es in-completa, si acaso de superación de los...

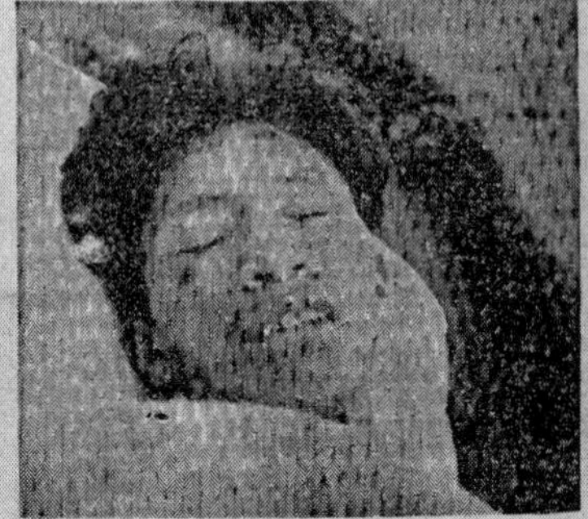

José Peralta Gonzáles en su lecho del Hospital Dos de Mayo

LLORO COMO UN NIÑO ANTE SUS PATRONES

Con la captura del mayordomo José Peralta Gonzáles, se esclarece en parte la muerte de Justina Ramos, que tanto ha intrigado a la policía.

José Peralta Gonzáles fue hallado ayer al mediodía en el fondo de uno de los barrancos que hay en la proximidad del cuartel San Martín, en estado inconsciente, siendo trasladado por la guardia civil del puesto de Surquillo a la Asistencia Pública, y de allí internado en el hospital Dos de Mayo, quedando alojado en la sala del Carmen, en la cama número 31.

El cabo Ulloa, comandante del puesto de Surquillo, no descuidó la vigilancia del herido, ordenando que se le mantuviera en estricta incomunicación.

En el primer momento, dijo llamarse Víctor Condorí Quispe, de oficio albañil y domiciliado en el Callao, en la calle Marco Polo.

En la mañana de ayer fué identificado como el autor de la muerte de la Ramos, comunicándose el hecho a la comisaría de Miraflores. Inmediatamente el jefe de investigaciones, oficial primero, señor Mendoza, y el investigador Alvarez, se trasladaron a esta capital, con el fin de tomarle declaraciones a Peralta.

Gonzales confesó ser el autor de la muerte de su amante, con la que, dice, sostenía relaciones maritales desde hacía algún tiempo, y que ante la imposibilidad de abandonar la casa de sus patrones, se vió obligado a tomar tal determinación.

Ha confesado que le golpeó con el martillo hallado junto al cadáver, y que es su precipitada fuga dejó abandonado.

Gonzales, agobiado por los remordimientos, trató de suicidarse, arrojándose al mar, y como le faltara, posiblemente valor para hacerlo, vagó por las calles de Magdalena del Mar, hasta que encontró a un sujeto llamado César Augusto, cuyo apellido no recuerda. Con él permaneció la mayor parte del día, hasta algunas horas de la noche, en que se separaron. Y como Gonzáles seguía obsesionado por la idea de la muerte, se arrojó desde lo alto del barranco, originándose heridas que seguramente lo retardrán algún tiempo en cama.

Con el fin de identificarlo en forma concluyente, se solicitó a la familia Barría que se acercara al hospital Dos de Mayo, a fin de reconocer a su ex mayordomo.

Cuando la señora Barría ingresó a la sala donde se asiste Gonzáles, y como éste la reconociese, se cubrió la cara con la frazada; pero como se le obligase a descubrirse, lloró ante su patrona, ocultando el rostro entre las almohada.

Una de las hijas de la señora Barría le increpó su conducta.

Los investigadores han continuado tomándole la instructiva a Gonzáles, con el fin de concluir el parte.

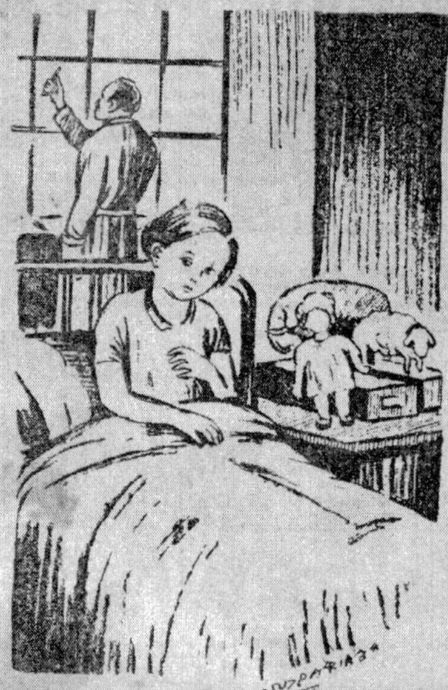

En el recinto donde se se tiene recluida, Lina Medina, pasa las horas, ajena a su tragedia. Al fondo, el médico jefe, contemplando la necesidad de colocar una tela metálica en la ventana. — (Reconstrucción de Atuparia).

The only image aimed at proving the truth of the girl's pregnancy during these early days of coverage anatomized her. This was the image published on April 15, four days after the story broke.[25] Atusparia here illustrated an X-ray of Lina's uterus. I have been unable to locate a photographic reproduction of this plate published anywhere. It is doubtful that readers could determine that this X-ray shows a fetus in utero; the illustration merely gestures to scientific proof of pregnancy rather than providing conclusive evidence. Months later, a histological study of microphotographs from a biopsy of Lina's ovaries was published, along with the microphotographs, in Peru's medical journal, *La Reforma Médica*, and then shared with a French medical publication.[26] These too anatomized Lina, never connecting the detailed images of postpartum ovaries to her body or face.

After the illustration of the X-ray of Lina's uterus appeared, readers of *La Crónica* were provided another image of Lina, lying in bed asleep, her midsection again strategically covered (by a blanket), and dreaming of her mother.[27] The image here marked a tension: Should Lina be viewed as an Indigenous subject or as a normative (whitened or unraced) child?

After a very early pronouncement that Lina was "of the white race," *La Crónica* went virtually silent on the issue.[28] Still, the question of the girl's racial background lurked in the illustrations in *La Crónica* and invaded international coverage. The hundreds of US papers that picked up the story tended to describe Lina as an "Indian." And savvier local readers in Peru would know that the region from which she hailed was a peasant community where lifeways were heavily contoured by Andean culture, regardless of her biological ancestry. Indeed, a recurring element of the story was that her parents had first availed themselves of a local *curandero* to diagnose her. His assessment involved traditional Andean notions of possession by snakes to explain her growing belly. In this illustration, the artist seems to have it both ways: Lina is somewhat unraced as in other pictures. Her hair is cut into a

(*Opposite*) This drawing of Lina's body covers her abdomen to drive up curiosity, underscores her young age by positioning her with toys, and heightens the sense that her pregnancy posed a mortal danger to her by placing the story beside another featuring a photograph of a dead man. The caption reads, "In the facility where she was placed, Lina Medina spends the day oblivious to her own tragedy. At the back, a doctor considers putting up a metal shade in the window." "Lina Medina debe ser traída a esta capital con intervención de las instituciones científicas," *La Crónica*, April 14, 1939, 14.

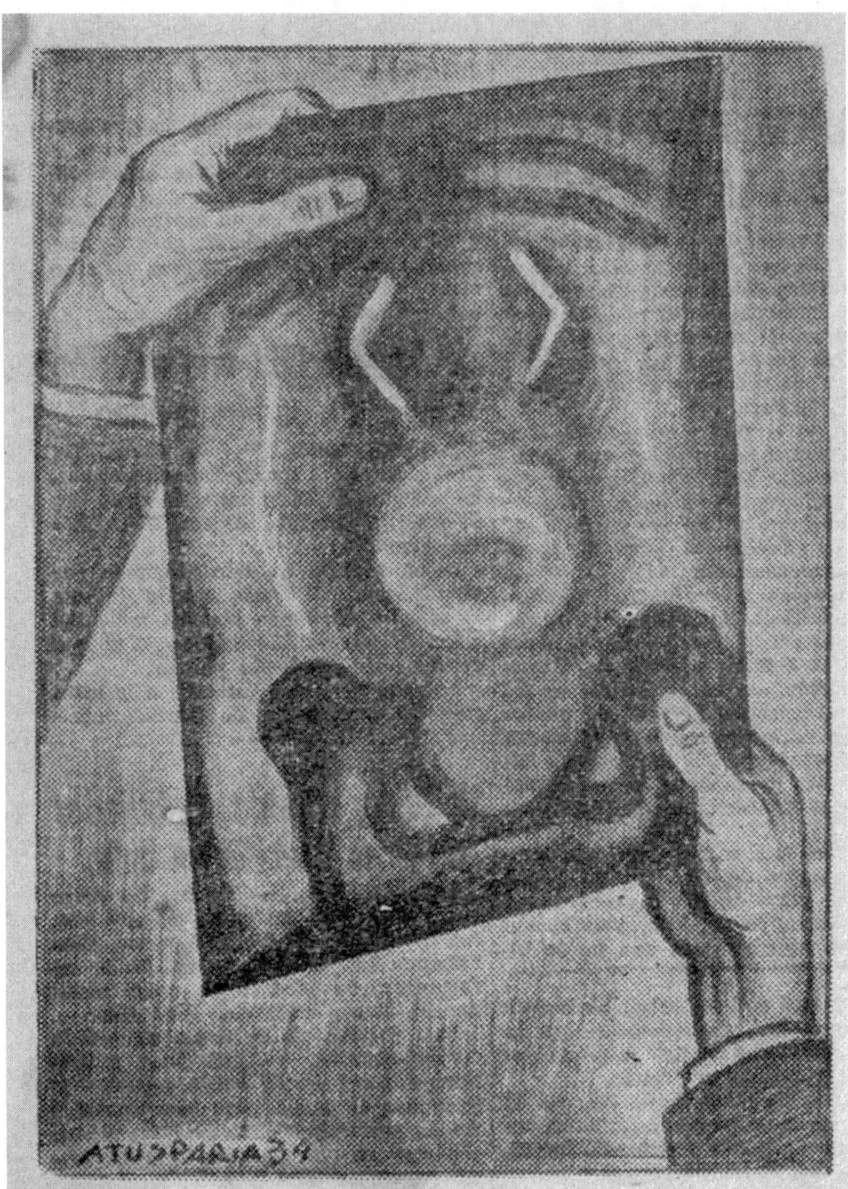

Drawing of a hand holding the plate or image from an abdominal X-ray taken of Lina in Pisco hospital, with the rounded shape in the center representing the fetal head. "Crea un problema complejo para la biología el caso de Pisco, dice el Secretario Perpetuo de la Academia Nacional de Medicina, *La Crónica*, April 15, 1939, 14.

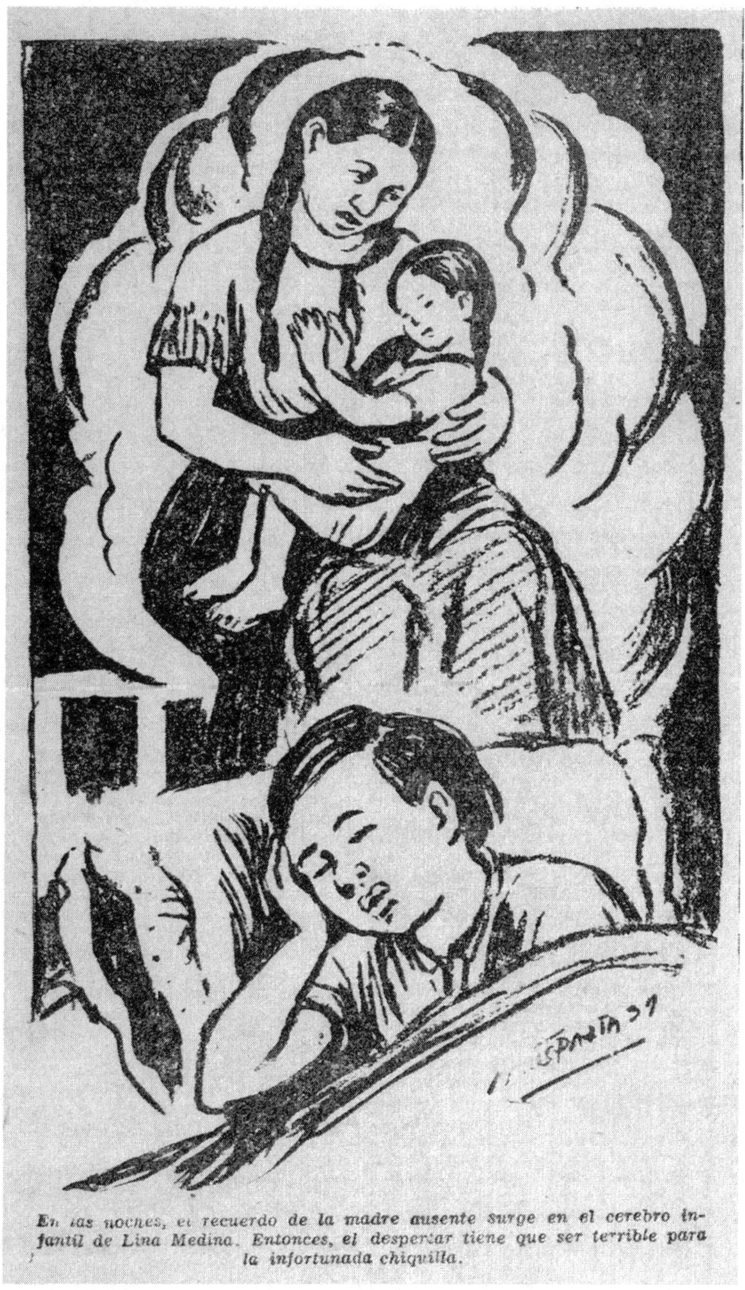

A short-haired Lina dreams, as shown by a "dream bubble," that her (Indigenous) mother holds her while she sleeps in the hospital. The caption reads, "In the nights, the memory of her absent mother rises in the infantile mind of Lina Medina. As such, waking must be terrible for this unfortunate little girl." "Destacados médicos de esta capital parten hoy rumbo a Pisco para comprobar el sensacional caso de Lina Medina," *La Crónica*, April 16, 1939, 15.

short bob but, as she dreams of her mother, both are clearly indexed as rural and Indigenous with long, black braids. She has literally been moved out of the category of "Indian"—braids cut, mother gone—through medical care.

Alongside the drawing, the text of this article followed a new strand of advocacy: bringing Lina to the capital city of Lima to give birth and placing her with state-approved physicians and agencies. The reporting began focusing on Lina's parents and her internment in the Pisco hospital under Dr. Lozada's care. Behind the attention to the adequacy of medical facilities in provincial Pisco was a growing demand among statesmen and physicians in the capital city to gain control of the case and, eventually, custody of the child. Soon, the questions of who Lina was and where she should be cared for began to elicit reflection about who, exactly, should be looking at her. The drawing accompanying a piece about the stir Lina's pregnancy was causing was one of several over the coming days that would visually focus on crowds or clusters of people looking.[29]

In this drawing, a notably unraced or white bourgeois crowd gathered outside Lina's hospital room in the dusty provincial city accompanies a headline announcing international attention from "Scientific Institutions in Paris and Río de Janeiro." The caption tells us that the crowd was composed of visitors from Lima as well as Pisco locals. Interest in Lina's case was quickly spreading both nationally and internationally, and this renown forced a literal and figurative self-examination among Peru's onlookers. It is notable that the illustration depicts two reactions at once: the crowd in the background is struggling to see in through a hospital window or door—shaded black to suggest opacity—while a distressed, blonde-looking woman sits on a step in the foreground. It's worth pausing together here to examine the contrast between the avid spectators shown in profile and the woman facing the reader.

The text of this article is filled with emotive keywords that urge action such as *afán* (eagerness) and *urgencia* (urgency). It also describes the "*magno interés por cerciorarse del fenómeno*" (great interest in verifying the phenomenon). But even with these insistent keywords and phrasings, the article portrayed the public fascination with beholding Lina as rational. People gathered to listen to Lina's attending physician deliver medical details about the girl's condition, as if they were part of a medical team. It was true, the paper admitted, that there were some "*gentes llevadas por sus supersticiones*" (folks carried away by their superstitions) who saw mystery in the pregnancy

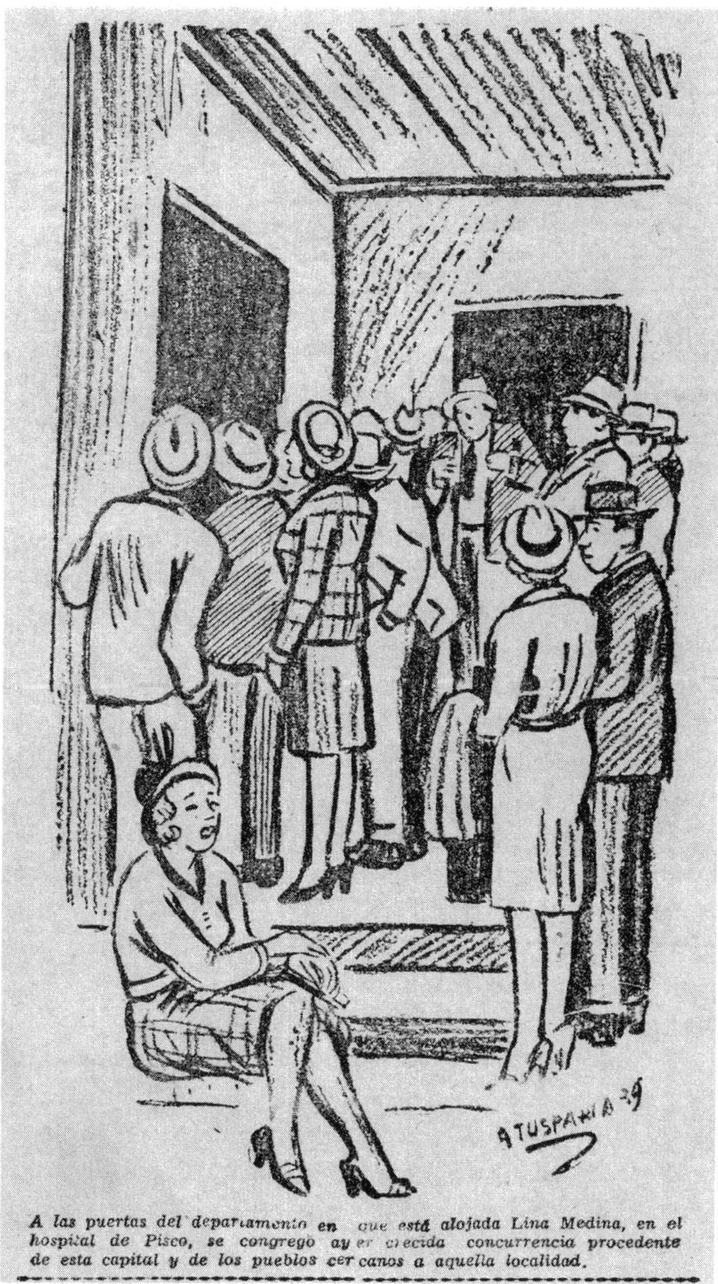

A las puertas del departamento en que está alojada Lina Medina, en el hospital de Pisco, se congregó ayer crecida concurrencia procedente de esta capital y de los pueblos cercanos a aquella localidad.

In this drawing, a well-dressed crowd from "this capital and nearby pueblos" gathers outside the black door to Lina's hospital room in San Juan de Dios Hospital in Pisco, while one woman sits on stairs in the foreground, in distress or overwhelmed. "Instituciones científicas de Paris y Rio Janeiro se interesan por el sensacional case de Lina Medina," *La Crónica*, April 17, 1939, 14.

and read it as a sign of the end of times. But readers were assured that the case *"no tiene nada de misterio"* (contains no mystery); it was a *"fenómeno biológico"* (biological phenomenon), even if one of extraordinary proportions.

Using the text as guide, we can look again at the woman's face in the illustration of the crowd not as a portrait of compassion—either the woman's own empathy for the violated girl or our own understandable distress at imagining the whole scene. Instead, if paired with the text, this is a depiction of irrationality and unproductive superstition. The overwrought woman is not modern enough for the kind of scientific looking, the "clinical gaze," of which the group gathered behind her is capable.[30] Eager public gawking and scientific observation were thus collapsed, and the desire to see Lina was rationalized. Looking away was stigmatized.

In the following day's paper, Atusparia took a break and a photographer took over. The headline again announced international attention and a bursting public desire to look at Lina: "North American Business Offers 5,000 Dollars to Film the Extraordinary Case of the Minor Lina Medina." Several features of the photos in this day's reporting are worth highlighting. Principal among them is the correspondence, or perhaps clash, between the text—in this case, the headline—and the images. The desire to behold Lina was presented as suspect when it emanated from *"determinados sectores"* (certain sectors)—namely foreign ones—that possessed a *"sentido práctico y comercial"* (practical and commercial aim). This was contrasted with the intentions of national spectators, whose interest was born of *"avidez"* (emotional avidity), a term that connotes anxious desire.

The article's text focused on the disapproval and outrage that the foreign offers of money to film Lina evoked among Peruvians. Its images focused on the concern of two sectors: feminized health care workers and an ordinary working man. The nurses from the downtown maternity ward of the Hospital Loayza in Lima who stayed past their long working hours to read the paper were the embodiment of avidez. Also representing avidez was a reclining working-class man, clad in boots and laid out on the grass, described as rapt, oblivious to the *"tiranía del calor"* (tyranny of the heat), and entranced by the question of whether Lina would be moved to Lima. Their interest in Lina, their desire to see her, placed Lima's diverse working classes as the subjects of the report, displacing the regional rivalries between the provinces and the capital as they wrestled to control the birth, even displacing the girl herself. This was a kind of triumph for the city of Lima, where caring parties

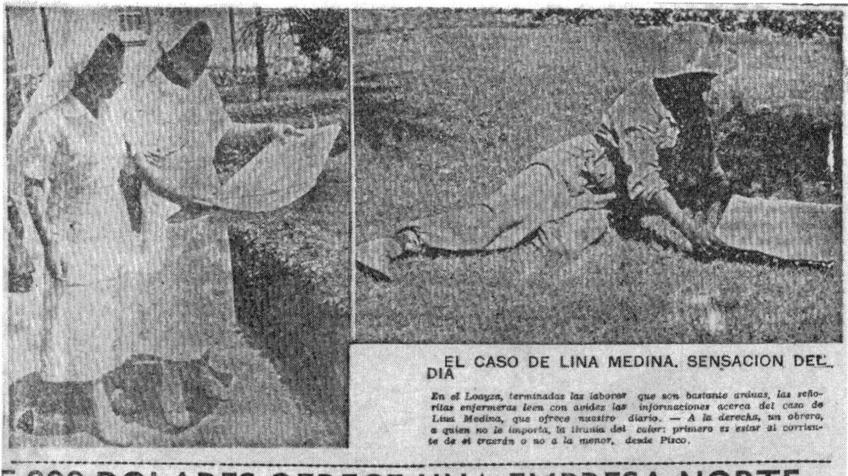

En el Loayza, terminadas las labores que son bastante arduas, las señoritas enfermeras leen con avidez las informaciones acerca del caso de Lina Medina, que ofrece nuestro diario. — A la derecha, un obrero, a quien no le importa, la ironía del color; primero es estar al corriente de si traerán o no a la menor, desde Pisco.

5,000 DOLARES OFRECE UNA EMPRESA NORTE-AMERICANA PARA FILMAR EL EXTRAORDINA-RIO CASO DE LA MENOR LINA MEDINA

Photographs of (*left*) nurses from hospitals in Lima hopeful to admit Lina for the birth and (*right*) an unidentified working man on a break, outside on hospital grounds, papers splayed before him, poring over the "sensation of the day." The headline below the photos warns about foreign offers to film the girl. "5,000 dolares ofrece una empresa norteamericana para filmar el extraordinario caso de la menor, Lina Medina," *La Crónica*, April 18, 1939, 14.

awaited her. One imagines the worker wondering whether Lina would be moved closer to him, increasing the chances that he could see her himself.[31]

Comparing these photos of working-class, caring Limeños reading about Lina with the drawing of the crowd in Pisco from the day before, we may discern a shift in just one day: In addition to the contrast between scientific and superstitious spectators, a new clash has emerged between the capitalist, profit-motivated foreign exploiter and the national, working-class producer-viewer-reader. This day's photographs also establish an interiority, a kind of looking from within that is not passively consumptive but rather compassionately productive, rooted in care, work, and affinity. During the month of April 1939, the paper also frequently ran allegorical depictions of Lina, such as one of her confronting a cluster of corpulent, cigar-smoking men whose suit pockets were stuffed with US dollars, and another, of her running for refuge into an oversized hand labeled "*patronato*," or patronage. These illustrations encouraged readers to center themselves, as protagonists and scientific caretakers, in the story unfolding, to see themselves as her salvation.

In the days leading up to the birth, the pressure from Lima's physicians and statesmen to transfer the girl from the provincial hospital in Pisco to the capital city was becoming too strong to resist. But looking at Lina was about more than her physical location. Dr. Lozada, Lina's obstetrician in Pisco, was seeking the equipment and crew to make his own film, focused on his "*estudios y experimentos*" (studies and experiments) and plans "*filmar el proceso científico*" (to film the scientific process). The "experiments" he was conducting involved intense looking at her "*características faciales y de otras partes de su cuerpo*" (facial characteristics and of other parts of her body). The purpose of creating images was asserted as scientific, and alongside that justification came acknowledgment that all this looking was meant to *comprobar* (prove) the reality of her pregnancy. Lozada prepared to go to the capital city of Lima to present his findings.[32]

On April 22, when Dr. Lozada arrived in Lima, his report prepared, the issue of looking created a scene. The National Academy of Medicine was to host an afternoon presentation by Lozada in its headquarters, in a converted republican-era mansion in the city center. Crowds packed into the tiny auditorium of the Academy, then overflowed into its halls, upper floors, and offices. In descriptions of the event, it seems women were in ample attendance. But soon there were simply too many spectators.[33]

La Crónica reported that the audience, "*invadido*" (invaded) by a crowd of hundreds who formed a "*compacta masa humana*" (compact human mass), had so exceeded the space's capacity that the presentation had to be postponed. Lozada retreated to his hotel room in the fancy Hotel Bolívar in Lima's central Plaza San Martín to await his rescheduled event, in the meantime entertaining only the upper-class ladies from charitable societies who had taken up Lina's case as a cause.

In the end, his presentation, delayed by five days, would be attended by only a select audience, "which was be technical [since] this concerns an event of such importance for scientific research. In reality, this is not about offering a spectacle, much less to satisfy collective curiosity" (*que debe ser técnico, tratándose de un hecho de tanta trascendencia para la investigación científica. En realidad, no se trata de ofrecer un espectáculo, ni mucho menos satisfacer una curiosidad colectiva*). Despite the earlier overtures about creating an expert scientific public, collective curiosity on the part of the (compact human) masses was thus again partitioned from scientific investigation: gawking was distinguished from examining, looking from knowing. The illustration capturing the presentation shows no women in attendance. The smaller crowd viewed a photo or film of a naked pregnant Lina, but the readers saw only this shadowed drawing, with her skin dark and her features blurred.[34]

The image on the film almost defied other depictions of Lina as an un-raced or whitened child, and it seemed to undo the work that had been accomplished by whitening Lina in other illustrations. When the public was replaced by experts, the child was replaced with an anthropological specimen. The contradiction revealed how tenuous the endeavor to create an ethos of state-centered collective care could be and how longer-held traditions of race-based gawking and spectacle remained right below the surface in *La Crónica*'s reporting.

And this was not the first full-length depiction of Lina's body. An illustration of Lina, posed fully from the front, had run two days prior to the report on Lozada's presentation. It is the only illustration not signed by the artist Atusparia. This unique drawing by an anonymous artist, depicting her at a two-thirds turn in a gown, with short hair, is, to my eye, is stylistically completely out of step with Atusparia's drawings. Gone are the images of Lina as a normative (whitened) child. Aesthetics of cuteness and youth are also gone, as are the attentive care workers and physicians.[35] Instead, Lina is depicted alone. Her features are portrayed in a manner reminiscent of depictions of dwarfism, with larger feet, full breasts, shorter arms, and a head, all of which evince adulthood, as if the actual image of a pregnant child in full, from head to toe, exceeded the artist's ability to represent it.

The image evokes a deeper history of fascination with Latin Americans, particularly those of Indigenous descent, as marvelously small. Dwarfism among Latin Americans had long attracted imperial attention. Nineteenth-century cases of smallness included another world record holder, the so-called smallest person on record, a Mexican girl with microcephalic dwarfism named Lucía Zarate, whom English physicians photographed, exhibited, and promoted as the "Mexican Lilliputian!" Around the same time, promotors measured the bodies and heads of so-called "Aztec children" Bartola and Máximo, on stage daily in New York City before public audiences to prove their links to disappearing Indigenous peoples.[36]

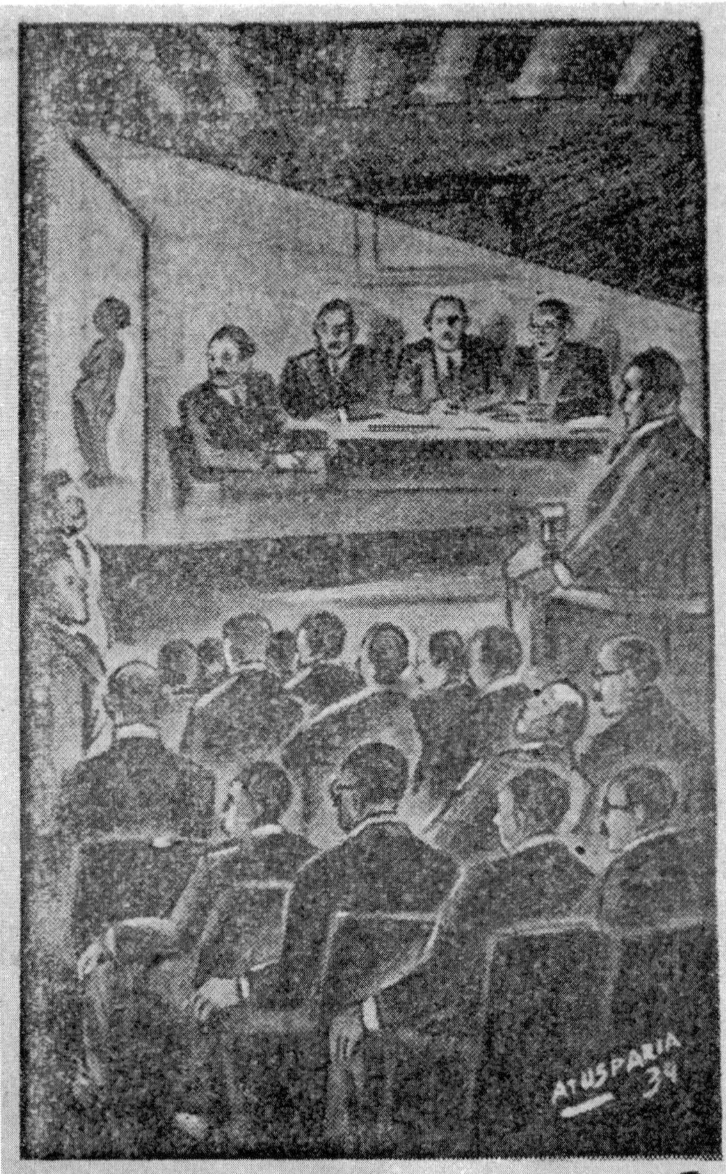

Dentro del ambiente austero del recinto, los señores académicos siguieron atentos la exposición hecha por el notable médico doctor Gerardo Lozada, sobre el sensacional caso de Lina Medina.

This artistic half-capitulation—Lina small but not a child, rendered into the stable category of "disabled" adult and thus rendered a "protagonist"—did more than merely reflect the possible artistic limits of the anonymous illustrator. Its genealogy in the fascination with unnaturally small, perpetually developing Latin Americans shaped the very categorization and archiving of Lina's history in the United States. Chicago businessman and sideshow promoter Leo A. Seltzer, who aggressively pushed to wrest control of Lina from the Peruvian state and bring her to the US for display, unsuccessfully sought a visa for Lina in the early 1940s. The US Immigration Office declined the application, noting that his ethically dubious bid fell into the cracks between "educational" travel and "labor." The paperwork was filed under the heading "Freaks."[37] The entry for her file is surrounded by foreign performers with dwarfism who sought entry as entertainers to fairs, expositions, and circuses.

This pull toward the more historically recognizable, permanent category of "freak" or "dwarf" remained a countervailing force even as the adults surrounding Lina tried to focus the public on themselves and their curative, collective effort to care for her as a prototypical, "normal" child. Accordingly, in the weeks before the birth, the tensions between popular gawking and scientific observation, between Lina as an object of care and as a protagonist, between seeing and believing all remained unresolved. But what was clear is that, as Peruvians strained to catch a glimpse of Lina, they were deeply aware that they were looking at themselves looking.

Conclusion

To conclude, let's look at one final allegorical illustration that captured how conscious Peruvians were of the question of consensus when

(*Opposite*) Dr. Gerardo Lozada, the diagnosing physician from Pisco, giving his delayed presentation to an expert audience at the National Academy of Medicine in Lima. The crowd, comprising men only, is in shadow, and the image the film projector emits is an indistinct, dark rendering of the photo of Lina, nude, that would become the only proof of her pregnancy. The caption reads, "Within the austere environment of the venue, distinguished academics intently follow the presentation made by the notable doctor Gerardo Lozada, about the sensational case of Lina Medina." "Nombra la Academia Nacional de Medicina una comisión para q' determine sobre el caso de Lina Medina," *La Crónica*, April 28, 1939, 14.

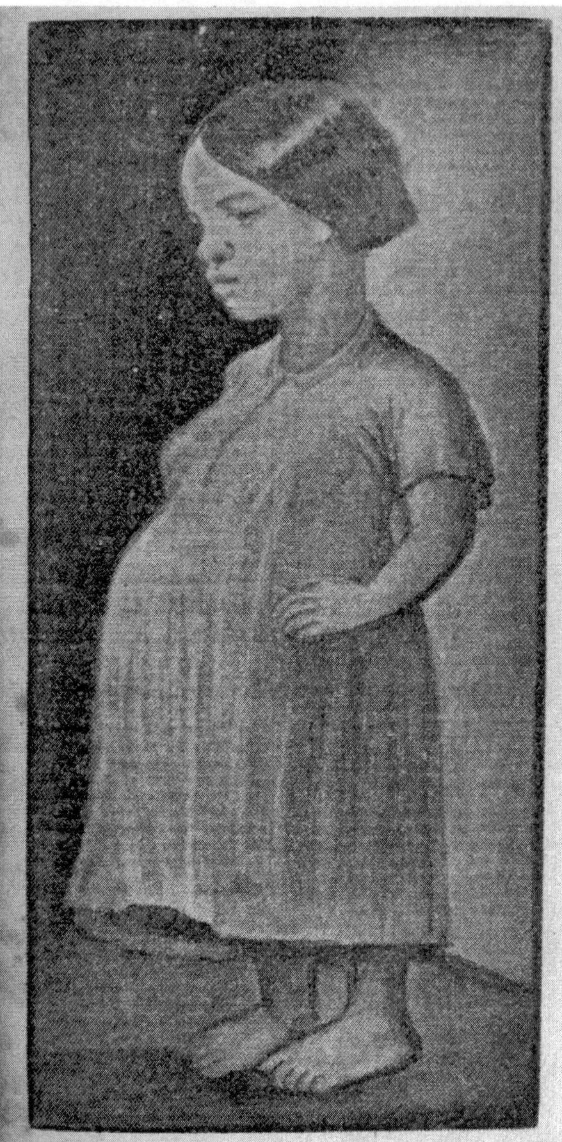

Estado en que se encuentra la menor *Lina Medina*, de cinco años y medio de edad, en el Hospital de Pisco y que, siendo protagonista de un suceso de tanta trascendencia científica, debe inspirar en la sociedad un elevado sentimiento humanitario para acudir en su auxilio. La organización de un Patronato formado por damas y caballeros es urgente. Hay que salvar dos vidas y el porvenir de la propia menor y la de su posible vástago.

```
Freaks                                          1-2-40 d

55,925-867   Sundry file - SINGER MIDGETS - engaged at
                SF - World fair - Golden Gate exposition.
56,036-229   LINA MEDINA   - 6 years old - algd to be mother
                of 15 mos old ALEJANDRO MEDINA - coming
                for scientific examination by doctors of
                the US and for public exhibition.
```

US National Archives defunct card catalog entry on the immigration of "Freaks," with Lina Medina's file listed alongside "Singer Midgets" who were to be featured at another World's Fair. Subject Index to Correspondence and Case Files of the Immigration and Naturalization Service, 1903–1952, January 2, 1940, INS reference number 56,036-229, microfilm roll 15, US National Archives and Records Administration.

looking at Lina, and how fragile this new, national way of looking was. In this illustration, (surgically) gloved hands reach out for a slightly off-center Lina, shown only in bust so that her pregnant belly is again out of view. The illustration displays both looking and reaching. This is curative looking. An eye, perhaps a woman's, peers at the girl; another eye peers through a telescope; physicians gather around data, rapt in reading or viewing, one with a

(*Opposite*) The caption for this full-length portrait rendering of Lina's body captures the ethos of care-based, urgent looking, even as the image itself adultifies, isolates, and "disables" her: "State in which the minor Lina Medina, of five and half years, is found in the Hospital in Pisco and in which, being a protagonist in a process of such scientific transcendence, should inspire in society an elevated humanitarian sentiment to come to her aid. The organization of a charitable board (*patronato*), formed of ladies and gentlemen, is urgent. Two lives must be saved, as well as her future and that of her possible descendant." "Lina Medina es bastante agil y sale a pasear a los jardines del Hospital de Pisco al medio," *La Crónica*, April 23, 1939, 15.

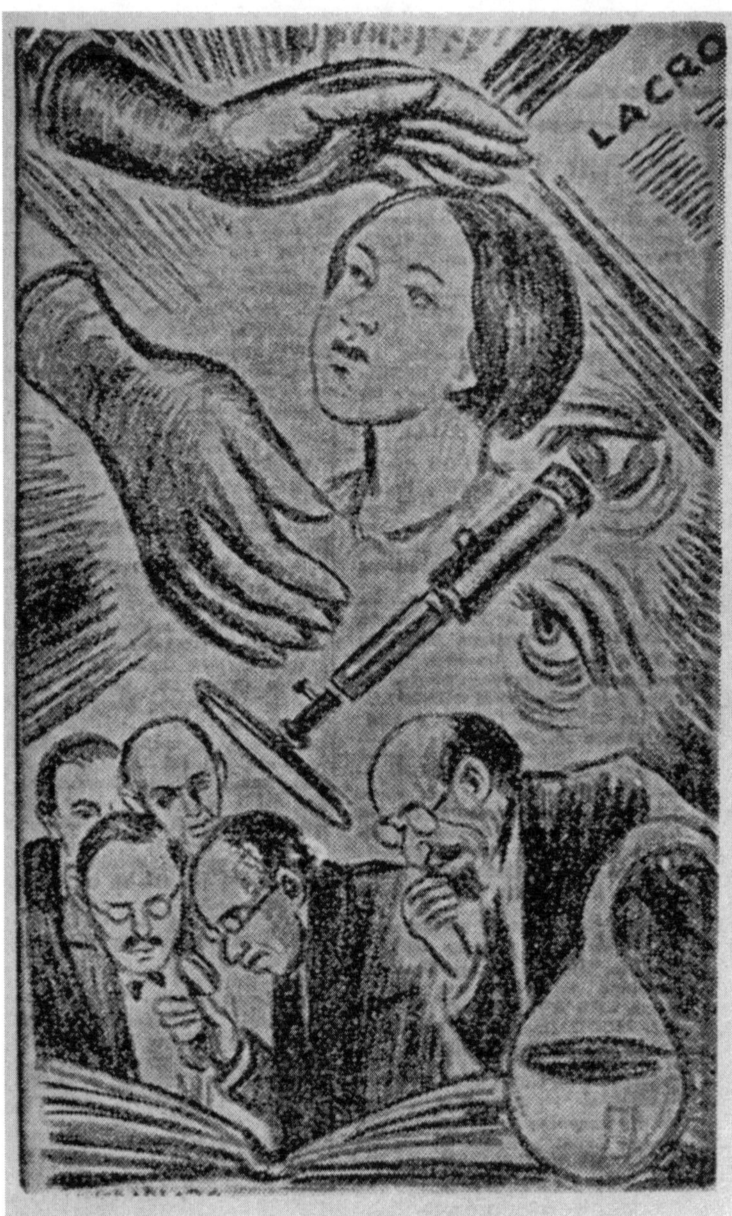

El mundo científico concentra su atención en el extraordinario caso de Lina Medina, con el interés de descubrir las causas del proceso biológico. — (Apunte de Atusparia).

magnifying glass, a beaker nearby. Notably, an issue of *La Crónica* itself peeks out from the upper right corner.[38]

As Garland-Thompson might have predicted, for *La Crónica* and its readership, looking at Lina meant literally turning its gaze onto itself. But the "self" of the paper was not singular, and the final image reveals that the distinctions between action and observation, between science and popular interest were unstable. In *La Crónica*, looking at an extraordinary body involved a continual tension and a constant drawing of boundaries of "normality" and "abnormality," of exteriority and interiority, within observers (expert and the public), within Peru (between Pisco and Lima), and beyond (between Peru and the US).

Furthermore, the newspaper—Peruvians' chief window onto Lina—could not fully center itself, its readers, or even Lina herself in this last illustration. This is because it is ultimately unclear who the subject of fascination was: Was it the girl, or was it the way her case was handled by the nation? Was it the patient or science itself? Was it ultimately the visual media through which we know others? At moments the images reached for medical respectability by signaling traditional social patronage and curative care, as when Gerardo Lozada, retreating from the throngs of popular interest, was flanked in the Hotel Bolívar by officials of government ministries and the ladies who ran the beneficence society. At other times it meant the careful inclusion of the popular classes or working medical professionals—including women—as legitimate possessors of knowledge and acting, caring spectators who would tend to the girl and her baby. And, at still others, the images defaulted to imperialist freakery, leaning on a long association of Latin Americans with dwarfism, erasing Lina's childhood.

There is no image—drawn, photographed, or beheld—that can witness what happened to Lina. We can only look at Lima's experts and spectators looking at her. And then look at ourselves. On the internet, comments sec-

(*Opposite*) An allegorical drawing of Lina's face, with men (presumably physicians) poring over texts and surrounded by medical instruments; a single eye peers and gloved hands reach, with the newspaper *La Crónica* itself captured in a corner. The caption reads, "The scientific world concentrates its attention on the extraordinary case of Lina Medina, with the interest of discovering the causes of the biological process." "El unico problema creado en el caso de Lina Medina es el endocrinico, dice el notable medico chileno Dr. Gmo. Caceres," *La Crónica*, April 24, 1939, 15.

tions of YouTube "films" that aggregate images of her from "weird news" websites are full of reactions. The comments typically fall into two camps: they lament what happened to her or express disbelief. As Garland-Thomas might predict, they are caught between staring and looking away. Yet seeing extraordinary bodies and, in turn, defining and normalizing a collective self are, while not automatically commensurate, the same process. And they are, and were, a process. Watching the images of Lina transform in the first two weeks of coverage in Peru forces us to recognize that the communal dimensions of looking at extraordinary bodies and their attendant ethics were dynamic in their moment and remain so as we continue to look for and at disabled bodies in Latin America's past.

While historians of disability and all of us interested in ethical practices of looking might strain to create "a belated alliance with the oppressed, whose resistance or repugnance and harm or injury could not be voiced," I propose that we pause with some humility before this restorative ethos.[39] By remaining faithful to the sequence and focus with which Lima's reading public was exposed to images of Lina Medina's improbable pregnancy and extraordinary body, it becomes clear that they were engaged in an ongoing, evolving attempt not to give voice but to turn staring into caring.[40] This involved an ultimately failed attempt to move her away from the category of freak by whitening her, showing her as an endangered child, playing games with illustrations of her body to render her a normalized object of charity, and rallying the nation to attend to her and her newborn son rather than to gawk. Of course, that attempt had become history by the time an elderly woman was furtively pursued returning home with groceries in 2018. But, given how unlikely any of us are to look away, perhaps the story is not yet over.

NOTES

1. In the twenty-first century, there appears to be a global incidence of the condition (called central precocious puberty) in 1 in 5,000 to 10,000 children, with a female-to-male ratio of about 20:1, though this ratio is debated. See Anne-Simone Parent, Grete Teilmann, Anders Juul, Niels E. Skakkebaek, Jorma Toppari, and Jean-Pierre Bourguignon, "The Timing of Normal Puberty and the Age Limits of Sexual Precocity: Variations Around the World, Secular Trends, and Changes After Migration," *Endocrine Reviews* 24, no. 5 (2013): 668–93.

2. The paper would show its first photograph of Lina on the day she was scheduled to undergo surgery to give birth. It placed a black bar over her eyes and cropped the original

photo from the shoulders up, though the original was later published elsewhere, showing her nude, including breasts and belly. "Los doctores Lozada y Busalleu intervendran en la operación quirugigica de la menor Medina," *La Crónica*, May 14, 1939, 14.

3. Catherine Kudlick, in exploring definitions of disability, notes that nondisabled (also called normate) people might experience a temporary disabling event or state but that "such visits only scratch the surface of living with a chronic condition and fail to introduce people to the real problems" faced by the permanently disabled. Kudlick, "Disability History: Why We Need Another 'Other,'" *American Historical Review* 108, no. 3 (2003): 763–93. Physicians' struggle to differentiate disease and disability based on projections of a future "cure." See Beth Linker, "On the Borderland of Medical and Disability History: A Survey of the Fields," *Bulletin of the History of Medicine* 87, no. 4 (2013): 499–535. Complicating this distinction, a compelling first-person account written by a US man who was treated for precocious puberty between the ages of 3 and 14 features recollections of the trauma of being medically photographed as well as sexualized because of his condition. Throughout his recounting, the idea that he would simply "[grow] out of" a condition that, for a time, was deeply similar to chronic illness and disability, falls apart. See Patrick Burleigh, "I Was a 4-Year-Old Trapped in a Teenager's Body," *The Cut*, January 16, 2019, https://www.thecut.com/2019/01/precocious-puberty-patrick-burleigh.html. See also Sami Schalk, "Disability," in *Keywords for Gender and Sexuality Studies*, ed. Kyla Wazana Tompkins, Aren Z. Aizura, Aimee Bahng, et al. (New York University Press, 2021), 43–46, https://keywords.nyupress.org/gender-and-sexuality-studies/essay/disability/. For more on precocity as a disability, see Holly N. S. White, "Judging the Bodies of Children: Racial Science and Double Age as Legal Strategy in the Early United States," *Journal of the History of Childhood and Youth* 15, no. 3 (2022): 399–409.

4. Martín Mucha, "Lina Medina, una madre a los cinco años," *El Mundo / Crónica*, February 11, 2018, https://www.elmundo.es/cronica/2018/02/11/5a7f22cf46163f2f158b4586 .html.

5. See the roundtable inspired by Sarah Maza, "The Kids Aren't All Right: The Problem of Childhood," *American Historical Review* 125, no. 4 (2020), 1261–85; and the ensuing responses, including Nara Milanich, "Comment on Sarah Maza's 'The Kids Aren't All Right,'" 1296–99; and Ishita Pande, "Comment on Sarah Maza's 'The Kids Aren't All Right,'" 1300–1305.

6. Roy Hanes, "Introduction," in *The Routledge History of Disability*, ed. Roy Hanes, Ivan Brown, and Nancy E. Hansen (Taylor and Francis, 2017), 3.

7. See Kevin Coleman, "The Right Not to Be Looked At," *Estudios Interdisciplinarios de América Latina y el Caribe* 25, no. 2 (2015): 43–63.

8. My relationship with Lina as a subject shares much in common with Françoise N. Hamilton's work on Anne Moody, "Finding Anne Moody: Historians and Ethics," *American Historical Review* 125, no. 2 (2020): 487–97. Rosemary Garland-Thompson makes "looking back" central to "mutual recognition," which is more difficult if the "staree" is dead, but perhaps not impossible. See Garland-Thompson, *Staring: How We Look* (Oxford University Press, 2009).

9. See Zachary M. Schrag, *Ethical Imperialism: Institutional Review Boards and the Social Sciences, 1965–2009* (Johns Hopkins University Press, 2010).

10. Jacques Rancière calls this ethical quandary the "duplicity of the abhorrent image": "For the image to produce its political effect, the spectator must . . . already feel guilty about viewing the image," and this guilt is magnified, it might be said, because the assumption is that the guilty spectator can never be moved to action by viewing. Rancière, *The Emancipated Spectator*, trans. George Elliot (Verso, 2011), 84, 86. The contradiction between guilt and action is also at the heart of Susan Sontag's *Regarding the Pain of Others* (Picador, 2004).

11. Rosemary Garland-Thompson, "Introduction," in *Freakery: Cultural Spectacles of the Extraordinary Body*, ed. Rosemary Garland-Thompson (New York University Press, 1996), 13; Pete Sigal, Zeb Tortorici, and Neil Whitehead, eds., *Ethnopornography: Sexuality, Colonialism, and Archival Knowledge* (Duke University Press, 2020).

12. Roland Barthes, in *Camera Lucida: Reflections on Photography* (Hill and Wang, 1982), placed death at the center of the photograph, observing that each mechanical image contains a "catastrophe that already has come to pass." See also Gerhard Richter, *Inheriting Walter Benjamin* (Bloomsbury, 2016), 126–27; and Susan Sontag, *On Photography* (1977; reprint, Picador, 2004).

13. Carla Rice, "The Spectacle of the Child Woman: Troubling Girls and the Science of Early Puberty," *Feminist Studies* 44, no. 3 (2018): 537.

14. Alison Kramer, *Feminist, Queer, Crip* (Indiana University Press, 2013), 27–28.

15. Erik Thamdrup, "Precocious Sexual Development: A Clinical Study of One Hundred Children," *Danish Medical Bulletin* 8, (1961): 141–42. Cf. Hugh Jolly, *Sexual Precocity* (Blackwell, 1955). It should be noted that Jolly, intervening in a spate of studies of precocious puberty from the 1920s and 1940s, attempted to show that many children who demonstrated precocity actually lived long lives and had longer periods of fertility, but his was somewhat of a lone voice.

16. Here we might consider the inclusion of Indigenous and pregnant subjects as exceptions in human subjects protocols and ideas of children as a "protected category" of research subjects. Tamar W. Caroll and Myron Guttmann, "The Limits of Autonomy: The Belmont Report and the History of Childhood," *Journal of the History of Medicine and Allied Sciences* 66, no. 1 (2011): 82–115; Michael Grodin and L. Glantz, eds., *Children as Research Subjects: Science, Ethics and Law* (Oxford University Press, 2004). On the ideas of the future embedded in Lina's pregnancy, see reference to her in Sarah Norgate, *Beyond Nine to Five: Your Life in Time* (Columbia University Press, 2006), 53.

17. Rosemary Garland-Thompson, *Extraordinary Bodies: Figuring Physical Disability in American Culture and Literature* (Columbia University Press, 1996); Andrea Zittlau, "The Freak-Show Act: Science and Spectacle in the Nineteenth Century," *The Routledge History of Disability*, 381–393.

18. Garland-Thompson, *Staring*, 6.

19. Rancière calls communal prohibitions "consensus" and the hesitation "dissensus." *Emancipated Spectator*, 90–92, 50.

20. Rancière, *Emancipated Spectator*, 25; Rancière, "Comment and Responses," *Theory and Event* 6, no. 4 (2003), https://dx.doi.org/10.1353/tae.2003.0017, accessed 6-10-2025.

21. Marcos Cueto has described social medicine as a "heterodox European current" that galvanized Latin American medicine in the twentieth century. Cueto, "Social Medi-

cine and Leprosy in the Peruvian Amazon," *The Americas* 1, no. 61 (2004): 55–80. More recent studies emphasize its origins in national and transnational thought. See, for example, Eric D. Carter, *In Pursuit of Health Equity: A History of Latin American Social Medicine* (University of North Carolina Press, 2023). In Peru, Carlos Enrique Paz Soldán, a key figure in Lina's story, created the curriculum for social medicine at San Marcos and in 1927 founded its Institute of Social Medicine. The stress on the "collective" in his vision of social medicine can be detected in *La Medicina Social (Ensayo de Sistematización)* (Imprenta SS CC, 1916), especially the definition he borrows from the Italian G. Tropeano (11) and his comments on the "collective life" (*vida colectiva*) that united different branches of science and social sectors, from charities to state enterprises, and particularly the contact between the "medical class" and the "proletariat," 15. On social medicine in Latin America, see Howard Waitzkin, Celia Iriart, Alfredo Estrada, and Silvia Lamadrid, "Social Medicine Then and Now: Lessons from Latin America," *American Journal of Public Health* 91, no. 10 (2001): 1592–1601.

22. For a suggestion about an ethos of "care" in the early programs in Peru, see Cueto, "Social Medicine and Leprosy," 56.

23. "Sensacional caso que produce un revuelo entre los hombres de ciencia ha realizado en Pisco," *La Crónica*, April 13, 1939, 14.

24. "La policía de Miraflores investiga la sospechosa Muerte de un menor de tres años," *La Crónica*, April 25, 1939, 14.

25. "Crea un problema complejo para la biología el caso de Pisco, dice el Secretario Perpetuo de la Academia Nacional de Medicina," *La Crónica*, April 15, 1939, 14. X-rays can be viewed as another form of violative looking, especially when considering anxieties around women's bodies during the advent of this technology. See Bettyann Kevles, *Naked to the Bone: Medical Imaging in the Twentieth Century* (Rutgers University Press, 1997); and Joel D. Howell, *Technology in the Hospital: Transforming Patient Care in the Early Twentieth Century* (Johns Hopkins University Press, 1995). For a patient-centered take on the experience of being X-rayed in the early twentieth century, see Matthew Lavine, "The Early Clinical X-Ray in the United States: Patient Experiences and Public Perceptions," *Journal of the History of Medicine and Allied Sciences* 67, no. 4 (2012): 587–625.

26. "El Caso Lina Medina," *La Reforma Médica* 25, no. 308 (1939): 445.

27. "Destacados médicos de esta capital parten hoy rumbo a Pisco para comprobar el sensacional caso de Lina Medina," *La Crónica*, April 16, 1939, 15.

28. "Sensacional caso que produce un revuelo."

29. "Instituciones científicas de Paris y Río Janeiro se interesan por el sensacional caso de Lina Medina," *La Crónica*, May 17, 1939, 14.

30. The phase is (famously) Michel Foucault's. See Garland-Thompson, *Staring*, 47, 48.

31. "5,000 dólares ofrece una empresa norteamericana para filmar el extraordinario caso de la menor, Lina Medina," *La Crónica*, April 15, 1939, 14. See also "Lina Medina debe ser traída a esta capital con intervención de instituciones científicas," *La Crónica*, April 14, 1939.

32. "5,000 dólares ofrece," *La Crónica*, April 15, 1939, 14.

33. "Postergase el acto en que el Doctor Gerardo Lozada iba a exponer sus estudios en el caso de la menor Lina Medina," *La Crónica*, April 22, 1939, 14.

34. "Nombra la Academia Nacional de Medicina una comisión para q' determine sobre el caso de Lina Medina," *La Crónica*, April 28, 1939, 14.

35. Lori Merish, "Cuteness and Commodity Aesthetics: Tom Thumb and Shirley Temple," in *Freakery*, 187; S. Ngai, "The Cuteness of the Avant-Garde," *Critical Inquiry* 31, no. 4 (2005): 811–47.

36. Judith G. Hall, "The Smallest of the Small," *Gene* 528, no. 1 (2013): 55–57. This article, drawing from a long genealogy of looking to mothers as the source of "abnormality," notes that it was likely that Lucía's mother, from the "country side [*sic*]," would have had "poor nutrition" that "compounded her small stature" (57). For more on mothers and normality, see Nora Jaffary, *Reproduction and Its Discontents in Mexico: Childbirth and Contraception from 1705 to 1905* (University of North Carolina Press, 2016). On the "Aztec children," see Zittlau, "Freak-Show Act."

37. Defunct card catalog entry, Subject Index to Correspondence and Case Files of the Immigration and Naturalization Service, 1903–1952, January 2, 1940, Entry A1 9, Subject and Policy Files, 1906–1957, Microfilm roll 15, Record Group 85, Records of the Immigration and Naturalization Service, US National Archives and Records Administration.

38. "El único problema creado en el caso de Lina Medina es el endocrino, dice el notable médico chileno Dr. Gmo. Cáceres," *La Crónica*, April 24, 1939, 16.

39. Ariella Azoulay, "Photography Consists of Collaboration: Susan Meiselas, Wendy Ewald, and Ariella Azoulay," *Camera Obscura* 31, no. 1 (2016): 196; Rancière, *Emancipated Spectator*, 103.

40. Sandy Grande, "Care," in *Keywords for Gender and Sexuality Studies*, 43–46, https:// keywords.nyupress.org/gender-and-sexuality-studies/essay/care/

2

Disability and the Heroic Creation
of José Carlos Mariátegui

Paulo Drinot

At the age of seven, José Carlos Mariátegui had an accident while playing. Little could he have imagined that the accident would aggravate latent health problems, cause a limp, and set him on a life trajectory shaped by disability. Even less could anyone have foreseen that the child would become the most important Peruvian intellectual of the twentieth century.

Described as the "first Marxist of Latin America," Mariátegui was to become a central figure of the Latin American left and the continental intellectual scene. During his lifetime he would publish more than 2,500 articles on a wide variety of topics, from World War I to the Russian Revolution, Chaplin's cinema, and psychoanalysis, but he would come to be known primarily for his reworking of Marxism in a Peruvian context. The magazine *Amauta*, which he founded in 1926, was a milestone in the cultural avant-garde of the 1920s. His book *7 ensayos de interpretación de la realidad peruana*, published in 1928, widely seen as the most important Marxist work written in Latin America, has been read by thousands, perhaps millions, of readers in multiple languages. He founded the Peruvian Socialist Party (renamed after his death as the Peruvian Communist Party) as well as the General Confederation of Peruvian Workers. In 1930, at the age of 35, Mariátegui died, leaving behind an unparalleled intellectual and political legacy that has influenced several generations in Peru and abroad.

Although much has been written about Mariátegui and his political and cultural work, the key role that disability played in his life has not received

This chapter is an abridged version of Paulo Drinot, *José Carlos Mariátegui o el "cojito genial": Historia y discapacidad en el Perú* (Planeta, 2023).

attention. Mariátegui's disability is both present and absent in studies of his life and work. When it is present, his biographers usually mention two key episodes. First, the accident at the age of seven (1902) in Huacho and his subsequent stay at the Maison de Santé, a clinic of the French Charitable Society located in Lima. Second, the amputation of his right leg in 1924. The childhood accident plays a particularly important role: It is a sort of "origin story" that triggers a singular life journey. It serves to mark a life experience in which disability, according to these accounts, becomes a daily struggle but also an identity. In such accounts, moreover, disability and illness appear as the source of Mariátegui's genius. In particular, it is said, the long stay at the Maison de Santé produces his fondness for reading and languages, bestows on him a certain cosmopolitanism, and sets him on a self-taught and idiosyncratic path, in a struggle for "agonizing life" as Alberto Flores Galindo suggests, toward the creation of the "Amauta" (a Quechua word for teacher or master) of Peruvian thought or the global heterodox Marxist thinker.[1] In other words, these accounts treat disability as a necessary condition for Mariátegui's own heroic creation.[2]

At the same time, Mariátegui's disability is absent in many of the studies dedicated to him, as they are in general perceptions of the intellectual. Like the Italian Marxist thinker Antonio Gramsci, Mariátegui is, as David Forgacs has put it, often "undisabled" in representation, perhaps because disability is not a desirable trait in Marxist or revolutionary icons.[3] The most famous image of Mariátegui, is a photograph, taken by the Argentine painter José Malanca and often reproduced, which gives no hint that it was taken with Mariátegui sitting in his wheelchair.[4] Likewise, the monument to Mariátegui on 28 de Julio Avenue in downtown Lima depicts him seated, but his legs are covered by a large blanket, under which Mariátegui's two feet are showing, so that his physical impairment is literally covered, while his amputated leg has grown back.

Perhaps Mariátegui's disability has not received the attention it deserves, because he himself did not address it in his writings.[5] From Italy, in 1921, he wrote about a house for the "war-blind" but said little about the blind themselves, whom he imagined to be mired in pain and "resigned to their misfortune."[6] A few years before his trip to Europe, he had written in the newspaper *La Prensa* about neurasthenia and suicide and their effect on Lima's youth.[7] In *Labor*, the magazine he founded in 1928, he published several articles on social security plans in different countries of the world, and public

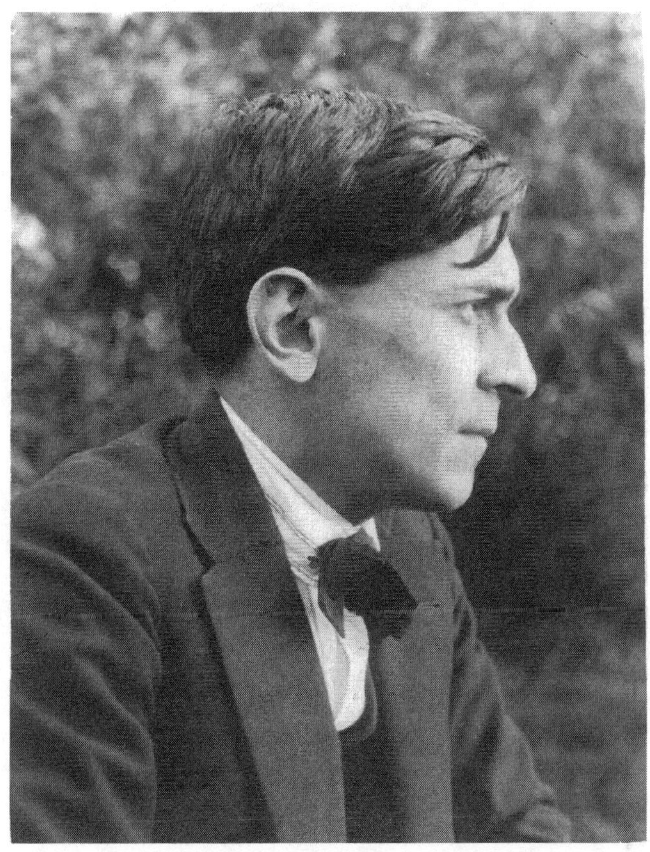

A black-and-white photograph of José Carlos Mariátegui taken by Argentine painter José Malanca (1897–1967), a close friend, in 1928. The image shows Mariátegui's face and torso in profile. He wears a dark jacket, a white shirt, and a black bow tie. The background, out of focus, consists of foliage, suggesting that the photograph was taken outdoors, quite possibly in Bosque Matamula in Lima, where Mariátegui and his friends and family regularly went for walks. Other photographs of these outings represent Mariátegui seated in his wheelchair. The wheelchair is not visible in this photograph because of the framing or cropping. Courtesy of Archivo José Carlos Mariátegui.

health was not absent from his concerns. But physical and mental disability did not occupy an important place in his work, nor was it a motive for political activism.

Perhaps the reason is that, in contrast to the "Indian question" or the "labor question," central themes in his intellectual production and political activism, Mariátegui did not understand disability in its proper social and political dimension, as did, for example, his near contemporary the US essayist and radical thinker Randolph Bourne. As Paul Longmore and Paul Steven Miller show, Bourne, in the essay "A Philosophy of Handicap," published in 1913, presented "a social analysis that explains the experience of disability by situating it within the larger patterns and structure of the unjust modern social order."[8] This approach to disability would not have been alien to Mariátegui, who, after all, drew on Marxist materialist analyses in his work to critique Peru's "unjust modern social order." However, he did not adopt it.

This chapter approaches the topic of Mariátegui and disability from two angles. First, it focuses on how Mariátegui's disability has been represented both visually and in texts. Second, it examines his experience of disability, using a variety of sources, in particular his correspondence. His letters reveal the extent to which he perceived disability as something that impacted his life trajectory, his intellectual production, and even his political work. Moreover, this analysis reveals that disability became a key element in the positive representation of Mariátegui by his contemporaries, by himself, and later by those who studied him. Mariátegui's ability to "overcome" disability became central to the value placed on his intellectual and political contributions. Ultimately, I propose that Mariátegui's disability was understood as the root of his exceptionality and inspiration.

Visualizing Disability

Mariátegui's visual repertoire allows us to think, first, about the visibility of his disability and, second, about the way he managed to give a meaning to disability other than its usual association with vulnerability and marginalization. Despite the central role that disability supposedly assumed in his formative years, Mariátegui's disability is not visible in the photographs of his childhood and youth. In the one of Mariátegui and his brother Julio César, taken in 1904—that is, two years after the accident that supposedly triggered or, at least, physically manifested his illness—it is not possible to glean his disability. According to María Wiesse, his biographer and contemporary, "He is seen, in the portrait, to be fragile, with a weak structure—one leg is badly shaped [*se advierte mal conformada*]."[9] However, none of that description is evident in the photograph, shown in the adjacent figure.

It is unclear whether Mariátegui used a cane. No cane is visible in any

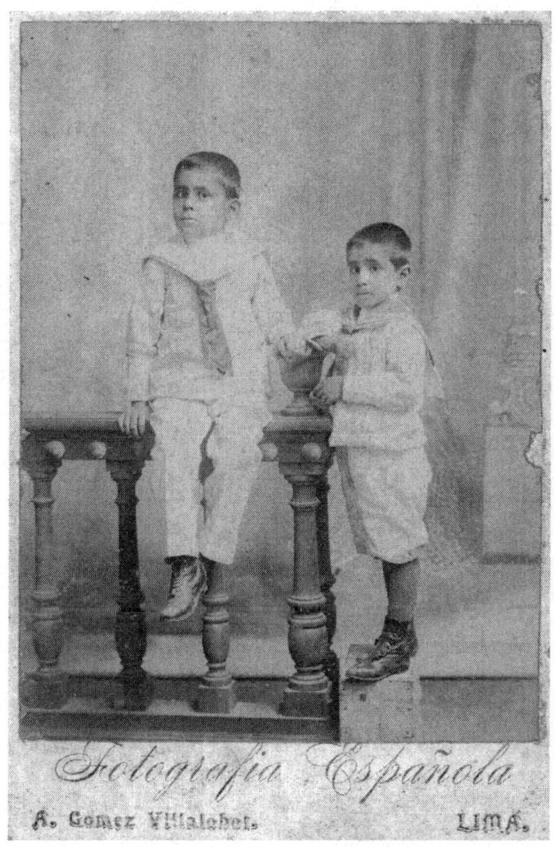

This black-and-white studio photograph (the original is in sepia), taken in 1904, depicts José Carlos Mariátegui seated on a railing, with his brother Julio César standing next to him. They both look directly at the camera. José Carlos is ten years old, and his brother is a year younger. Both are wearing light-colored clothes with dark ties and leather shoes. José Carlos's legs are crossed at the bottom, so that only one of his shoes is visible. The lower part of the photograph includes text identifying the photographer (A. Gomez Villalobos), the studio (Fotografía Española), and the city (Lima). Courtesy of Archivo José Carlos Mariátegui.

of the photographs that survive from before the amputation of his right leg, nor is there any visual suggestion that Mariátegui limped. Luis Alberto Sánchez, an intellectual and Alianza Popular Revolucionaria Americana (APRA) politician, noted: "Mariátegui had a crippled leg since he was a child; he limped when he walked. But he did not [even] need a cane."[10] However, in

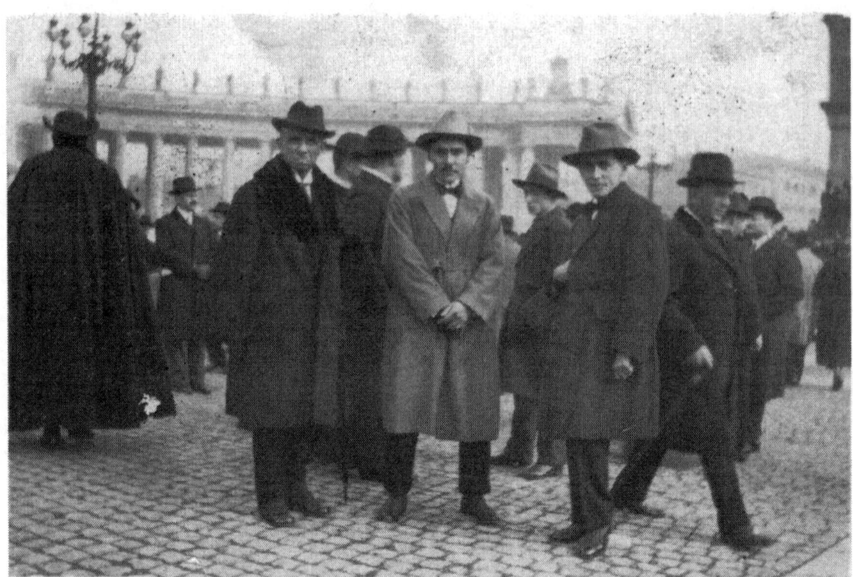

A photograph of José Carlos Mariátegui and two friends in St. Peter's Square, the Vatican, taken in 1922. Mariátegui stands to the right of his two companions. They are all looking at the camera. They are wearing heavy coats and hats, as the photograph was taken in winter. Several men, also wearing coats and hats, appear in the background, standing around or walking. In the far background, the columns of the Vatican are visible. The context is the election of Pope Pius XI, who succeeded Benedict XV in February 1922. Courtesy of Archivo José Carlos Mariátegui.

his memoirs, Sánchez portrayed him with a cane: "Mariátegui was angular, pale, with a semitic nose, bold and slightly curved; his black and penetrating eyes a little close together; small, limping, with a crippled leg, always leaning on a cane."[11] What is important, ultimately, is not so much whether Mariátegui used a cane but that the photographic nonrepresentation of disability suggests an attempt by Mariátegui to challenge the vulnerability and marginalization associated with disability and to control how his image was represented.

In contrast, following the amputation of Mariátegui's right leg in 1924, the visual repertoire makes his disability overtly visible. The photograph that shows Mariátegui in bed surrounded by his doctors, friends, and colleagues is particularly important.[12] Mariátegui is represented in a manner that expresses a clear state of vulnerability: The photograph shows an ex-

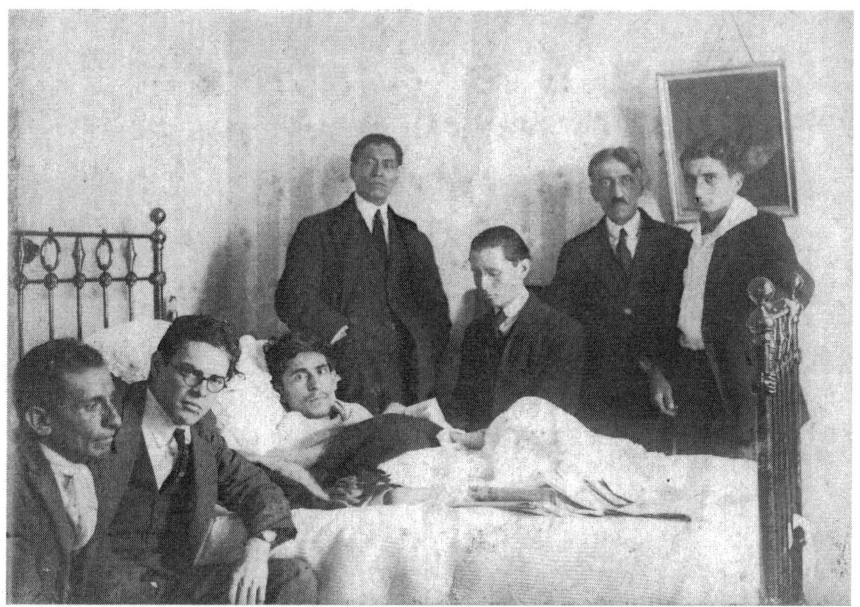

This photograph shows José Carlos Mariátegui, in bed, surrounded by his doctors and friends at his home in the district of Miraflores, Lima, in 1924. Mariátegui, whose body is covered by a blanket, looks directly at the camera, as do some of the men. He has an uncharacteristic mustache and looks weary. The men around him appear concerned, even despondent, conveying the gravity of the situation. The photograph was taken shortly after Mariátegui underwent an operation that resulted in the amputation of his right leg. Courtesy of Archivo José Carlos Mariátegui.

tremely weakened man, with an unusual moustache that suggests that the patient has not been able to shave because of the seriousness of his condition. This gravity is also conveyed by Mariátegui's gaze at the camera, a gaze that suggests a state of alertness and fear. Finally, both the gazes of the four men looking at the camera and, even more clearly, those of the two men not looking at the camera, convey the extreme gravity of the situation. This vulnerability is perhaps also conveyed by the homosocial character of the photograph—men appear in the photograph, but with heteronormative masculinities diminished by the situation.

This image of vulnerability in turn contrasts with a series of images that show Mariátegui in his wheelchair. While Mariátegui's disability is clearly visible in these images, both because of the wheelchair and the fact that the

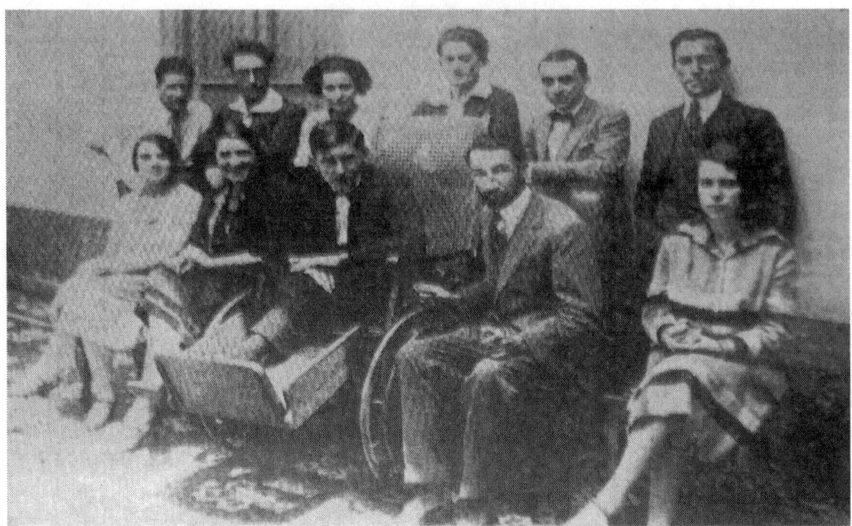

The photograph shows José Carlos Mariátegui, in his wheelchair, and (to his right) the Bolivian leftist intellectual Tristán Marof, with friends and family in 1928. The group is aligned in two rows. Mariátegui and Marof appear in the front row and lean slightly forward, looking at the camera. Ana Chiappe, Mariátegui's wife, and Marof's wife, are seated to the left of Mariátegui. Ángela Ramos, the poet and journalist and future major figure of the Peruvian Communist Party, is seated to the left of Marof. Behind them stand six people, including Noemí Milstein and Miguel Adler, the Jewish couple who worked closely with Mariátegui, and Ricardo Martínez de la Torre, a close collaborator of Mariátegui and an important figure in the socialist party that Mariátegui founded. Courtesy of Archivo José Carlos Mariátegui.

photographs clearly show that his right leg has been amputated, they do not express vulnerability. On the contrary, Mariátegui appears in these photographs as a fragile figure, protected by those who surround him, but at the same time as someone dominant and important. In most of the photographs, he appears in the center of the composition, flanked on either side by his companions. By placing him at the focal point, the composition clearly establishes his importance and relegates his companions to subordinate, supportive, and, as I suggest, protective roles. The position of his companions in relation to him indicates their relative importance. This is the case in the photograph with Tristán Marof, the Bolivian Marxist intellectual, seated next to Mariátegui and leaning forward like his Peruvian comrade, repro-

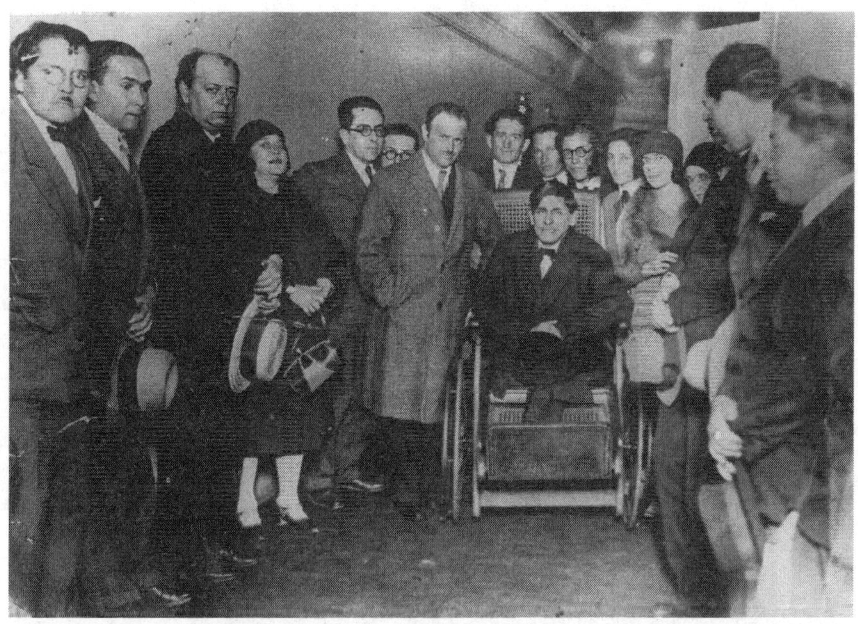

This photograph shows José Carlos Mariátegui, in his wheelchair, together with the US writer Waldo Frank and the Peruvian academic and APRA figure Luis Alberto Sánchez, both to his right, with a group of friends and family, 1929. Mariátegui, positioned at the photo's focal point, looks directly at the camera, smiling. The photograph was taken during Frank's visit to Lima in 1929, when the US intellectual gave several talks. Courtesy of Archivo José Carlos Mariátegui.

ducing his gesture, but to a lesser extent, as if acknowledging his subordinate status.

This is also the case with the photograph of Mariátegui with Waldo Frank, the US writer, and Luis Alberto Sánchez, who together, though standing and therefore in a position that might denote superiority relative to Mariátegui, are relegated to a subordinate position by the composition, which undoubtedly centers Mariátegui as the most important figure in the photograph.

These photographs show how, despite, or perhaps because of, the visibility of his disability, Mariátegui was represented in a way that reflected his undoubted importance and thus denied, or at any rate called into question, the association between disability and vulnerability or marginalization. It is interesting in this sense to also highlight the existence of several photographs that show Mariátegui in a wheelchair in a family environment. His

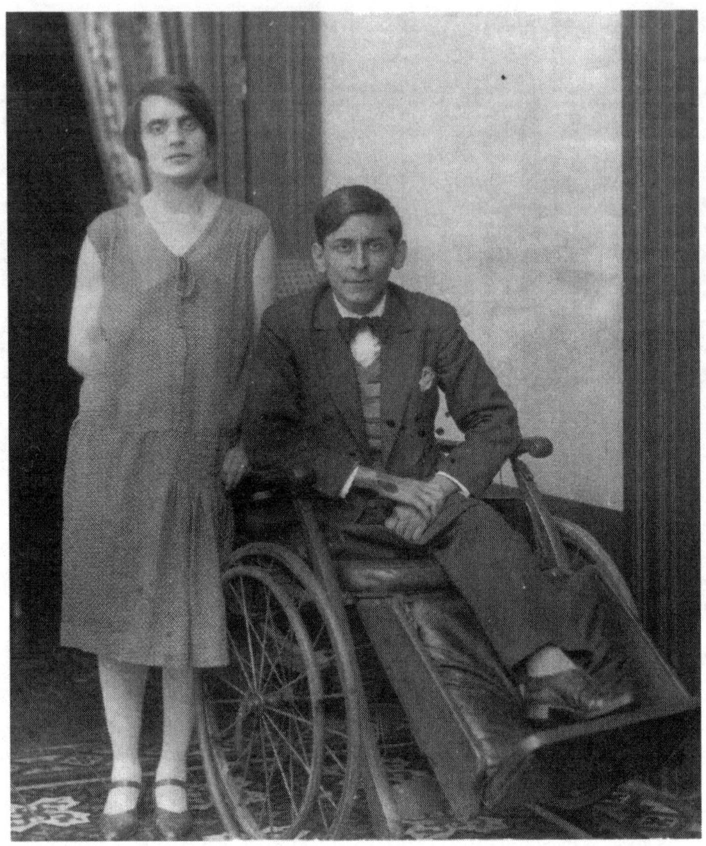

This photograph shows José Carlos Mariátegui, in his wheelchair, and his wife, Anna Chiappe, in the interior courtyard of their home at Washington Street in Lima in 1928. Both look directly at the camera. Mariátegui wears a suit and bow tie. Chiappe, standing to his right, wears a dress and leans on the wheelchair. In this, as in the previous two photographs, it is evident to the viewer that Mariátegui has had a leg amputation. Courtesy of Archivo José Carlos Mariátegui.

disability in these photographs again is not associated with vulnerability. In the photograph with his wife, Anna Chiappe, she is represented leaning on Mariátegui's wheelchair, thus suggesting that Mariátegui's gender role as the paterfamilias who supports his wife and family remains intact. Similarly, a series of photographs show Mariátegui with his children. In these, the wheelchair becomes a space that welcomes the children, protects them, and serves as a medium in which a father's affection toward his children can be manifested (the children appear to be sitting on Mariátegui's lap or sharing the space of the wheelchair with their father). Thus, these photographs, while making Mariátegui's disability visible, serve at the same time to reaffirm his ability to fulfil his gender role as husband and father.

The presence of Mariátegui's wheelchair in the photographic collection opens a window on a key issue in disability studies: its relationship to technology or, more broadly, to the material culture of disability.[13] But it also allows us to look at the ways people with disabilities like Mariátegui sought to adapt to an "ableist" world. Mariátegui's biographers mention that he used the streetcar to get around Lima.[14] Perhaps access to this mobility technology allowed him to dispense with the cane; another technology, which made his disability visible. In the case of the wheelchair, the available evidence suggests that Mariátegui considered it indispensable. In the last years of his life, he gained access to another key (and expensive) technology: an automobile. Although he had previously used cars that belonged to acquaintances, in 1929 he bought, with his friend and Socialist Party cofounder Hugo Pesce, a Chrysler. This allowed him to move around the city with some ease, though for a short time, as he would die a few months later.

Mariátegui also had a telephone installed at home, which allowed him to communicate with many people and, in particular, with the editors of *Variedades* and *Mundial*, two weeklies for which he wrote. The visual repertoire shows that the car allowed him to access spaces far from his home on Washington Street in downtown Lima, such as the beach of La Herradura, in the district of Chorrillos, while the telephone made it possible for the city and its inhabitants to get closer to him without his having to travel. Another fundamental technology related to Mariátegui's disability was the longed-for orthopedic leg or prosthesis, which, as we will see, became very important in the last years of his life and in his decision to emigrate to Argentina.

As David Hevey has suggested, disabled people are photographed usually to celebrate the work done by others in seeking or achieving their "inclusion," or to highlight their disabled status.[15] Most photographic representations of people with disabilities in the first decades of the twentieth century in Peru likely conformed to this idea. However, this is not the case of Mariátegui. Unlike most disabled people, he appears to have controlled his image (at least in photographs). He achieved this before the amputation by making the limp in his left leg invisible and also, afterward, by resignifying his disability by eliminating, or at least reducing, the association with vulnerability and marginalization, representing himself, rather, as a paterfamilias and as an intellectual figure. In short, photography was another technology—like the streetcar, the wheelchair, the automobile, or the telephone—that Mariátegui used to attach to his experience of disability a sense contrary to the hegemonic one.

The Textual Representation of Mariátegui's Disability

Mariátegui's disability also appears in documents written by various people who knew him. In a letter written to him in 1918, for example, the writer, poet, and close friend Abraham Valdelomar, from the city of Trujillo, comments on the talks he has given in that city and his imminent trip to Cajamarca. In the letter, Valdelomar signs off: "I embrace you with all my soul, *cojito genial.*"[16] The figure of the "cojito" reappears in several documents written after Mariátegui's death (the Spanish noun *cojo* refers to a person who walks with a limp; the use of the diminutive *-ito* in Spanish often denotes affection or endearment). In a biographical sketch written in July 1930, two months after Mariátegui's death, Luis Alberto Sánchez writes: "In 1912, el cojito Mariátegui was about to turn seventeen."[17] But whereas in Valdelomar's phrase the adjective "genial" (genius) and the context of the sentence (an affectionate farewell: "te abrazo con toda mi alma") attach to the mention of Mariátegui's physical impairment a humorous but friendly tone, in Sánchez's more purely descriptive comment we can glimpse a more contemptuous tone (suggesting that a more accurate translation in this case might be "the cripple Mariátegui"). In short, depending on the context, Mariátegui's disability could be represented in different ways and thereby given different meanings. Still, as I argue in this section, although there was no lack of those who used his physical impairment for mockery or attack, what prevailed was the valorization of his disability.

Sánchez's biographical sketch inaugurated a leitmotif in the representation of Mariátegui's disability: the determining role in his life of his childhood illness and the disability that resulted from it. Mariátegui, Sánchez writes, "lived thirty-four years, from June 14, 1895 to April 16, 1930. He was from Lima, and since his childhood, spent partly in Huacho, he suffered from an ostensible physical weakness. He suffered his first serious crisis at the age of seven. From then on, he was crippled with a shrunken leg."[18]

The exact nature of Mariátegui's condition is unclear. Whereas Sanchez speaks of a shrunken leg, Wiesse points to an "infection that was located in the leg."[19] According to Flores Galindo, Mariátegui suffered from osteomyelitis.[20] According to a medical certificate signed by Doctors Carlos E. Roe and Eduardo J. Goicochea, who attended Mariátegui at the San Bartolomé Hospital, the military facility where he was confined following the alleged "communist plot" of 1927, Mariátegui suffered from "articular tuberculosis."[21] It is most likely that Mariátegui, like many Peruvians at the beginning of the twentieth century, had tuberculosis, a disease that in his case manifested mainly in his bones, causing him a limp in his left leg, and that, in the opinion of his doctors, made it necessary to amputate his other leg—the right one—to save his life when he suffered a health crisis in 1924.[22]

What happened in the childhood accident and the sequence of events that resulted in Mariátegui's limp are also unclear. Several contemporaries mention a blow received while playing with other children. Some indicate that the accident occurred at school. According to Mariano Larico Yujra, who worked in Mariátegui's home, the blow occurred during a soccer game.[23] But it is far from clear why a blow in a soccer match, or a rough game with schoolmates, would have triggered the series of events that resulted in the need to transfer him to Lima, particularly if we consider that, as Humberto Rodríguez Pastor argues, the El Carmen Hospital in Huacho was relatively new and therefore probably well equipped to care for a child with a leg hematoma. This suggests that either the accident was serious or that it made evident an undiagnosed underlying condition that could not be treated locally. Either way, Mariátegui's mother must have thought that her son would receive the treatment he needed only in Lima.[24]

The surgical operation that Mariátegui underwent in Lima, performed by a French surgeon named Félix Larré, and his stay of several months in the Maison de Santé appear in these accounts as a key moment in the origin story of Mariátegui's disability. In her biography, Wiesse narrates this episode in manner that evokes physical and psychological trauma:

> His martyrdom began very early. . . . From the age of seven he becomes familiar with the smell of chloroform, the cold whiteness of the hospital rooms, the painful touch of the doctors' hands, the immobility, the solitude, the silence. He learns to see in his mother's face the process of the disease; to guess, in the tone of her voice, the course of his ailment.[25]

But Wiesse presents this trauma as an experience that makes possible Mariátegui the intellectual:

> But if the little boy cannot romp and frolic, like the other boys, he can, however, find joy and happiness in books. . . . The world of letters has opened up for him, wide, cordial, friendly, and the sick child, who already frequents hospitals, has in books his most constant and loyal companions.[26]

In the end, Wiesse suggests, it is the illness and disability that engenders Mariátegui. The martyrdom of the operation and its outcome is a necessary sacrifice so that the genius Mariátegui is born from the weak child.

This relationship between disability and genius is present in several texts. In Wiesse's biography, as in Valdelomar's phrase, Mariátegui's limp is directly associated with his intellect. Recalling his beginnings in journalism, Wiesse writes, "When people talk about him, this phrase jumps out: 'El cojito Mariátegui? He is very intelligent.' Thus, the intelligence of the 'cojito' was established in Lima. It is known that he is one of the finest and most modern writers in the Lima press."[27] In this formulation, the emphasis on his intelligence serves to compensate for his lameness. According to Eudocio Ravines, an APRA militant of the 1920s who would become the leader of the Peruvian Socialist Party after Mariátegui's death, he did not mind being called "cojo": "When he walked, he limped because of an absurd operation performed on him in childhood. His close friends nicknamed him 'el cojo,' which did not seem to bother him in the least: he had undoubtedly overcome victoriously the inferiority complex that his limp must have caused him."[28]

We do not know why Ravines considered Mariátegui's operation "absurd." But, as far as the inferiority complex is concerned, the evidence indicates that although Mariátegui did not suffer from it, he did seek to "overcome" his disability. We will see later that the possibility of acquiring a prosthesis and access to better treatment motivated his decision to move to Buenos Aires in the late 1920s.

The relationship between disability and genius also appears in Armando Bazán's 1939 biography. A poet who edited the first avant-garde poetry magazine in Peru, Bazán was a member of Mariátegui's intellectual circle. In the book, he compares Mariátegui's experience to that of Beethoven:

> Mariátegui's life shares more than one similarity with that of that poor boy who in a German city learned to play piano under the implacable iron rule of his fa-

ther, and who, already a brilliant musician, lost the ability to hear the sounds of the world and the voices of men. I, who had the perhaps undeserved privilege of living with Mariátegui from the moment he became forever invalid [*inválido*], prostrate, know to what depths and to what height his pain reached to transform itself, as in the case of the divine deaf man, into joy, into a source of inexhaustible work and absolute happiness.[29]

In this interpretation, genius not only compensates for disability. For Bazán, disability makes genius possible. Mariátegui's pain, he tells us, was transformed into a source of work and happiness, which, as in the case of Beethoven, bore fruit for the good of humanity. The Peruvian intellectual was a product of his disability, which, in this reading, became a kind of martyrdom and a necessary sacrifice.

We find a similar interpretation in comments of political leaders close to Mariátegui. Shortly after his death, Manuel Seoane, an important figure in the APRA, wrote:

> Even though José Carlos Mariátegui suffered from a physical ailment [*dolencia física*] that deprived him of mobility, he never resigned his spirit to immobility or defeat. On the contrary, he was always a fighter in the field of ideas. . . . His illness did not discourage him even though death was lurking in his half-ankylosed organism.[30]

Similarly, Antenor Orrego, another APRA leader, argued in a brief article:

> Few existences passed with greater human dignity and goodness and, almost none, with more resounding vital affirmation, notwithstanding his weakness and physical ailments (*males físicos*). His life was marked by bodily suffering, but he was emboldened, inflamed with a historical passion and faith that arose from his apostolic clairvoyance. You could see him in his armchair, always smiling, as if he were filled with an extrahuman energy that seemed, at every step, to stop the lightning bite of death. He was a permanent survivor of his acerbic ills, thanks to the lucid awareness of his personal mission.[31]

Thus, the suffering caused by disability, both APRA leaders tell us, not only did not prevent genius from emerging but contributed to its construction in a definitive way.

The praise expressed by some of Mariátegui's political opponents contrasts with the words of APRA leader Víctor Raúl Haya de la Torre. The two had maintained a close friendship and had collaborated intellectually since the late 1910s; however, the relationship broke down in 1928 when Haya de la Torre decided to establish a political party in order to run for the presidency.[32] On more than one occasion, the APRA founder referred to Mariátegui's disability so as to mock and stigmatize him. For example, in March 1929, in a delirious letter to Ravines, Haya de la Torre calls Mariátegui "the most dangerous individualist and opportunist of the movement" and directly mocks his disability: "Peruvian fascism will build a monument to Mariátegui . . . with a leg." He then suggests that Mariátegui, in alliance with President Leguía, takes advantage of his disability to undermine him: "When he had his leg, he wanted power; now that he lacks it, he wants to appear as a puritan." Finally, in a handwritten postscript, he notes: "I will take Mariátegui by the stump and will [——] in all his ugliness before smashing him against his own filth."[33]

In a September 1929 letter to César Mendoza, Haya de la Torre distinguished himself, "a man of action," and the APRA, "a work of action," from Mariátegui: "I have always sympathized with Mariátegui. He seems to me an interesting figure of romanticism, of faith and of the intellectual exaltation of a revolutionary. But Mariátegui has never been in the struggle itself. . . . But I believe that no more can be demanded of him. Mariátegui is immobilized and his work is merely intellectual . . . in our milieu only action teaches the path of revolution."[34] Similarly, the poet and APRA leader Magda Portal referred to Mariátegui's disability in an article published shortly after his death. She contrasts a physically limited Mariátegui, "forced by his disability to look at life from an armchair" and unable to carry out a transcendent political work, to a vigorous and dynamic Haya de la Torre. The APRA leader had traveled all over Peru, "living with the Indian," and had gone "into the pores of his homeland to extract that truth which is now the banner of his struggle," while Mariátegui "continued to rehearse topics on European affairs," She concludes: "José Carlos, of Peru, only knew Lima. And this is the great difference. While J.C.M., because of his physical tragedy and his special inclination, dreamed and wrote, Haya acted. History will tell which of the two built on firmer ground."[35]

But while Portal sought to belittle Mariátegui's political role, accusing him of being an ally of the *civilistas* and the Partido Civil (the oligarchic political party that had ruled Peru during the so-called Aristocratic Republic, 1895–1919) and of not understanding the country because he identified "too much with the European mentality" and had never left Lima, she did not fail to stress his genius: "This does not tarnish the brilliance of Mariátegui's intellectual work, which is undoubtedly the most notable produced in Peru—of such weak intellectual standard—and one of the most outstanding in America."[36]

Mariátegui and the Figure of the "Supercrip"

The narratives discussed in the previous section reflect what in the field of disability studies is called the supercrip—that is, a representation of disabled people that emphasizes overcoming, inspiration, and exceptionality.[37] Both Bazán and Wiesse narrate Mariátegui's beginnings in journalism as a teenager from this perspective. Both highlight the fact that Mariátegui was forced to walk extensively in order to do his work; that is, they highlight precisely what his disability supposedly prevented him from doing. According to Wiesse, Mariátegui "has to walk—difficult walks for his ailing leg—all over Lima."[38] Similarly, Bazán notes, "So with his injury already causing him discomfort when walking, he had to walk incessantly inside and outside of the workshop and covered on foot all the streets of Lima."[39] In both cases, this way of narrating Mariátegui's capacity to overcome the limitations imposed by his disability has the function precisely to point out his exceptionality and to underscore his experience of overcoming as an inspiration for others.

The notion of Mariátegui as a supercrip is particularly present in the narration of the amputation of his right leg in 1924. From the outset, Wiesse presents this episode as a process of overcoming: "Every human existence has to undergo some trial, which will temper and purify it." However, the operation, which Wiesse stresses was performed without anesthesia, created a conflict between Mariátegui's mother and Anna Chiappe, his wife. Doña Amalia was opposed to the operation for religious reasons. According to Wiesse, "Rather than surgical intervention, she wanted a priest to confess her son";[40] Bazán points out that the mother, "Catholic to the point of fanaticism, . . . considered that the mutilation of the body was an attack against nature."[41] Chiappe saw the matter from a different perspective, Wiesse reports: "She loved her companion deeply and knew all the reserves of spiritual energy that were hidden in José Carlos's weak body. Amputated, mutilated, invalid? What did it matter, if his intelligence and his spirit remained intact, alive, luminous, powerful!"[42]

Similarly, in relating the fact that Mariátegui had "a truly pathetic crying crisis" when he awoke from the operation, Wiesse adds that after being calmed by his wife, "Mariátegui never complained again. He endured his fate with manly fortitude, and, in his wheelchair, he was an example of heroic and simple joy."[43]

Bazán's account of the operation is very similar. This crisis, far from aggravating the disability, created the conditions for the emergence of a marvelous creative intellect. Bazán recounts Mariátegui's reaction when he awoke, four days after the operation, and realized that his leg had been amputated: "Then the pallor of his face increased mortally, and he began to cry between sobs. . . . It was the only time he was seen to cry. It was the only time he was seen to be truly bowed down by grief." Like Wiesse, Bazán converts this moment of apparent weakness and pathos into a transcendental turning point in Mariátegui's life:

> The road ahead of him would be strewn with great setbacks, privations and sufferings of all kinds, but the temper of his spirit resisted everything with a magnificent silent nobility. Then America had one of the most beautiful and exciting spectacles: that of a prostrated man, who turns his pain into an inexhaustible source of life and creative optimism.[44]

At the end of his account, Bazán asks rhetorically:

> What does health consist of? How was it possible that a human body reduced to invalidity [*invalidez*] and continually beset by illness could be a creative source, giving a light of optimism and joy capable of eclipsing the optimism and joy of the healthiest body? Mariátegui was for me the revelation of a marvelous mystery of life.[45]

In this account, as in Wiesse's, we see how Mariátegui's disability serves to establish his character as a worthy or valuable disabled person. It is a rhetorical operation that has an explicit gender dimension: Wiesse contrasts Mariátegui's desperate weeping with the "manly fortitude" with which he faced the rest of his life, and both biographers insist that it was the only time Mariátegui cried (the implication being that men do not cry). Thus, these narratives attribute to Mariátegui a diminished body but a whole masculinity and, above all, an intellect, a "creative source" that not only compensates for the physical impairment but also allows Mariátegui, with his body "reduced to invalidity," to overcome, to surpass, the contribution of a non-disabled person.

This narrative of overcoming serves to establish Mariátegui as a source of inspiration at not only a personal but also a political level. In 1946, the leader of the Peruvian Communist Party, Jorge del Prado, wrote:

> Nothing [is] more expressive of the profound concept he had of his responsibility than that anecdote referring to the first crisis of his illness. Everyone believed that Mariátegui had to die then; but he did not believe it, and he did not believe it because he considered that he had not yet fulfilled his mission. And we all know the superhuman efforts he then made to continue living to continue his "arrow" path until he hit his target, until he cemented his fundamental work. . . . [The] magnitude and importance of the work initiated by Mariátegui make it seem to us not only that the life—so fruitful and brilliant—of the man who laid the first foundations of socialism in Peru, but also that of all of us who want to follow his example and continue his work with dignity, is a short one.[46]

There is, undoubtedly, in these textual representations of Mariátegui's disability an evident allusion to Christian notions: terms such as "sacrifice" and "martyrdom," as well as the very idea of Mariátegui's life as agony developed by the historian Flores Galindo, allude to the saints and to the figure of Christ itself. But, as I suggest here, at least as important are the allusions to exceptionality and overcoming, central to the figure of the supercrip. Mariátegui's example for socialism was to be found not in his martyrdom but in his ability to overcome adversity.

Alongside the narratives of exceptionality and overcoming these texts also offer an explanation of Mariátegui's condition in more structural terms that highlight his poverty and, in doing so, inscribe his disability with a broader social reality. "Mariátegui, like all poor children in the world, did not have a childhood," says Bazán. He lacked clothes and food, he adds. The impairment caused by the blow to the leg he received as a child was "insufficiently cured because of the ignorance and poverty of his relatives." For Bazán, this reality is part of a larger social problem that he describes as "this spectacle of children, crawling, dirty, their eyes sunken by anemia, through the streets of our big cities."[47] Wiesse, meanwhile, explains the health crisis that resulted in the amputation by referring to Mariátegui's poverty and the need to work nonstop, among other factors: "And now that his intelligence was fully deployed, when Peru expected so much from his talent, his culture, his will to work and organize, once again the disease assaulted Mariátegui's organism, weakened by excessive intellectual work, the climate of Lima, the privations imposed by his poverty as an austere and idealistic writer."[48] In these accounts an identification of illness and disability with material factors, amounting to a social critique, is thus not entirely absent. However, as we have seen, the accounts pay much more attention to Mariátegui's disability as a personal tragedy and to his overcoming of this condition as evidence of his genius, exceptionality, and exemplarity.

Mariátegui's Experience of Disability

Several of the themes already mentioned are present in Mariátegui's self-representation of his disability. His operation in 1924 occurred shortly after he took over the direction of the journal *Claridad*, founded by Víctor Raúl Haya de la Torre. In issue 6, published in September 1924—an issue that came out late, partly because of the operation—Mariátegui included a letter entitled "Palabras de Mariátegui" (Words of Mariátegui) accompanied by a reproduction of the hospital room photograph. The issue also includes an editorial that mentions "the painful illness of José Carlos Mariátegui, which momentarily deprives us of his vigorous and intelligent collaboration" and a short, unsigned article, in the section titled "Página del Proletariado," that refers to the illness and operation as the "tragedy of Mariátegui." The unsigned article establishes the tragedy of Mariátegui as the tragedy of the Peruvian proletariat: "His tragedy, our tragedy, murmured, beside the bed of the dying, the depth of our silence." The article compares the imagined death of Mariátegui to the struggles of the proletariat—except that in this case "we lived the mute tragedy of being close to being defeated without fighting. We have never had such collective pain." The article presents Mariátegui's recovery as a rebirth: "That is why perhaps the conversations with the dear convalescent now have a taste of spring morning, the flavor of a furrow that germinates again, the sprouting of holy heritages."[49]

These texts clearly establish Mariátegui's centrality to the Peruvian proletariat. If illness and disability are believed to marginalize individuals, diminish their capacity to serve society, in this case the rhetorical operation ensures that this will not happen. In his letter, Mariátegui participates in this exercise. He writes that he does not want to be absent from this issue of the magazine, because "if [. . .] it were to reappear without my signature, I would feel my physical brokenness [*quebranto físico*] all the more." Like his biographers, Mariátegui turns to the notion of overcoming:

> My greatest yearning at present is that this illness that has interrupted my life may not be strong enough to divert or weaken it. May it not leave in me any moral imprint. May it not deposit in my thoughts or in my heart any germ of bitterness or despair. It is indispensable for me that my words retain the same optimistic accent as before. I want to defend myself from any sad influence, from any melancholy suggestion. I feel more than ever the need for our common faith.[50]

Mariátegui adds that he writes in "the *estancia* where I spend my long convalescent days" and that his intention is to greet his *Claridad* colleagues and reaffirm his "fervor" and the hopes of his colleagues. As if to show that the disease cannot stop him, he dedicates the rest of the text to discussing "our cause," which he understands as the "great human cause" and the establishment of "a new social order." Although "it is clear that the world is moving toward socialism," he regrets that "our bourgeoisie does not understand or realize any of this."[51]

As we have seen, the amputation was traumatic for Mariátegui and undoubtedly marked a turning point in his life. Before the operation he had been able to "pass" as nondisabled, dispensing with a cane and relying on available technologies, such as the tram, which allowed him to operate in a way that conformed to a certain ableist normativity. After the operation, however, the need to use a wheelchair meant that his disability became not only visible but defining: the "cojito genial" was now an amputee who had been saved from death and who could not disguise the wheelchair on which he depended. At the same time, as I argue in my analysis of visual representations, Mariátegui was able to give new meaning to his disability in a way that avoided the most common associations, particularly marginalization and vulnerability. Despite the many economic hardships he faced, Mariátegui had access to certain assets and advantages derived in part from his role as a leading intellectual figure, and to certain networks of influence and support. In other words, his experience of disability was not that of most Peruvians with disabilities in the early twentieth century.

There are no studies on disability in Peru during this period, but we can assume that the disabled represented a high proportion of the total population. This cohort would have been composed of three main groups: (i) people with disabilities caused by war (both the War of the Pacific [1879–1883] and the Civil War of 1895 must have left many men with physical disabilities resulting from combat and with mental disabilities resulting from war-induced trauma); (ii) those with disabilities caused by work accidents (both in urban and rural contexts, especially in industries involving heavy machinery or the use of explosives); and (iii) those with disabilities caused by diseases of various kinds (from poliomyelitis to tuberculous arthritis and including mental and congenital diseases of various kinds). Although some people with disabilities, such as war veterans, received financial assistance in the form of pensions, and although benevolent societies provided charitable aid to the poorest, in general disability likely meant not only social marginalization but poverty. The Work Accidents Law of 1911, one of the first laws of its kind in Latin America, to some extent helped those who, because of work accidents, acquired a disability that prevented them from working. But the law applied only to a small group of workers—mainly those who worked with machinery—and its application was always deficient.

Mariátegui's experience of disability, therefore, was not that of most people with disabilities in early-twentieth-century Peru or anywhere else for that matter. To start with, despite his relative poverty, Mariátegui had access to renowned doctors. As mentioned, after his accident at age seven, he was attended by the French surgeon Félix Larré. The surgeon who operated on him in 1924 was Guillermo Gastañeta, one of the most renowned physicians in the history of Peruvian medicine. Later, the doctor who attended him when he was hospitalized at the Villarán Clinic, toward the end of his life, was Fortunato Quesada Larrea, a distinguished physician: He had been president of the Federation of Students of Peru in 1918, was professor of anatomy at the University of San Marcos, and became minister of health during the government of Óscar Benavides. Moreover, Hugo Pesce, a specialist in Hansen's disease (leprosy), was a close friend of Mariátegui and was one of the people who participated in the founding of the Socialist Party in 1928. According to Rouillon, Sebastián Lorente Patrón, President Leguía's health minister, was a childhood friend of Mariátegui. In short, Mariátegui had access to the cream of the Peruvian biomedical "establishment," unlike the majority of the disabled, who had to rely on so-called *empíricos* (quacks) or simply had no access to medical care.

Beyond access to doctors, Mariátegui was able to count on the solidarity and support of individuals and collectives. Unlike many disabled people, he was not isolated or marginalized by his physical impairment, particularly after his return from Europe. Although he lost mobility, which limited his ability to travel in- and outside the country, the photographic record shows that Mariátegui maintained some mobility in Lima, thanks to his access to automobiles. Thus, he was able to maintain contact with the groups he sought to relate to, such as the workers of the textile town of Vitarte during the Fiesta de la Planta (Plant Festival), a yearly working-class festivity. He also access a certain level of leisure, in places such as the Bosque Matamula and the beach at La Herradura.

On the other hand, his home on Washington Street became a meeting place for intellectuals, artists, workers, and Indigenous peasants, who converged on the so-called red corner. Thus, his lack of mobility was compensated for by the members of his networks of influence and support, who visited him regularly. As the *indigenista* intellectual Luis Valcárcel recalls:

> Until 1924 José Carlos could still walk leaning on a cane, then he worsened and lost his healthy leg. But neither his precarious health nor the limited mobility to which the wheelchair condemned him prevented him from doing work of fundamental importance to understanding the deep drama of Peru. Moreover, he knew how to take advantage of this limitation, for he turned his house on Washington Street into a lively meeting place, frequented by workers, students, politicians, and intellectuals, both from Lima and the provinces and, eventually, foreigners.[52]

These networks not only provided emotional support and solidarity but also helped Mariátegui to pay for some of the expenses caused by his illness. As Wiesse mentions, following the operation "the situation of Mariátegui and his family was truly distressing." He could not afford to pay for the operation, the clinic, and his convalescence. However, the support networks came to his aid, as Wiesse noted: "A beautiful movement of fraternal solidarity is produced, then, among the intellectuals and artists of Peru. Writers of the most diverse ideologies, artists of different tendencies, students, workers, contributed their help to the comrade, in the difficult hours he was going through."[53] Luis Alberto Sánchez claims that he initiated this act of solidarity. Thanks to this support, Mariátegui was able to spend his convalescence in Miraflores, "where sea breezes invigorated his organism," and in Chosica, a town outside Lima known for its pleasant climate.[54]

Finally, Mariátegui had a more intimate support network as well. At home, in addition to his wife, children, and mother, he had the support of close friends such as Miguel Adler and Noemí Milstein, but also of domestic servants, who—as was quite common in Peruvian middle-class families, even those in relative economic decline—lived in the house of their employers.[55]

Thus, it is possible to conclude that, in contrast to the experience of most disabled people in the early twentieth century, Mariátegui's disability did not significantly affect his trajectory of the "normative progression through the stages of life (marriage and children)."[56] He was able to enjoy, to a greater extent than most people with disabilities, a life that corresponded to ableist normativity and, particularly after his return from Europe (and notwithstanding the political persecution he suffered), middle-class or bourgeois respectability. In fact, as Magda Portal lets it be understood in her posthumous critique, Mariátegui enjoyed a comfortable situation: "Seen from the bourgeois point of view, Mariátegui was poor; from the point of view of many of the intellectuals and Apristas who were with him until our deportation, Mariátegui enjoyed a comfort that none of us had."[57]

However, this does not mean that disability did not have an important effect on Mariátegui's life. His correspondence reveals that illness and disability affected him in two main ways: First, they affected his daily life and his ability to work and thus to carry out his intellectual and political projects. As Nielsen points out: "Disability and manifestations of ableism can also result in daily tasks, such as personal maintenance, commuting, or eating, taking longer than considered normal; illness or fatigue can disrupt the rhythm of the workday or career."[58] Second, they had a clear impact on his plan to migrate to Buenos Aires with his family. As we will see, behind this will was the desire to "overcome" his disability.

A recurring theme in Mariátegui's correspondence after his operation is the effect of illness and disability on his capacity to work, including answering his correspondence, and to cover his expenses. On August 22, 1924, for example, Mariátegui wrote from Miraflores to Victoria Ferrer, the mother of his daughter Gloria María, to whom he was sending money: "I am not well yet. My convalescence is slow and the expenses that my illness has caused me and continues to cause me [are] innumerable and substantial."[59] A couple of years later, in November 1926, he wrote her again: "I am not well yet and my illness, which does not allow me to attend to my work as before, has me behind in my payments."[60] It is a theme also present in his correspondence with people who were not part of his family circle. In April 1927, he wrote to Samuel Glusberg, the Argentine writer and publisher with whom he kept a regular correspondence, apologizing for having taken so long to reply: "I wanted to answer without delay your pleasant message of friendship and sympathy. But for some time now I have been forced to neglect my correspondence almost completely. My health is unstable. Three years ago, I saved myself from death at the cost of an amputation and until now I suffer the consequences of that crisis that left me mutilated and sick. Fortunately, for a few months now, I have been improving. My work, however, is still beyond my strength."[61]

In fact, Mariátegui's health and disability were topics also addressed by those who wrote to him. Thus, in May 1927 Luis Carranza, the editor of *El Tiempo*, a newspaper in the northern city of Piura, wrote to Mariátegui:

> Believe me that for me one of your greatest successes consists precisely in the poor health that I know you enjoy and that, nevertheless, you work intellectually more than any other writer from Lima. This is an example and an exception to the habits of laziness, which we "criollos" [creoles or whites] generally suffer.[62]

In a February 1928 letter, the Uruguayan poet Blanca Luz Brum advised: "Be aware that you teach all of us to support each other and to stand up straight. Precisely you, the materially handicapped [*el incapacitado materialmente*], are the only one with the correct and definitive attitudes."[63] A few months later, the *indigenista* writer Gamaliel Churata wrote from Puno:

> I am very happy to know that the doctors have found a definitive way to cure the illness that mortifies you so much. This way we will all win. You because your work will be celebrated and we [because we] will learn from it.[64]

Tristán Marof, in a similar vein, stated:

> I have your letter of July 10 in my possession, and I answer it immediately with great pleasure. I have learned from some friends of yours that you were already ill, and several times we have lamented your situation. But I rejoice immensely at the news you give me that a happy operation will, perhaps, put you in a better condition. Everything that happens to you—your triumphs and your ailments concern us—not because of mere sentimentality, but because, stuck there in Lima, you are carrying out revolutionary work with a clear vision and within reality.[65]

These letters clearly show how members of Mariátegui's networks contributed to the narratives linked to the supercrip figure and the notions of overcoming, inspiration, and exceptionality that characterize it. They confirm Simi Linton's argument that overcoming disability often does not emerge from within the disabled community but "is wish fulfilment generated from outside."[66] Despite his disability, Mariátegui worked harder than everyone else, according to Carranza. Brum observed that Mariátegui was physically disabled, but he surpassed others, even the nondisabled, by his "correct and definitive attitudes." Mariátegui's overcoming of his illness, affirmed Churata, would be an example for others, for humanity. Marof repeated the idea: overcoming disability would be a step toward the realization of Mariátegui's revolutionary vision.

These narratives express an attempt to show solidarity with Mariátegui, to demonstrate affection and support. But they also contribute to rooting the idea of the "worthy" disabled by assigning to Mariátegui, just as many of his biographers do, aptitudes and capacities that, in society's view, compensate for and, in a way, cancel out disability. Luis Valcárcel, for example, takes up this idea in his memoir:

> From a very young age a relentless disease—tuberculosis—gave José Carlos no respite. But everything in him remained faith. It is extraordinary to see someone so strong spiritually and so weak physically.[67]

As we have already seen, Mariátegui himself contributed to establishing this narrative of overcoming. For example, in a text addressed to the students of the Universidad Popular González Prada in 1927, he wrote:

> The physical disability [*invalidez física*] that prevents me from taking my place in your meetings and classes does not separate or exclude me from the Universidad Popular, because, conceiving its mission and understanding its effort to create a revolutionary culture, I know that I have given to this work, integrally, my energy and my capacity, in these two and a half years. A few hundred articles, in all of which I have tried to contemplate and define facts and things with socialist criteria, represent my contribution during this time, in which I have not spoken, but I have written, and in which I have the satisfaction of having written as I would have spoken.[68]

Thus, Mariátegui takes up the idea of compensation. The "invalidez física" limits his ability to be physically present in the activities of the Popular University, but this absence is compensated by his intellectual work and the contribution that this activity represents for the construction of socialism. The obstacles of physical disability are overcome by the intellectual contribution.

Buenos Aires

Several contemporaries and scholars have discussed Mariátegui's planned trip to Buenos Aires.[69] Although we cannot specify when the idea of emigrating to Argentina first surfaced, following the so-called communist plot of 1927, which resulted in the closure of *Amauta*, the arrest of Mariátegui, and his confinement in the San Bartolomé Hospital, the idea was already sprouting. This is evidenced in a letter that Óscar Herrera wrote from Buenos Aires in October of that year in which the Peruvian student leader deported by Leguía in 1924 confirmed to Mariátegui that "in Buenos Aires you would not only have assured your success as an intellectual but also your home life."[70] The subject also appears in the correspondence with the poet Alberto Hidalgo, who lived in Buenos Aires, who assured him that "contrary to what is believed, here you can live with very little, with almost nothing";[71] and more extensively in the correspondence with Samuel Glusberg, to whom Mariátegui confided in January 1928: "If *Amauta* were to suffer a new closure, I would give up the task of rectifying the judgment of these people [he refers both to the police and, by extension, the Leguía regime] and head for Buenos Aires, where I believe my work would find a better climate and where I would be free from espionage and absurd stalking."[72]

As Flores Galindo has indicated, what motivated Mariátegui's plan to emigrate to Buenos Aires was both the increased political repression in Peru and the fact that he was fed up with the polemics with Haya de la Torre and the Apristas.[73] However, the correspondence also shows to what extent Mariátegui's disability was a determining factor in the relocation project. Already in July 1928, a letter from the Peruvian writer César Miró from Buenos Aires alluded to this circumstance:

> We are quite worried about your health. We learned of your illness first from *Amauta* and then from news of you. We seriously think that you should come. It is necessary that you come. But we think you must be very much needed there. What would it [mean] if you were missing in Peru? *Anyway, if your health needs this sacrifice, it is necessary to make it.* The Revolution needs you and this is the

main thing. It does not matter where you are. What is essential is that you be completely restored [to health] to be able to steer our rudder.[74]

This is a subject that Mariátegui had discussed with Miró and probably with Blanca Luz Brum, at that time Miró's lover. At points in the correspondence, disability appears as an element that motivates the desire to emigrate but also impedes it. Thus, Mariátegui wrote to Glusberg in June 1929, "I am often seized by the urgent desire to breathe the atmosphere of a freer country. If I do not hasten to satisfy it, it is not so much because of my physical invalidity [*mi invalidez física*], of which I have not yet been cured, than because I do not want to give the impression that I am abandoning my struggle, tired and defeated."[75]

Just as Mariátegui related being able (or unable) to work to his illness and disability, he also related it to his treatment. Towards the end of 1929 and the beginning of 1930, he went regularly to the beach at La Herradura, as several photographs and his correspondence show. On January 26, he commented to Ernesto Reyna: "I am doing a beach cure at La Herradura, where I spend my afternoons. This takes up a lot of my time, but I have no choice but to avoid a crisis in my health, which has been quite weakened in recent weeks. I have almost no moments available for my correspondence."[76] On February 9, he apologized to Glusberg for not having answered his letters; he had not had time to write, he explained, "because of a beach cure at La Herradura which takes up the whole afternoon and happens before my bedtime, leaving me only the indispensable time for my most urgent daily work."[77] In the early twentieth century, doctors who believed that the salty sea air had a therapeutic effect used these beach cures to treat tuberculosis in children and adults.[78] According to Mariátegui, the treatments worked: "My beach season has been very good for me, after the fatigues of 1929," he told Glusberg.[79]

However, Mariátegui hoped not only to alleviate his ailments with treatments such as beach cures but to be cured definitively and to "overcome" his disability, perhaps precisely because the treatment he was following, even when it alleviated his condition, did not allow him to work as he wished. As historians Daniel Blackie and Alexia Moncrieff suggest, "Rather than resisting medicalization, disabled people have often promoted it for their own benefit."[80] As we can see, this is precisely the case with Mariátegui. Already in March 1927, he had written to Esteban Pavletich, another intellectual deported by Leguía:

Since I received your first [letter] I would have liked to write to you at length; but in January I suffered an attack of rheumatism in my right arm that has prevented me from writing for a month. And this has not been, strictly speaking, the last failure of my health. Later I had another minor one. But now I feel optimistic. The fistula that remained to my stump has closed. And if this is definitive, I will be able to walk with crutches and use an orthopedic leg.[81]

The emotion conveyed in a letter to Glusberg in July 1928 is palpable:

Fortunately, the doctors are very optimistic about the treatment I am currently undergoing. Quesada, a great surgeon here, is convinced that he can cure me within eight to ten months and to put me in a position to walk with a prosthetic leg. His confidence has rubbed off on me.[82]

We do not know what effect the beach cures had on his health but, in contrast to his initial optimism, Mariátegui gradually lost confidence that Quesada's treatment would work. Hence, the possibility of a more effective treatment and access to a prosthesis in Buenos Aires converged with the plan to escape the increasing repression of the Leguía regime, a plan that gained new strength after the police "raid" on Mariátegui's house in November 1929. This police intervention, part of a larger raid in response to an alleged Jewish-Communist plot, seems to have convinced Mariátegui to finally undertake his plan to emigrate to Argentina. As he wrote to Glusberg: "My intention to leave Peru with my wife and children is affirmed by these events. I cannot remain here. I will stay only as long as necessary to prepare for my journey. I will leave Peru whatever happens."[83]

As potent a threat as the repression of the Leguía regime was, then, the decision to migrate owed to the fact that Mariátegui believed that in Argentina he would have access to better treatment and, above all, to a prosthesis. "I have reaffirmed my intention to go to Buenos Aires," he wrote Glusberg in December 1929, indicating that he had decided not to leave his children in boarding school in Lima. In the same letter, he surprisingly attributed health and weakness to countries and cities: "The contact with a healthy and strong country will do me a lot of good, spiritually and physically. In Buenos Aires, the convalescence that the weakness of Lima has delayed will end."[84] He recounted a discussion with the US writer Waldo Frank, who had just been in Lima: "Frank thinks that in Buenos Aires the problem of my mobility can be solved just as well as in Europe by the adaptation of an orthopedic leg. I believe that surgery and orthopedics are perfectly developed there. I would leave that for after my first stage of work. But it is very important for my future."[85] As this passage suggests, the treatment that Dr. Fortunato Quesada had envisioned, and that had filled Mariátegui with hope, was not accessible or possible in Peru. It was necessary to obtain it outside the country, in Europe or in Buenos Aires.

In his reply, Glusberg calculated what Mariátegui would need to earn to live "modestly" in Buenos Aires (about 500 pesos a month), and confirmed: "I believe that the matter of your mobility can be arranged in Buenos Aires and that you will even have [access to] the best doctors free of charge. Of course, the orthopedic device will have to be paid for and it is expensive. However, we will get it."[86] The importance of the trip for Mariátegui was undeniable. It is clear from his correspondence with Waldo Frank that the latter had promised to help him so that he would be able to travel. Frank indicated in December 1929 that he had written twice not only to Glusberg, "telling him the importance of achieving your visit to B.A.—a truly American importance," but also to Victoria Ocampo, the writer and founder in 1931 of *Sur* magazine, "who may be able to help you."[87] On February 9, Mariátegui confirmed to Glusberg that the trip was "totally decided" and that he needed only to arrange some matters such as "the continuation of *Amauta* in Lima for as long as this is possible."[88] On March 16, to Juan Marinello, the Cuban poet, he emphasized the medical dimension of the trip, "I am preparing my trip to Buenos Aires, where I hope that by resolving the problem of my mobility, by means of an orthopedic application, I will resolve that of my health."[89] Exactly one month later, on April 16, Mariátegui died.

In his influential history of disability, French historian, anthropologist and philosopher Henri-Jacques Stiker suggests that, in the medicalization of disability, reintegration has appeared as a way of erasing, of disappearing, people with disabilities. Reintegration, he writes, is a social death that reflects a desire to make difference invisible. In this conception, prostheses contribute to this process of making difference invisible: "There's more to prosthetics than the pieces of wood, iron, and now plastic that replace a missing hand or foot. It's the very idea that something can be replaced. The image of the mutilated person and of the society that surrounds them becomes prosthetic. Replacement, reestablishment of the same situation as before, substitution, compensation: this becomes a possible language."[90]

As I argue in this chapter, however, through the use of various technol-

ogies, Mariátegui sought to resignify the visibility and meaning of his physical disability; he wanted to give it a meaning contrary to the hegemonic
one, which emphasized marginalization and vulnerability. And, as this section shows, he understood the rehabilitation he hoped to achieve in Buenos
Aires not as a social death but as the opportunity to achieve a new life that
would allow him to continue his cultural and political work. Mariátegui's
experience seems to confirm Catherine Kudlick's idea that the medicalization of disability "created a special role for disabled people in society and
for disability as a social variable." But at the same time, as multiple studies
show, people with disabilities "challenged these classifications, often introducing not only a different interpretation, but an alternative narrative about
how they fit into history."[91]

Conclusion

What effect did disability have on Mariátegui? He did not suffer systematic discrimination, vulnerability, or isolation because of his disability
to the same degree as most of his contemporaries, even though, as we saw,
some of his political opponents mocked his physical impairment. Unlike
Gramsci's, Mariátegui's disability does not appear to have made him particularly reserved in public or introverted.[92] His experience contrasts with
that of Randolph Bourne, discussed in the introduction, whose "deformity"
marked his life in such a way that "handicap formed the core of [his] perspective on society."[93] For Mariátegui, in contrast, disability was absent from
his view of society, perhaps in part because the impact of disability on his
lived experienced was alleviated by the technologies and networks to which
he had access.

If Bourne included disability within a social and political critique, Mariátegui did not; it was not a space that allowed him to reflect on, as Kim Nielsen
suggests, "the role of ableism—built structures and social systems that favor
the non-disabled—in shaping relationships, systems of power, ideals, dis-
paragements and the multiple ways of being in the world."[94] Mariátegui experienced disability as a personal misfortune and not as a social and political
condition; as we have seen, he was convinced that it could be addressed with
medical interventions and a prosthesis. In this sense, Bourne anticipated
what is called the "social model of disability," while Mariátegui's perspective
corresponds more to the "medical model of disability," which conceives of
disability as a pathology that requires a cure and overcoming.

That, perhaps, is why the figure of the "cojito genial," resonated in the collective imaginary of his time. A representation that he and, to a greater extent, his entourage cultivated as demonstrated by the visual and written repertoire that I analyze. This representation presented Mariátegui's disability as the origin and trigger of his intellectual genius and, more generally, as the central element of a narrative of heroic overcoming: the supercrip who in the face of adversity achieves exceptional accomplishments and becomes an inspiration to others. The narrative of Mariátegui's experience of disability and his attempts at overcoming it served to shape a notion of Mariátegui as a "worthy" disabled person from whose example others, on the left and beyond, were to learn. This component was central to the "heroic creation" of the "Amauta" of Peruvian socialism.

NOTES

1. Alberto Flores Galindo, *La agonía de Mariátegui: La polémica con la Komintern* (DESCO, 1980).

2. I use "heroic creation" here to refer to Mariátegui's famous phrase according to which Marxism in Latin America would be "neither trace nor copy. It must be heroic creation." See "Aniversario y balance," *Amauta* 3, no. 17 (1928): 2–3.

3. David Forgacs, "Gramsci Undisabled," *Modern Italy* 21, no. 4 (2016): 345–60.

4. This image and all the others I discuss in this essay can be found in "Sección 4—Documentación Visual" in the online Mariátegui archive Archivo José Carlos Mariátegui, https://archivo.mariategui.org/index.php/documentacion-grafica. The letters may be found in "Sección 5—Correspondencia JCM" in the same archive, at https://archivo .mariategui.org/index.php/correspondencia-5. All translations from Spanish and French are mine.

5. I have chosen to use the category "disability" (anachronistic for the period under study, when, as we shall see, other terms, such as *invalidez* and *inválido*, were used) to refer to both the biological and the social dimensions of this condition. Also I have not sought to reflect the distinctions that exist in the field of disability studies between what is usually called "impairment" and "disability," distinctions that characterize the "social model of disability" by differentiating it from the "medical model of disability," which perceives disability as "unchanging, pathological, rooted in individual bodies, and always in need of cure, correction or elimination." See Michael A. Rembis, Catherine J. Kudlick, and Kim E. Nielsen, "Introduction," in *The Oxford Handbook of Disability History*, ed. Michael A. Rembis, Catherine J. Kudlick, and Kim E. Nielsen (Oxford University Press, 2018), 4. As Carolina Ferrante and Karina Ramacciotti pithily explain, "Disability is not reduced to what is called 'impairment' or 'deficit,' an organic or behavioral particularity that implies a departure from normal or capable body and majority functioning, justifying the total or partial suspension of general social expectations. On the contrary, for the social model, disability is a form of socio-political oppression born of a social organization that systematically, and not randomly, excludes people who are called 'disabled' and devalues them

because it is only designed according to the parameters of an able or normal body, which meets the dispositions and values exalted by modern societies, especially capitalist ones." Ferrante and Ramacciotti, "Potencialidades y obstáculos para analizar las discapacidades desde el abordaje sociohistórico," *Pasado Abierto* 7, no. 13 (2021): 9–10.

6. See José Carlos Mariátegui, "La casa de los ciegos de guerra," in *Cartas de Italia* (Empresa Editora Amauta, 1969).

7. See "El mal del siglo," *La Prensa*, April 29, 1915, reprinted in José Carlos Mariátegui, *Escritos Juveniles (La edad de piedra)* (Empresa Editora Amauta, 1991), 235.

8. Paul K. Longmore and Paul Steven Miller, "'A Philosophy of Handicap': The Origins of Randolph Bourne's Radicalism," *Radical History Review*, no. 94 (2006): 71.

9. María Wiesse, *José Carlos Mariátegui* (Empresa Editora Amauta, 1971), 9. Wiesse, a poet, was married to the *indigenista* painter José Sabogal. Both were close collaborators of Mariátegui, particularly in publishing the journal *Amauta*.

10. Luis Alberto Sánchez, "Datos para una semblanza de José Carlos Mariátegui," in *El APRA y Mariátegui*, ed. M. Arroyo Lozada (Centro de Documentación Andina, 1990), 164.

11. Luis Alberto Sánchez, *Testimonio personal*, Vol. 1: *El Aquelarre 1900–1931* (Mosca Azul Editores, 1987), 168.

12. Published in *Claridad* 2, no. 6 (1924).

13. See Katherine Ott, "Material Culture, Technology, and the Body in Disability History," in Rembis, Kudlick, and Nielsen, *Oxford Handbook of Disability History*, 125–35.

14. See Armando Bazán, *Biografía de José Carlos Mariátegui* (Zig-Zag, 1939), 40.

15. David Hevey, "The Enfreakment of Photography," in *The Disability Studies Reader*, ed. Lennard J. Davis (London: Routledge, 2013), 432–46.

16. Abraham Valdelomar to José Carlos Mariátegui (JCM), June 1918. This letter, and all the others cited in this chapter, are available in the Archivo José Carlos Mariátegui.

17. Sánchez, "Datos para un semblanza."

18. Sánchez, "Datos para una semblanza," 153. In fact, Mariátegui was born in 1894.

19. Wiesse, *José Carlos Mariátegui*, 34.

20. Flores Galindo, *La agonía de Mariátegui*, 104.

21. Certificado médico, June 11, 1927, Archivo Mariátegui. In June 1927, the government denounced a "communist plot" to overthrow President Augusto B. Leguía. In a context of increased repression of the workers' movement by the authorities, Mariátegui was arrested, and the printing press where *Amauta* was published was closed. On the communist plot, see William Stein, "José Carlos Mariátegui y el complot comunista de 1927," *Anuario mariateguiano*, no. 7 (1995), 113–34.

22. According to Guillermo Rouillon, the doctors who knew Mariátegui, from Sebastian Lorente to Hugo Pesce, agree that he had *"artritis tuberculosa."* See Rouillon, *La creación heróica de José Carlos Mariátegui*, Vol. 2: *La edad revolucionaria* (Editorial Arica, 1984), 45.

23. José Luis Ayala, *Yo fui canillita de José Carlos Mariátegui: (Auto) biografía de Mariano Larico Yujra* (Kollao Editorial Periodística, 1990), 149.

24. Humberto Rodríguez Pastor, *José Carlos Mariátegui La Chira: Familia e infancia* (SUR Casa de estudios del socialismo, 1995).

25. Wiesse, *José Carlos Mariátegui*, 10.

26. Wiesse, 10.

27. Wiesse, *José Carlos Mariátegui*, 14.

28. Eudocio Ravines, *La gran estafa: La penetración del Kremlin en Iberoamérica* (Libros y Revistas S. A., 1952), 68.

29. Bazán, *Biografía*, 34.

30. Manuel Seoane, "Contraluces de Mariátegui," *Claridad* (Buenos Aires), May 1930, reprinted in *El APRA y Mariátegui*, 35.

31. Antenor Orrego, "El hombre de una pasión y fe," *La Tribuna*, April 16, 1959, reprinted in *El APRA y Mariátegui*, 77.

32. On the breakdown of the relationship, see Flores Galindo, *La agonía de Mariátegui*.

33. Víctor Raúl Haya de la Torre to Eudocio Ravines, March 2, 1929 (word missing in transcription), in *Los inicios*, ed. Armando Villanueva del Campo and Javier Landázuri García (Fundación Armando Villanueva del Campo, 2015), 246–57.

34. Haya de la Torre quoted in Ricardo Luna Vegas, *Contribución a la verdadera historia del APRA, 1923–1988* (Editorial Horizonte, 1990), 41.

35. Magda Portal, "Haya De la Torre y José Carlos Mariátegui," *APRA: Organo del frente único de trabajadores manuales e intelectuales*, no. 2 (October 20, 1930): 4.

36. Portal, "Haya De la Torre y José Carlos Mariátegui," 4.

37. Sami Schalk, "Reevaluating the Supercrip," *Journal of Literary and Cultural Disability Studies* 10, no. 1 (2016): 71–86.

38. Wiesse, *José Carlos Mariátegui*, 13.

39. Bazán, *Biografía*, 40.

40. Wiesse, *José Carlos Mariátegui*, 33.

41. Bazán, *Biografía*, 105.

42. Wiesse, *José Carlos Mariátegui*, 33.

43. Wiesse, *José Carlos Mariátegui*, 36.

44. Bazán, *Biografía*, 104.

45. Bazán, *Biografía*, 104–105.

46. Jorge del Prado, *Mariátegui y su obra* (Ediciones Nuevo Horizonte, 1946), 112–13.

47. Bazán, *Biografía*, 39–40.

48. Wiesse, *José Carlos Mariátegui*, 34.

49. "La enfermedad de Mariátegui," *Claridad* 2, no. 6 (1924): 10–11.

50. "Palabras de Mariátegui," *Claridad* 2, no. 6 (1924): 1.

51. "Palabras de Mariátegui," 2.

52. Luis E. Valcárcel, *Memorias* (Instituto de Estudios Peruanos, 1981), 239.

53. Wiesse, *José Carlos Mariátegui*, 36.

54. Sánchez, "Datos para una semblanza," 164–65.

55. On the middle class and domestic servants, see D. S. Parker, *Idea of the Middle Class: White-Collar Workers and Peruvian Society, 1900–1950* (Pennsylvania State University Press, 2010). See the plans of Mariátegui's house, which clearly show the domestic servants' quarters, in Claudio Lomnitz, *Nuestra América: My Family in the Vertigo of Transition* (Other Press, 2021), 102.

56. Kim E. Nielsen, "The Perils and Promises of Disability Biography," in Rembis, Kudlick, and Nielsen, *Oxford Handbook of Disability History*, 27.

57. Portal, "Haya de la Torre y José Carlos Mariátegui."

58. Nielsen, "The Perils and Promises of Disability Biography," 27.

59. JCM to Victoria Ferrer, August 22, 1924.

60. JCM to Victoria Ferrer, November 15, 1924.

61. JCM to Samuel Glusberg, April 30, 1927.

62. Luis Carranza to JCM, May 12, 1927.

63. Blanca Luz Brum to JCM, February 1, 1928.

64. Gamaliel Churata to JCM, July 30, 1928.

65. Tristán Marof to JCM, August 6, 1928.

66. Linton quoted in Nielsen, "The Perils and Promises of Disability Biography," 22.

67. Valcárcel, *Memorias*, 254.

68. See Mariátegui's contribution to the *Boletín de las Universidades Populares González Prada*, no. 1 (January 1927), reprinted in Servais Thissen, *Mariátegui: Nuevos aportes* (ARGOS, 2021), 143.

69. Flores Galindo, *La agonía de Mariátegui*; Horacio Tarcus, *Mariátegui en la Argentina: O las políticas culturales de Samuel Glusberg* (Ediciones el Cielo por Asalto, 2001).

70. Óscar Herrera to JCM, October 29, 1927. See also Herrera's letter of December 6, 1927, where he discusses the possibility of working for a "great bourgeois newspaper" funded by "an important English firm" and edited by Alberto Gerchunoff, the famed Argentine journalist.

71. Alberto Hidalgo to JCM, n.d., 1927.

72. JCM to Glusberg, January 10, 1927 [1928].

73. Flores Galindo, *La agonía de Mariátegui*.

74. César Alfredo Miro Quesada to JCM, July 2, 1928 (emphasis mine).

75. JCM to Glusberg, June 10, 1929.

76. JCM to Ernesto Reyna, January 26, 1929 [1930].

77. JCM to Samuel Glusberg, February 9, 1930.

78. Meghan Crnic and Cynthia Connolly, "'They Can't Help Getting Well Here': Seaside Hospitals for Children in the United States, 1872–1917," *Journal of the History of Childhood and Youth* 2, no. 2 (2009): 220–33.

79. JCM to Samuel Glusberg, February 26, 1930.

80. Daniel Blackie and Alexia Moncrieff, "State of the Field: Disability History," *History* 107, no. 377 (2022): 803.

81. JCM to Esteban Pavletich, March 8, 1927.

82. JCM to Glusberg, July 4, 1928.

83. JCM to Glusberg, November 21, 1929.

84. JCM to Glusberg, December 18, 1929.

85. JCM to Glusberg, December 18, 1929.

86. Glusberg to JCM, December 28, 1929.

87. Waldo Frank to JCM, December 30, 1929.

88. JCM to Glusberg, February 9, 1930.

89. JCM to Juan Marinello, March 16, 1930.

90. Henri-Jacques Stiker, *Corps infirmes et sociétés* (Dunod, 2013), 215, 172.

91. Catherine Kudlick, "Disability History: Why We Need Another 'Other,'" *American Historical Review* 108, no. 3 (2003): 773.

92. Forgacs, "Gramsci Undisabled," 355.

93. Longmore and Miller, "'Philosophy of Handicap,'" 63.

94. Nielsen, "Perils and Promises of Disability Biography," 22.

3

Border Conceptions

Anencephalic Births and Geographies of Bodily Difference in the Rio Grande Valley

Emily Xiao and Elizabeth O'Brien

In March 1991, in the border city of Brownsville, Texas, Teresa Salazar was five months' pregnant when an ultrasound detected something concerning. The baby boy she was carrying had anencephaly, a fatal neural tube defect (NTD) in which major portions of the brain and skull are missing.[1] A month later, anencephaly was found in three other pregnant women at Valley Regional Medical Center within a 36-hour period. Alarmed, hospital epidemiologist Connie Riezenman contacted the Texas Department of Health (TDH), which in turn alerted the Centers for Disease Control and Prevention (CDC).[2] An occupational health specialist named Margaret Diaz simultaneously learned that a colleague had recently performed sonograms on several pregnant women in Brownsville, all of whom were carrying children without brains. Diaz, too, sounded the alarm, reporting six affected infants within a six-week period. These surprising findings prompted "full-blown investigations" by the CDC and TDH. Epidemiologists discovered 31 cases of NTDs in Brownsville in just two years, whereas the national average should have yielded only 6 during this time frame.[3]

Newspapers nationwide dramatized the cluster as a medical "mystery."[4] When the *South Florida Sun Sentinel* introduced its readers to the unfolding anencephaly drama in Cameron County, whose seat is Brownsville, Texas, the reporters wrote: "The affliction is a tragic mystery. A baby, normal in every other way, is born without a brain."[5] In the months following the discovery, the media buzzed with each resurgence of stillbirths, generating anxiety about the potential of periodic recurrence.[6] For years the cases bewildered physicians, epidemiologists, journalists, and parents themselves. They speculated about innumerable culprits that spanned the gamut from poverty to pollution, and from diet to diabetes. Health officials eventually discovered that neural tube defects had occurred, undetected, for years in this community near the Rio Grande, where they primarily affected Mexican-origin women. Despite years of investigation, the cause remained, and is still, an epidemiologic "mystery."

Yet it was also much more than a mystery, and there is much to learn from how politicians, physicians, and the media told and retold this story and how they imbued it with beliefs about race, citizenship, and pathological maternity. Approaching neural tube defects through disability, borderlands, and environmental studies, this chapter reexamines the cluster's social and political implications by arguing that authorities ascribed anencephaly within an imagined geography of race, poverty, and pollution at the border. Some authorities blamed Mexican-origin women for their children's bodily aberrations while claiming that cultural factors caused their children's disabilities. Our discussion demonstrates that ableism reified ethnonational stereotypes at the same time that racism exacerbated pathologizing depictions of mothers and their debilitated children. These dynamics fit in a longer history of the social construction of racialized bodies as devious and monstruous.[7] The chapter also explores the ways local activists contested the vilification of women's bodies and the products of their wombs. Community members made a distinct spatial argument for the cases' clustering along lines of pollution at the Rio Grande, pointing to toxic water and land pollution by US corporations that exploited local workers while capitalizing on lax environmental regulations.

The crisis of anencephalic babies prompted the establishment of a state birth defect registry as well as a federally sponsored folic acid distribution campaign. Mexican women's bodies may not have been welcome as part of the greater body politic, but the knowledge gained from their tragedies was extrapolated for the benefit of the nation. Here we explore the terms under which a border community—seen as marginal, unmanageable, and undocumented—became a flashpoint for public health surveillance, despite long-standing disinvestment in its social and environmental welfare. By examining how distinct stakeholders viewed the anencephalic babies, we embrace Bianca Premo's call for historians of disability to cast their critical gaze onto onlookers, "seeing them as more than mere passive consumers in structured (capitalist) relations of power, inured to violence and instinctively bent on consumption or domination of unexpected bodies."[8] Anencephaly held a range of meanings for the public, for scientists, and for families. Mexican researchers and activists made anti-imperialist arguments, placing the harms done onto border families within the US's long-standing eugenic-inspired mistreatment of Mexicans. In their eyes it was US greed and racism that made the border, as Gloria Anzaldúa famously wrote, "an open wound," "where the first world grates against the third world and bleeds."[9]

Anencephalic Babies, Environmental Toxicity, and Disability History: Discussion of the Literature

That the Brownsville babies did not survive the condition of anencephaly is relevant to the way their stories fit into the history of disability and debility. For a condition like congenital rubella, as Leslie Reagan has shown, middle-class parents sought educational access and inclusion for their children.[10] In contrast, anencephalic fetuses who survived to birth died shortly thereafter. They were here, all too briefly, on the periphery of life and citizenship, and then gone.[11] Narratives around their existence were created by other actors, and the significance of the babies' lives was always unstable and contested. As such, anencephaly does not fit neatly under identity categories that are, as Robert McRuer says, "legible beneath the universal access symbol for disability."[12]

These tensions point to the broader limitations of Western disability studies, which has generally sought to reclaim disability experiences by rejecting associations with tragedy in favor of empowerment and rights.[13] A social approach has been enormously valuable for challenging the medical model of disability, which assumes that biomedical progress can, and should, improve disabled people's lives and their bodies through technocentric cures. Because the elimination of disabilities also results in the erasure of disabled people, the medical model is well worthy of critique. At the same time, an individual-centric discourse can sometimes obscure the state-sponsored violence that debilitates vulnerable populations, disabling people's bodies through corporeal harm and subjugation, including environmental harms. Jasbir Puar's use of the term "debility" encompasses these political dislocations, which tend to be flattened by mainstream connotations of "disability."[14] Globalized disability theory attends to the historical and spatial junctures that not only produce impairment in different contexts but also shape its interpretation by communities.[15]

Brownsville's anencephaly cluster is a rich site to interrogate the intersections of environmental history and disability history. On one hand, people are disabled by the built environment and debilitated, in the case addressed in this chapter, by toxic poisons. As Alison Kafer has so eloquently explained, in Texas "social arrangements" were quite literally "mapped onto 'natural environments.'"[16] Yet, when we decry the poisoning of people's bodies and their environments, we sometimes run the risk of ontologically devaluing those people's worth by using biologized and medicalized language to describe the effects of harm on their bodies. Kelly Fritsch contributes to this critique by pointing out that environmental activism has sometimes reified ableism through the language of "individual health problem[s]."[17]

While toxic environments produce forms of disability, we must resist the urge to frame this harm in neoliberal terms that emphasize productivity and value, given that, as Fritsch puts it, "biocapitalism and the economization of life marks a way of talking about more and less valuable lives." It is possible to value disabled people's lives "while still critiquing neoliberal economies that produce disability." One way to advance this critique is to recognize that "toxins and disability are not individual health problems of bodies or environments gone astray but rather shared continuities of each other." In other words, scholars can view toxins and contamination as not static but relational; not limited to any one community or region, but affecting us all.[18] Because we live in a toxic world, toxicity is in everyone. Authorities in Texas attempted to trace and contain it, but to no avail: toxicity results from environmental harms both foreseen and unforeseen.

In his critique of seeing environmentally wrought health problems as individual-level failures of the body, Eli Clare addresses incommensurable loss of life in environmental and disability histories by posing a question relevant to this chapter: How do we "deal with bodily and ecological loss when restoration in its various manifestations is not the answer?"[19] In Texas there was no answer to the anencephaly crisis; no solution to the poisoning of the children. Restoration was not an option. This chapter responds to Clare's call by looking to the mothers of anencephalic fetuses, and by taking their cues on how to situate narratives about disability and impairment. Although the mothers referenced herein seem to have been born as able-bodied people, they came to be seen as corporeally defective due to their wombs' production of disabled children. This was an ableist and gendered social debilitation, reproduced by racist authorities who blamed women for birthing children who were incompatible with life. When the state turned to blame and surveillance, Teresa and others like her were not silent: They challenged xenophobic ableism by resisting the demonization of their lifestyles, their diets, and their sexual reproduction. They also grappled with the emotional complexity of having birthed a baby with anencephalia, especially in way they countered media depictions with their own commemorative practices. This chapter centers the women who conceived these babies and retraces their expressions of care, embodiment, and meaning-making around their babies.

The anencephaly cluster in the Rio Grande Valley thus challenges us to consider what debility means to disability history when its subjects cannot live to claim a related identity. It similarly casts light on the contingencies of nonnormativity in a borderlands context, a site of imperialistic and racialized exclusion from US citizenship. This is a disability history in which many of the central subjects cannot speak, but whose lives were, nonetheless, deeply significant and meaningful for myriad reasons. We also seek to highlight how individuals, families, communities, and transnational groups resisted the conditions that disparaged perceived racial and bodily differences. Tragedy, ambivalence, and grief were meaningful responses to debilitation and political marginalization. With their responses, women and families affirmed a space in disability discourse and history.

The Mothers of Anencephalic Babies
Maternal Blame

The national panic about anencephaly coincided with increased public awareness of health issues caused by industrial hazards. We now understand these toxins through the frame of structural violence, as capitalists and state leaders harmed communities of color and impoverished people by relegating contaminants disproportionately to marginalized residential areas. A 1985 article in *Ladies' Home Journal*, for example, decried birth defects occurrent in Jacksonville, Arkansas, a town "next to an industrial area where 23,000 barrels of the highly toxic substance dioxin are stored."[20] Communities critiqued environmental injustice and birthed the second wave of the environmental justice movement.[21] For instance, an article in *Essence* noted a high incidence of birth defects in Carver Terrace, a Black subdivision in Texarkana, and issued a rallying cry: "Corporations choose poor areas, areas where Blacks, Hispanics, and Native Americans live. We have got to fight back."[22]

When coming from above, however, concerns about industrial hazards joined with biologically essentialist rhetoric that made a mother's body responsible for protecting her fetus, while also casting doubt on marginalized women's ability to do so. The *Ladies' Home Journal* article warned that "the fetus—and indeed the reproductive system—is more vulnerable than was once theorized." Citing "abundant" statistical evidence from the CDC showing that the incidence of birth defects was on the rise, the article stressed the need for action from federal agencies and the scientific community. On one hand, this was true: As discussed below, environmental toxins are particularly damaging to a fetus's developing brain. On the other hand, this approach urged readers to take personal steps to ensure a safer pregnancy, including educating themselves about teratogenic toxins.[23] Women living with poisoned water, soil, and air had little individual agency over their surroundings. Yet mothers still tasked themselves with the personal duty to ensure the health of their babies.

In this context, authorities sometimes blamed unexpected gestational outcomes on maternal negligence, and especially outcomes involving women of color. As Dorothy Roberts has shown, during the Reagan years Black mothers faced legal convictions for exposing their babies to drugs in utero, with the first such case decided in 1989.[24] Related accusations played out at the border. Reader Ruth Key wrote to the McAllen, Texas, *Monitor* inquiring whether anencephaly was "confined to one social group (e.g., the poor, and say, barrio dweller)." She raised the "simple" possibility that these defects occurred among the "glue and paint-sniffers set. There is considerable abuse right there in the Brownsville area." Key added, "It would save the worrying public a lot of distress (and yes, the taxpayer a lot of money) if the investigators first determine whether these anomalies were self-inflicted through abuse of any kind of harmful substance from A to Z . . . from admixture (of any kind) to Zacatecas pulque."[25] Key's accusation was at once broad ("A to Z") and simultaneously charged with specific racial overtones: not only were these parents engaging in illicit behavior, she alleged, but their indulgences reflected their cultural deviance (perhaps particularly strong among Zacatecanos, according to the misinformed Key). If people and their culture could be blamed, then anencephaly could be cordoned off from the Euro-descendent population and did not merit a claim to the state's resources.

For would-be parents in Cameron County, the mystery of anencephaly imposed a heavy emotional toll as individuals were left to speculate on what, if anything, they had done wrong. "Some of us believe it was something we ate or drank. I do," Janet Ramirez told the *Fort Worth Star Telegram*. "My husband took it real bad. He had a nervous breakdown."[26] Some women, like Teresa Salazar, internalized a feeling of blame. "I felt very guilty. I told my husband to go away so he could have children [with someone else]," she told *Newsweek*.[27] At the June 1992 CDC-TDH press conference, Teresa Salazar spoke to the crowd: "I came here with some hope that I would know something more than what I did."[28] Apparently she wept as she continued, "I'm afraid that the same thing will happen again. But I'm going to try it, even though I know it will be a nightmare until the end of my pregnancy."[29]

Racist and ableist discourses about so-called defective reproduction cast a shadow on mothers' decision making about future pregnancies. Prior delivery of an anencephalic baby was one of the few known risk factors for recurrent NTD; this prognosis seemed a rare grain of truth to cling to, but it conferred an additional burden on women who had been affected by the cluster.[30] In statistical terms, their previous medical experience marked their bodies as posing higher risk and justified future reproductive surveillance. It mattered less what the original cause may have been, whether environmental or social. The ableist language of biorisk now located pathology in their wombs.

Women, for their part, questioned official assessments and demanded greater accountability from experts. At the press conference mentioned above, 22-year-old Janet Perez spoke out: "I'm still angry. My baby should have been almost a year [old] now. I want to know why it happened."[31] Janet Ramirez, who was part of a class action against toxic factories on the border, received a letter from General Motors claiming that the primary cause of NTDs was insufficient dietary intake of folic acid. The letter implied that her self-care was to blame, despite flimsy supporting evidence. One could even interpret the misinforming document as a form of intimidation. Countering General Motors, she shared the following at the press conference: "I was always watching my diet. They're just trying to blame the victim."[32] Judy Guerrero, who gave birth to a daughter with spina bifida, pointed out, "Sometimes they say it's bad prenatal care, but I had three sonograms."[33] When their bodies became subject to debate, and their prenatal management was called into question, mothers spoke out about their own health agency. They made their voices heard, contributing to the epidemiologic discourse around anencephaly in the Valley.[34]

Reproductive Dilemmas

Media portrayals hint at women's reproductive decisions around anencephaly. Abortion was not always named as such; newspaper accounts sometimes alluded to these choices euphemistically, eliding the politics of reproductive rights. Indeed, abortion narratives in the public sphere have long been linked to respectability, which in turn is shaped by considerations of race and class.[35] It is important to acknowledge here that media accounts can offer only so much insight into subjective experiences. Thus, related interpretations are necessarily circumscribed and mediated by the language available in journalistic portrayals, which pursued their own narrative aims. Sensationalistic media seemed to normalize and encourage expressions of disgust and horror toward anencephalic babies and their families.[36]

Anglocentric editorial choices sometimes make it difficult to recover the language that mothers used. One *CNN Evening News* segment featured four women, three of whom were dubbed from Spanish in English. The newscast muted their original voices, creating a language barrier for Spanish-speaking viewers in their own communities while making their words accessible to a mainstream English-speaking audience. The dubbed voices were also accented, an artifice that marked the Mexican American mothers as "foreign" inhabitants. But there is also much to glean from the firsthand experiences expressed in these sources, as evidenced by above examples of women who harnessed media visibility to challenge epidemiologic and legal narratives. Careful reading, beyond pity and pathos, offers glimpses into the emotional complexities of families with anencephalic births.

In the 1980s, screening for neural tube defects prior to 20 weeks of gestation had become feasible with detection of a substance called α-fetoprotein in maternal serum.[37] After the first trimester, neural tube defects could be detected later by ultrasound, as was the case for many of the affected mothers discussed below. The subsequent decline in the incidence of NTDs created a sense of optimism in the medical community that these conditions could soon be eradicated. Dr. Shlomo Shinnar and Dr. John Arras opined in a 1989 article that "the issue regarding anencephalic infants will probably become moot in the next few years."[38] But the means by which this could occur, pregnancy termination, did not exist in a political, social, or cultural vacuum; therefore prenatal technologies were a site of discourse and contention relating to abortion, disability, and gendered caregiving.[39] An article in *Morbidity and Mortality Weekly Report* demonstrated that the rate of spina bifida, which was highest among Hispanics, had been declining since 1985. Dr. Jon Aase suggested that this might be explained by a decreased rate of survival at birth rather than decreased incidence: in other words, a higher number of abortions. However, he stressed that he would "hate to condone that or make it a recommendation."[40]

Communities, meanwhile, varied in access to prenatal care and abortion services.[41] A 1991 study suggested that the declining incidence of anencephaly reflected a trend in white infants much more so than in nonwhite infants, suggesting the former communities' greater access to pregnancy termination services.[42] The Texas Department of Mental Health and Mental Retardation provided genetic screening at some locations throughout the state, including three in the Rio Grande Valley. The state charged patients on a sliding scale based on family income, but it is unclear from the available evidence whether these services were well utilized or the degree to which they addressed issues of access.[43] Women also navigated a fraught political landscape of abortion restrictions. In Texas, a 1987 law had prohibited all abortions in the third trimester, except in cases where the life of the mother was in danger or the fetus had a severe abnormality.[44] It is unclear whether the mothers of anencephalic babies were likely to know of this exception.

Some Catholic women carrying anencephalic fetuses grappled with additional religious considerations.[45] Physicians recommended that they speak with priests who were "known to grant forgiveness for the sin" of abortion, which could otherwise lead to excommunication from the Church. The particular circumstance of anencephaly may have mitigated the moral weight of abortion for religious leaders like the bishop of the Diocese of Brownsville, who affirmed his sympathy for the affected women. Bioethicists like John Fletcher, the director of the Center for Biomedical Ethics at the University of Virginia, weighed in: "What makes us human is what goes on upstairs in the brain."[46] These attitudes indicate a more flexible stance on abortion exceptions for severe medical abnormalities or disabilities—reflecting, to some degree at least, an ableist assessment of the purported value of those lives. "If you lose a baby that is normal in any other way but dies, people give you a couple of months to get over it," Alva Nelms told *The Monitor*. "But when the baby has some sort of disability, they don't even give you that long."[47] Nelms's testimony illustrates how societal attitudes toward bodily non-normativity could place mothers in a lonely position. Women considering whether to abort their anencephalic fetuses knew that their babies would not survive for long after delivery, but social and cultural constraints meant that their choices were still daunting and painful.

Teresa Salazar, for example, learned from a sonogram at five months that her baby had anencephaly. Told by her doctor to choose between a stillborn delivery or an abortion, she opted for the latter. A journalist alleged that Salazar felt "compelled" to terminate the pregnancy after having had two miscarriages. One wonders if she felt internally compelled, wishing to avoid the shock and disappointment of another miscarriage, or whether there were social, familial, or medical pressures.[48] Luz Perez shared a similar story: Her baby was nearly seven months when a sonogram detected that he had anencephaly. Doctors explained that continuing the pregnancy could be dangerous, and Perez consented to early labor induction after "two days of agonizing."[49] "Early labor" is not semantically the same as abortion, but historically the two categories have been collapsed in order to mitigate religious or legal prohibitions on pregnancy termination.[50]

Emotional displays in media accounts invite sympathy but likewise suggest that medical judgment was inadequate for navigating the distress of fetal loss. In these accounts, the media juxtaposed the allegedly "morally neutral" reasons for abortion with those that did not involve severe disabilities. As straightforward as medical logic may have seemed, it also constrained decision making so that it was not entirely volitional. Janet Ramirez, to take another example, learned of her baby's diagnosis five months into her pregnancy. As one article described her situation, "The pregnancy was terminated, and Ramirez became another piece in a puzzle that has plagued medical investigators."[51] Another source reveals in greater detail that Ramirez delivered her baby stillborn after undergoing induced labor at six months. The journalist described Ramirez's eyes "misting over" as she recalled the ordeal, stating, "I didn't want the termination. But the doctors said if I was going to go through the nine months I was going to suffer and so was the baby."[52]

Virginia Listman, a white woman, endured the controversy that could be ignited by public discourse around abortion. An article in the *Austin American-Statesman* printed a photo of her standing by an empty swing set, as if to highlight her childlessness. Listman, a state employee, had been forced to appeal her insurance company's refusal to pay for the medical costs related to her pregnancy after her "voluntary interruption," a euphemism for abortion. Listman's self-advocacy had not emerged from a pro-choice political stance; ironically, she emphasized that she and her husband were "totally against abortion," seemingly not understanding that she had chosen one.[53] Nevertheless, her case became politicized as an abortion issue. Lisa Salcedo of the Texas Right to Life Committee co-opted the language of disability inclusion, arguing that Listman's insurance company should have paid— not, in her opinion, because abortion is an unavoidable part of healthcare but rather because hers had been a "case where a helpless and unborn child in the womb was discriminated against because of his disability."[54]

These stories reveal an ambivalent picture. For women of color especially, the history of reproductive care has entailed significant tensions between choice and coercion.[55] A broadly inclusive history of reproductive justice also comprises those, like Virginia Listman, who did not claim their choices politically. In addition, the timing of sonograms meant women were sometimes making difficult choices during what has been described as "late-term" pregnancy. As these cases highlight, the concept of late-term abortions is as much a political construct as a medical definition, shaped by attitudes around pregnancy, reproduction, and the normative value of fetal bodies. Across the spectrum of political and spiritual views, decisions concerning anencephaly had profound emotional and medical effects. And in the aftermath of their ordeals, authorities gave women few answers as to why these birth defects had occurred.

Care and Kinship

In July 1994, a discovery was made near a gravesite in Brownsville's Santa Rosalia Cemetery: the remains of a premature baby girl. The ensuing investigation added yet another chapter to the story of the anencephalic births, further dramatizing the sense of mystery they had come to embody. The deceased fetus, wrapped in a green blanket from AMI Brownsville Medical Center, wore a knitted cap on her underdeveloped head. The plastic bands on her wrist and leg identified the physician who had delivered her, Dr. Juan Mancillas, who told reporters he had not delivered such a baby since 1991. Authorities investigated the case as a potential infanticide.[56]

Details continued to emerge, but they shed little light on the enigma. It turned out that the fetus, Victoria Gonzalez, had been stillborn at Valley Regional Medical Center on April 24, 1991. She was one of the three babies born within a 36-hour period that had set off the initial alarm bells about anencephaly. A funeral home gave her a proper burial a day later. Sometime later, her body had been exhumed and apparently frozen for three years before being "dumped unceremoniously" five feet from her original grave.[57] Victoria's mother, a native of Mexico, was described by the sheriff as "very indigent and very humble," and she had neither attended the burial nor visited the grave.[58] It is unclear whether the case was ever solved. Justice of the Peace Tony Torres remarked to reporters, "That little baby's a mystery."[59]

Victoria's story led to open speculation about personal and often unsettling topics, such as early-pregnancy loss and the handling of fetal remains. Established social procedures served to contain and ritualize the charged emotions arising from these misfortunes. Yet one of those rituals, professionalized disposition by a funeral home, had been disturbed by some unknown culprit from whom the fetus had elicited strong interest, whether scientific or spiritual. Beyond that is silence, as we cannot know with any certainty what she signified to the person who exhumed and held onto her remains for three years. Victoria's mother is also a figure in the background, initially difficult to track down by investigators. We know little about her feelings or motivations, such as why she did not attend her daughter's burial.

Maternal responses to anencephalic births ranged from ambivalence to deep sorrow. We may draw insight on these topics from medical anthropologist Lynn Morgan, who has delved into the cultural construction of the unborn, as well as fetal relationality and the relative silence around fetal remains.[60] A discussion of anencephaly and grievability is further enriched by Miriam Rich's and Julie Livingston's work on affective responses to nonnormative bodies, as mediated by seeing, emotion, and physical touch.[61] Newspaper stories, while sensationalized, reveal important details about how mothers performed affective rituals on their babies' remains. Centering these experiences allows us to retrace the ways mothers made meaning from their infants' brief lives.

"Two of the babies were stillborn. The third [baby] hung on for three days, doomed by a gruesome, fatal defect that leaves infants with an open skull and only the rudiments of a brain," wrote John McClintock for the *Baltimore Sun*.[62] His vivid description is representative of the terminology attached to the anencephalic births by outside observers. The media often used the phrase "brainless babies" as a shorthand, focusing, arguably excessively, on what made these tiny bodies different.[63] Anencephalic births were "tragic," "horrifying," and "haunting.[64] Sometimes the descriptions veered so far from the realm of the clinical that they were jarring. Dr. Manuel Guajardo, a Brownsville physician, said that the condition made babies appear as if "somebody took a knife and just whacked the top of the head off."[65] TDH epidemiologist Judy Henry spoke of anencephaly in dehumanizing terms, referencing "such a horrifying, disfiguring defect" and speaking of babies that did not "even look human."[66] One article metaphorized birth defects as "early symptoms" of pollution: "The warning is graphic. Many of the newborns have frog-like eyes or misshapen heads. The effect on families is devastating."[67] There was no shortage of terms to describe these so-called "Brownsville horrors."[68]

Yet these births had names, stories, and hopes attached to them. Janet Ramirez had decided on the name Maria Guadalupe long before her first baby was due, and she made weekly visits to her baby's gravesite.[69] Rosa Salinas named her baby boy Jaime, after his father.[70] Norma and Gilbert Olvera took pictures of their deceased infant and named her Amy Keiko, which to them meant "beloved" and "adored."[71] Mothers' attitudes sometimes stood in stark contrast to reporters' descriptions. A *Time* article contained the following description: "The photo is at once sad and gruesome, but Janet Ramirez treasures it. Dressed in a white hospital gown, an IV hooked up to her arm, the mother clasps her newborn baby, Maria Guadalupe. Only if you look closely can you see that the baby's face is a death mask; a white cap discreetly covers the gaping hole in the back of her skull."[72] At first glance, everything is arranged as it should be: the mother, cared for in a professionalized clinical setting, cradling her child. To the reporter, however, this claim to love and intimacy was "gruesome," an aesthetically challenging distortion of normative caregiving.

Janet Ramirez was not the only mother who engaged in rituals of maternal-infant bonding, even using photography as a commemorative tool. For babies who survived a few hours after birth, mothers sometimes had the opportunity to pose with their infants, pulling caps over their skulls.[73] This impulse to memorialize, or at least to mark the passing of a life, could also be seen in the disposition of remains. A *CNN Evening News* segment included a clip of an infant whose remains had been carefully arranged in a casket, the top of its head obscured by cloth.[74] The bodies of anencephalic fetuses were not just medical specimens or sources for sample collection; they were also touched and displayed by loved ones as objects of mourning. This visible claim to grievability or, in Judith Butler's words, "a presupposition for the life that matters," contrasts notably with dominant attitudes toward anencephalic births.[75]

Medical care teams sometimes inscribed restrictive boundaries around maternal expressions of care, whether out of paternalism or necessity. Indeed, whether mothers were allowed to see their babies often constituted an important moment in anencephaly narratives. Teresa Salazar asked to see her son, but her care providers would not show him to her.[76] They evidently interfered to spare her from the perceived horror of the situation, but in so doing they used their medical authority to dictate the terms of intimacy between mother and child. Judy Guerrero, whose daughter was born with spina bifida, had a similar experience. After 24 hours of labor and a cesarean section, her baby was "whisked" away for emergency surgery before she could bond with or caress the newborn.[77] Although the surgery needed to be performed as quickly as possible, doctors also refused to tell Guerrero what was happening. These stories offer an opportunity for health practitioners to reflect on how medical interventions impact maternal experiences of nonnormative births.

This chapter uses the phrase "anencephalic birth" as a conscious departure from the terminology employed by the media. As a fatal condition, anencephaly produced a situation in which mothers came to know their babies primarily in death. Yet this circumstance did not lessen their embodied relationality. Families' affective interactions, including the act of giving birth, were no less generative or meaningful for being centered on fetal remains. Indeed, this approach considers personhood in the context of relational care and kinship, rather than the animacy of an individual body.[78] A range of meanings proliferated around anencephalic births, seen as objects of horror by the public, of scrutiny by scientists, and of care and kinship by their parents. In the midst of all this, they were not abstractions or monstrosities. They were loved, and they were mourned.

Constructing the Border as an Insalubrious and Mysterious Region

For many readers, newspaper stories about the anencephaly cluster served as an introduction to the border itself. Local and national media associated the cluster with a dismal picture of life in the Rio Grande Valley: families living in poverty, surrounded by ramshackle structures and waste. Epidemiologists initially recognized that the affected mothers seemed to have little in common to connect their cases: They differed in economic background and access to prenatal care and shared no "telltale occupational trend."[79] Yet media stories collapsed these distinctions into stereotypes of the Valley as "one of the nation's poorest regions," with "more women who fall into the high-risk category here" than elsewhere.[80] Poverty does not automatically lead to poor prenatal healthcare: The situation becomes so when policy makers choose which communities to neglect.

Anencephaly's spatial association with the border became one of its defining characteristics in the popular eye. News stories included maps acquainting readers with the lay of the land in South Texas, constructing a visual argument for anencephaly's clustering along the Rio Grande. The front page of the *Baltimore Sun* featured a photograph of Dr. Carmen Rocco, a local pediatrician, holding a large map of Brownsville with black dots indicating individual cases. Dr. Rocco stands in front of another map in the background. If such geographic imagery was not suggestive enough, the reader could turn the page to find a third map demonstrating the relationship between Brownsville and Matamoros, its sister city across the Rio Grande.[81]

For environmental activists and local residents, geography provided evidence for industrial pollution as the culprit, as when John McClintock wrote in the *Baltimore Sun*, "Brownsville residents now fear that an environmental time bomb has gone off."[82] He was referring to Brownsville's proximity to the maquiladoras of Matamoros and the hazardous waste they spawned. Since the 1960s, US and foreign corporations operated these low-cost plants along the Mexican side of the border, capitalizing on a cheaper labor force, favorable tariff regulations, and loose enforcement of waste-handling protocols. Community members like Margaret Diaz, the occupational health specialist, saw a link between the stillbirths and toxic exposure. She declared these births "atrocities committed by two uncaring governments," the product of "years of neglect."[83] Diaz viewed reproductive aberration as the embodied manifestation of environmental aberration.

The US press packaged that sentiment for public consumption, narrating vivid "scenes of environmental destruction" while devoting less attention to political accountability.[84] A *CNN Evening News* segment described "Mexican Texas, or Texaco," as being "more Third World than first," with voice-over narration about openly dumped waste and water turned pink from factories.[85] "In a downpour," wrote one journalist for the *Philadelphia Inquirer*, "the privies spill their contents into the back yards where children play."[86] A

Newsday article described the home of Janet Ramirez, one of the affected mothers. From her "torn screen door," Ramirez could gaze across the Rio Grande at distant smokestacks "looming" over agricultural fields.[87] Suspicions about chemical toxicity may well have been correct. Most industrial chemicals have never been tested by the Environmental Protection Association, and "fewer than 20 percent of the eighty-four thousand chemicals registered with the EPA in 2008 have had any substantial safety testing." On this issue Kelly Fritsch quoted Philippe Grandjean (an environmental scientist) and Philip Landrigan (an epidemiologist and pediatrician), who testify that "the developing nervous system of the fetus is particularly vulnerable to chemical toxicity." The fetal brain requires the precise movement of neurons along pathways during the developmental process, in which the brain goes from "a single strip of cells" into a "complex organ consisting of billions of highly interconnected specialized cells." There are "windows of unique susceptibility to toxic interference" with "little potential for later repair." To make matters worse, "most chemical toxicity testing is done in relation to adult humans."[88] As discussed below, pollution was all too real at the border. However, the press perpetuated a narrative of the Valley that dramatized anencephaly, inscribing it in a legible geography of race and poverty.

The media characterized both anencephaly and its unknown etiology as insidious, mobile menaces. Journalists sometimes anthropomorphized the condition, describing it as a "killer lurking near this border city."[89] Such potent language alluded to the border's permeable nature. One newspaper warned that a breeze might bring welcome relief on a hot Texas day, but "maybe, just maybe, it should also be considered dangerous," for it could carry toxins from Matamoros's industrial zone.[90] The border was merely an imagined political boundary, porous to wind and water.

In the spring of 1992, in the midst of this media attention, the CDC and TDH launched a joint study to investigate a range of hypotheses, including environmental hazards, diet, genetics, lifestyle, and occupation.[91] Their epidemiologists initially seemed open to considering industrial hazards such as aflatoxin. For example, Dr. Jean Brender, the director of TDH's Environmental Epidemiology Program, pointed to her own case-control study that had found a link between paternal exposure to solvents and anencephaly.[92] But as the investigation progressed, critics wondered whether the agencies downplayed environmental factors by neglecting to test air, water, and soil samples.[93] State and federal officials expressed skepticism about environmental theories, sometimes openly deriding local opinion in the press. Dr. James Cheek of the CDC declared: "We aren't sucked into thinking that all problems are environmentally generated."[94] Others warned that there were too many unanswered questions to establish a causal "smoking gun," or direct evidence linking birth defects to industrial practices.[95] The agencies may have been reluctant to release a finding of toxic waste in the border zone because negotiations were under way for what would become the North American Free Trade Agreement.[96]

Alternative theories turned away from industrial pollution to possible localized defects intrinsically in the bodies of mothers. Some proposed that Mexican American women had a genetic predisposition to anencephaly, even though border populations in California, New Mexico, and Arizona had not experienced similar outbreaks. This theory also conflated nationality with race, ethnicity, and biology.[97] The language of heredity even made its way from the scientific to the legal realm in the form of the so-called Mayan Theory: In a class action suit brought by 28 affected families against maquiladoras, the attorneys for General Motors argued that the anencephalic fetuses' ancestry traced back to the ancient Maya of central Mexico, among whom a higher incidence of NTDs could be found.[98]

Investigators also turned their attention to diet, which could be rooted in both individual behavior and ethnocultural proclivities. They claimed that the "typical Hispanic diet" was lower in folic acid and that chemical, environmental, or genetic exposures might play a role only insofar as they were thought to exacerbate preexisting deficiency.[99] This preoccupation with diet persisted even as new data about environmental hazards continued to be published. In fact, some who proposed mechanisms for a link between industrial pollution and disease still racialized anencephaly by identifying cultural dietary habits as the mediator. "The corn in their tortillas is susceptible to infestations of mold," read a 1992 *Newsweek* article explaining how tortilla consumption might be the vehicle for hazardous exposure due to fumonisin, a fungal toxin that may have been exacerbated in corn crops due to pesticide use.[100]

Journalists spun these debates into an intricate scientific drama, pitting activists against outsider experts. Dissatisfied with the progress of the TDH-CDC joint investigation, a group of local physicians, attorneys, health workers, and activists launched its own study in January 1992. This group included Dr. Carmen Rocco and other health workers at the Brownsville

Community Health Center. Although the team struggled with funding and methodological limitations, they uncovered some compelling evidence of industrial hazards: Around the time that the anencephalic babies had been conceived, xylene and toluene had been detected in soil and water samples taken near a US-owned auto plant in Matamoros. Toluene had also been reported in air sampling in Brownsville. However, no autopsies had been performed on babies from the initial cluster, so they lacked access to samples of kidney tissue, for example, that might have revealed traces of toxins. This led some journalists to cast doubt on the local investigation's scientific grounds, implying that they lacked "hard evidence."[101] One newspaper suggested that the investigators' concerns were hysterical and amounted to "heresy in Brownsville where many are convinced a mysterious and deadly environmental cause exists."[102] R. Daniel Cavazos, the editor of *The Monitor*, called local activists "shrill critics who will seize on the tragedy of anencephaly to push their image of border plants that have brought mixed results to regions in desperate need of jobs."[103]

CDC-TDH officials maintained their credibility in part by employing a professional attitude of skepticism. But disagreement from other experts highlights how the agencies' omission of environmental data could be, and was, seen as methodologically unusual. Local physicians had specifically requested studies of environmental hazards, and Margaret Diaz criticized the agencies for having "absolutely ignored" them.[104] Dr. John Harris, chief of California's Birth Defects Monitoring Program, shared in a private letter that his team certainly would have tested for water contamination in response to community concerns.[105] Later that summer, Amalia Rodriguez-Mendoza, who chaired Texas governor Ann Richards's Commission for Women, wrote to the state health commissioner to point out that environmental testing had been "spotty or nonexistent." "As time passes, memories grow dim," Rodriguez-Mendoza wrote. "The parents of these children may not be available, and records of chemicals in the area might be lost."[106]

In June 1992, after almost a yearlong investigation, the agencies released their findings in a 70-page report. At a press conference, they revealed a failure to find a "smoking gun"; no convincing links had been found to the environment, occupational exposures, or even dietary issues.[107] Dr. David Smith lamented, "We are still groping around looking for the light switch."[108] Audience members were also troubled when TDH epidemiologist Dr. Dennis

Perrotta announced: "We no longer have an epidemic."[109] The Coalition for Justice in the Maquiladoras, an activist organization, accused Perrotta of making a "political decision" to defuse public alarm by downgrading the cluster to a mere "elevated rate among Hispanics and border residents." To them, Perrotta's conclusion struck "a chord of environmental racism."[110] Benedictine nun Susan Mika called the categorization a "political ploy" to avoid devoting resources to an environmental solution.[111]

This is not just a narrative about scientific uncertainty and how knowledge is contested. It also raises questions about the limitations of epidemiologic language and the process by which a bodily condition is labeled, counted, and understood. The cluster was constructed as a medical "mystery" as the borderlands itself evolved into a site of epidemiologic difficulty, seemingly resistant to scientific expertise. Although state and federal agencies devoted considerable energy to identifying a cause, they struggled to elucidate an answer with the tools available to them, or the ones they were willing to use. This difficulty calls into question why public health officials focused so heavily on identifying a single "smoking gun," and whether this paradigm was adequate for addressing the complex historical circumstances of environmental abuses, health inequities, and resulting debilities in the border region.[112]

For those writing from Mexico, there was no mystery at all. Mexican physicians, activists, and journalists fiercely criticized US officials' refusal to pinpoint corporate irresponsibility for the cases of anencephaly. Journalists focused intensely on the environmental effects of toxic waste. They also supported a large lawsuit of affected families against 36 maquiladoras on the border, tracking its progress and celebrating its settlements. Many of the details and critiques found in Mexican media were absent from US press coverage.

For commentators in Mexico, pollution at the border was an economic problem born of the imperialist and racist dynamic in which US and transnational corporations exploited Mexican labor while neglecting basic health and safety conditions for workers, much as the bracero worker program had done from 1942 to 1964. In their 2000 monograph on the topic, researchers Miriam Alfie Cohen and Luis Méndez wrote that the "relationship between the environment and development, as expressed in the industrial realm," was "contradictory, harmful, explosive, and threatening" and that the "successful" model of economic growth "came at a steep price for environment and health." The economic gains of neoliberalism were accessible only to some and left the rest behind.[113]

One of the largest and most dynamic activist groups to address the crisis was the Comunidad Ecológica de Matamoros, or Matamoros Environmental Group, which began in 1987 and was formalized in 1990 with the goal of demanding environmental justice in the border community and protecting the environment. Cofounder José Magdaleno had previously been employed in a maquiladora, where he was disturbed by the health problems and lack of accountability he witnessed. Magdaleno soon organized an interdisciplinary group of twelve people who worked horizontally to educate other factory workers and build a grassroots movement, eventually "becoming the communities' microphone."[114] Their first legal target was a local company called Kemet y Química Flúor, a chemical solvent company that eventually paid US$25 million in a class action to compensate families affected by the factories' pollution.

The Matamoros Environmental Group brought attention to the fact that overall rates of anencephaly were 60 percent higher along the border than in other locations, and that the rate in Brownsville had been three times higher than the national average (30 in 10,000) since 1990. Yet it was not until 1992, when a physician noticed that three disabled babies were born in 36 hours in one hospital, that the alarm bells sounded.[115] The number of cases was high on the Mexican side of the border from Brownsville, too: from 1987 to 1992, the Mexican state of Tamaulipas registered 386 cases, with 68 in Matamoros. The statistics changed when the border lines blurred.

Magdaleno and others believed that the cases of anencephaly were caused by toxins because they and their coworkers frequently experienced nasal hemorrhages, headaches, allergies, skin rashes and conditions, earache, miscarriages, airway infections and other respiratory problems, gastrointestinal problems, increased incidence of cancer, nervous system damage, impotence, respiratory failure, and chemical burns when working in or near factories. For more evidence they pointed to dark and polluted lakes and rivers, the common practice of burning factory trash in open air, unpermitted or underregulated dumping of toxic waste, and the improper transport of industrial waste, all of which exacerbated poor urban planning and a lack of social support.

The Matamoros Environmental Group believed that the US and Mexican governments should both be held responsible for establishing and enforcing environmental safety regulations. The group tracked recent problems to corporations' failure to adhere to agreements by the Programa Integral Ambiental Fronterizo (PIAF), which obligated the state of Texas to establish three safe dumping sites for toxic and radioactive matter. Companies insisted on constructing these along the border, and in the last three decades of the twentieth century more than 2,000 factories were constructed along the US-Mexico border. By the 1990s, the anencephaly cases were like the match that lit a tinderbox of rage in communities whose well-being had long been subsumed to corporate profit.[116] Critics pointed to the many scantly populated places throughout Texas where they could have put the chemicals instead, whereas the border is fairly populated and its citizens made especially vulnerable by marginalization. Protesters took a more direct approach, at one point interrupting a 1992 gubernatorial press conference to chant "'Bush and Reilly, you can't hide. We charge you with genocide.'"[117]

The toxic history they protested ran deep. In the early 1990s the company TEXCOR constructed a dumping ground for radioactive waste with capacity for 3.5 million tons of uranium just across the border from Texas; meanwhile, in the same vicinity, Chemical Waste Management constructed a storage place for 15 million tons of "extremely toxic" active chemical residue.[118] As Ana María Ohem Ochoa points out, "Environmental destruction on the Mexican side of the border is completely due to the growth of the maquiladoras. The relocation of highly contaminating industries to the Third World is a corporate policy resulting from Free Trade agreements."[119]

TEXCOR tried to block Mexican participation in Texas legislative hearings on the dumping grounds, but finally authorities from Coahuila were admitted to a discussion about the issue in May 1992. The Texas Water Commission could have blocked plans to dump the toxic waste, but it declined. One person testified to having seen 100 barrels of waste abandoned, and a public health test around this time showed that residents had 80 micrograms of lead in each 10 milliliters of blood, twice the acceptable upper limit.[120] In 1993, 16 families sued 88 factories on the border between Tamaulipas and Texas, arguing that they could be responsible for the anencephalia outbreak.[121] Of particular concern was the company Química Flúor, which produced sulfuric acid and hydrofluoric acid, used to make refrigerants, herbicides, pharmaceuticals, high-octane gasoline, aluminum, plastics, electrical components, and fluorescent light bulbs.[122] In response, the EPA classified the border zone as "dangerous," and SEDESOL, a Mexican regulatory agency, imposed sanctions and fines on four maquiladoras in Matamoros that dumped unpermitted toxic waste in the community dump as well as rivers.[123]

Such regulations met bitter resistance from free trade associations that advocated for increased movement of goods within and across the border. The early 1990s saw this goal advanced by the proposed construction of a land-bound canal in the state of Tamaulipas, which united 438 kilometers of canal infrastructure and connected the important economic ports of Madero and Matamoros. The canal would cost US$750 million up front, but was projected to increase the efficiency of transportation in the region. At the same time, however, it would also increase the flow of heavily polluted water to other locations—most notably, from the US to Mexico. All of this contamination was exacerbated by inadequate trash collection, sewage systems, and limited availability of potable water in the region, leading Mexico's secretary of the environment to declare the border town of Ciudad Juárez as the second-most polluted city in Mexico, right behind the megametropolis Mexico City.[124] The link between neural tube defects and contaminants has arisen elsewhere, too: just one example comes from the Brazilian city of Cubatão, where an unusually high number of anencephaly cases have frequently been attributed to the contamination of the Amazon with mercury.[125] By 1995, there was some recognition of harm done—on the Texas side of the border, at least. A number of maquiladoras settled with families harmed, for amounts ranging between US$100,000 and US$2 million. In total, 80 families received more than $US17 million from companies including General Motors, Kemet Electronics, and Mallory Capacitor Company. At least three people refused to settle out of court, hoping that publicity from their cases would result in lasting change to environmental policies.[126]

The public, the press, and scientific authorities came to view a bodily condition as a distinct product of the borderlands, though as we have just seen, they did so quite differently in the US and Mexico. Yet, in both places, anencephalic births came to signify a particular geography of bodily difference, whether traced to an external toxin or mapped instead to an inherent defect in a border population. Meanwhile, CDC-TDH investigators failed to speak the same language as the residents who lived, worked, and breathed in the Valley.[127] They also failed to see what was obvious to a transnational group of activists and to many representatives from Mexican government and business: that international agreements to dump historic amounts of highly toxic waste on the border was an act of corporate irresponsibility and environmental injustice against individuals, families, and Mexican sovereignty. Reproductive justice includes the right to raise children in safe environments; toxic dumping is a clear contravention of these principles. And both the search for an answer to families' struggles and anger over their neglect continued.[128]

No Magic Pill: The Search for Public Health Solutions

Establishing a Birth Defects Registry

In February 1992, a white woman named Anne Andis gave birth to an anencephalic baby girl in The Woodlands, an affluent community near Houston. The child, Emma Nicole, survived only five days. The *Houston Chronicle* ran a story about Andis's plight, describing her circumstances as a "far cry from the squalid border colonias."[129] Andis was not the first woman to have her child's birth defect publicized in the media, but she set herself apart from the Brownsville mothers, telling the *Chronicle,* "It's not just something that happens to poor women who don't have plumbing." The article's headline, "Baby Tragedy Has No Bounds," suggests that while anencephaly in Brownsville was problematic, the condition became truly troubling once it transgressed the boundaries of geography and, more implicitly, racialized differences. Neural tube defects were indeed occurring outside the Rio Grande Valley. The article represented an attempted remapping of the public health crisis beyond its material geographic impact, highlighting the potent imaginative divide between "White Texas" and "Mexican Texas."

Dividing these "two Texases" was a history and ongoing reality of political, infrastructural, and public health–based neglect. Before 1991, Texas was one of 13 states lacking a birth defects registry.[130] The March of Dimes Foundation and a "cadre of doctors, state officials, and parents" had campaigned for such a registry for years, but the state legislature was unwilling to provide the necessary funding.[131] In this absence, Andis took on the remarkable labor of documenting cases on index cards to demonstrate the spread of anencephaly.[132]

Public health was especially inadequate in the border region. Cameron County, surrounded by 5 towns and 18 colonias, was home to a large population of migrant agricultural workers.[133] Health institutions and authorities believed young women in the Valley posed a challenge to reproductive monitoring, as many fell beyond the reach of hospital-based obstetric care. A 1985 report from the Brownsville Community Health Center found that 40 percent of births in Cameron County occurred outside the hospital setting. Only half of these were delivered by lay midwives, meaning that the other half must have been unattended by a health aid.[134] Dr. Gregg Sylvester, a CDC epidemiologist, lamented the number of births that went unreported outside hospitals and noted that lay midwives were not always registered with local agencies.[135]

Authorities interpreted women's lack of access to prenatal healthcare through the lens of racialized blame and narratives about irresponsible maternity, as in media coverage that emphasized the difficulty of locating affected mothers. Unable to reach two of the mothers in his investigation, Dr. Sylvester was told that they had returned to Mexico after giving birth.[136] He took this news as confirming a broader phenomenon in which women "cross over from Mexico who deliver their babies here—those babies get US citizenship—then they go back home."[137] His speculations echo dog whistles painting Mexicans and Mexican Americans as untethered and undeserving of national belonging, and assessing the borderlands as an under-territorialized, epidemiologically unstable space. Dr. Sylvester accused these women of evading public health surveillance and gaming the system of citizenship, thereby presenting a dual threat to the state by their mere presence as well as their tendency to birth disabled citizens. Advocates of surveillance held an uncritical faith in data as the "foundation [of understanding] for all sorts of things," including anencephaly as well as birth defects caused by "crack" cocaine and other illicit substances.[138] Surveillance was linked not only to care but also to managing the dangers that could arise from a medically and administratively unmonitored population.

The state legislature soon became persuaded of the need for new law. In November 1991, state senator Carlos F. Truan contacted acting TDH commissioner Robert MacLean, requesting his help in planning for a birth defects tracking system.[139] Momentum continued to build over the next year, and the Texas senate approved a birth defects registry bill in March 1993.[140] Governor Ann Richards signed the bill into law in June, and preparatory work began in January 1994 in the Rio Grande Valley and gulf coast counties.[141]

The South Texas cases did provide the initial impetus for the state legislature to fund the birth defects registry, but stories like Anne Andis's played an instrumental role in pushing them toward action. The *Chronicle* piece contextualized the story of the birth defects legislation within Andis's narrative, highlighting her special status as a mother-turned-activist. The story concluded with a plea for readers' sympathy. Countering the depiction of anencephalic infants as "repulsive freaks," Andis asserted, "They're just sweet babies." In her renegotiation of anencephaly in the public eye, race and class shaped which expressions of love and kinship gained greater media visibility.

State senator Truan later stated bluntly that Andis's case had led to the legislation. "What helped me pass the legislation," he divulged, "was not so much what had happened, although that was important on the border, [but that] it was happening in the Houston area." It was testimony from individuals outside the border that "raised some eyebrows."[142] Andis's contribution to the registry's establishment should not be diminished. Yet it is also clear that as she marshalled political will for reform, she had access to narrative strategies not available to mothers at the border. The success and resonance of her story can be seen even today on the Texas Department of State Health Services' website, which spotlights Andis in its commemoration of the registry's twenty-fifth anniversary.[143] The Mexican-origin mothers in Brownsville are silenced by means of exclusion from this public memorialization.

The state's long-standing marginalization of the borderlands belies its self-congratulatory claim to progress, thus forcing us to ask what work monitoring performs and whom it neglects. In a region that was invisibilized by—and therefore invisible to—the state, the Valley's anencephalic fetuses had developed undetected for years before being discovered.[144] Yet postmortem, these babies' disabilities became hypervisible. Officials catalogued their death certificates from the periphery and incorporated them into a central registry, while their mothers were designated to a category of higher risk.[145] Instead of providing the mothers with the healthcare and other social supports they needed, public health authorities increasingly viewed their bodies and lifestyles as national threats. "Budget woes" subsequently forced the TDH to slash the registry's geographic scope.[146] Even as the celebrated initiative was diminished, officials still chose to focus its limited resources on the border region. The bare-bones registry preserved its original purpose: maintaining heightened surveillance of bodies that remained unproblematic as long as they were contained, and generating fear once anencephaly leaked outside the borderlands.

Folic Acid Distribution

The foreign or immigrant body has been a specter of contagion throughout the history of US hegemony, settler colonialism, and imperial expansion.[147] Here, too, the public feared the threat of anencephaly's transmission beyond the racialized confines of the border region. But this condition soon became interpreted through the distinct medical paradigm of nutritional deficiency. By the winter of 1992, CDC-TDH officials homed in on folic acid as a plausible etiology. Studies provided increasing evidence of the B vitamin's importance in neural tube development, and its hypothesized role in the South Texas cluster quickly gained the support of the federal government.

At first glance, nutritional deficiency seems a wildly different category from infectious disease or industrial toxins. There are also illuminating continuities; for authorities, both could be traced back to a unique susceptibility in the foreign body, whether through a so-called ethnic diet, unhygienic practices, or unconventional behavior. And both created powerful justifications for certain types of state intervention. As Julie Livingston has documented in her study of disability in Botswana, colonial medical frameworks of malnutrition in that context shifted blame away from starvation as a technology of colonial rule and toward individuals' dietary choices. Conceptualizing health in terms of specific micronutrients invited "narrow technological solutions."[148] In the Valley, community activists linked birth defects to political and environmental abuses that necessitated genuine political reform. The concept of nutritional deficiency was far less radical in contrast, and it invited a more facile solution.

The pathophysiology of folic acid deficiency implied that disrupted development did not arise de novo within the embryo but rather originated in an absence in the mother. Controlling this outbreak therefore necessitated effective management of all susceptible women's wombs. In the summer of 1992, despite their inconclusive research, TDH recommended that expectant mothers take folic acid to prevent neural tube defects.[149] They announced the launch of a pilot program in the Valley in which free multivitamins would be distributed to women of reproductive age via community health centers, family planning clinics, and county health departments. Folic acid began to "arrive in droves" at the border, with over a million multivitamins shipped to the TDH regional office.[150] An accompanying campaign included bilingual public service announcements educating women about the importance of the B vitamin.[151]

In September 1992, the US Public Health Service (USPHS) formally recommended that all women of childbearing age consume 0.4 milligrams of folic acid daily. This seems to have been the first time that the federal government recommended usage of a vitamin supplement to the general population.[152] At the time, the available body of evidence for this recommendation was small and relatively recent. Just a year prior, the only randomized controlled trial, the gold standard for clinical evidence, had been completed in British women who had already conceived a child with an NTD. However, it did find a significant 72 percent reduction in the rate of recurrence.[153] There were also preliminary results from a Hungarian trial of women who had never experienced such a pregnancy, but these data were not published until after the USPHS's recommendation.[154] Additional data on women without prior NTDs had been collected through observational studies.[155]

Whether or not evidence constituted enough for an official recommendation, it is striking that the state committed to such an ambitious distribution campaign even before federal guidelines existed.[156] Health officials admitted there was much to learn about folic acid. Dr. Scott Simpson, TDH's director of women's health, noted that they did not know what caused NTDs or the mechanism by which the vitamin worked.[157] At a press conference, the TDH representative found himself unable to describe the evidence supporting supplementation in women without prior NTDs.[158] Community members criticized TDH's lack of a plan following the outcomes of its pilot program and accused the agency of using local residents as "guinea pigs" without any way of judging the vitamin's effectiveness.[159] Some local physicians also remained unconvinced by the existing research; Dr. Carmen Rocco, for example, pointed out that there was scarce evidence and warned that folic acid should not be touted as a "magic bullet." Still, she added, "it's not going to hurt anybody." Dr. Gary Tamex echoed this sentiment, noting that folic acid was inexpensive and posed few side effects.[160]

Although folic acid offered an attractive panacea, an actual link between it and the specific cases in South Texas remained elusive. A retrospective review of the Texas Neural Tube Birth Defects Project found that among Mexican American women at the border, there was no significant difference in median serum and red blood cell folate levels between those affected by NTDs and controls.[161] John Harris, director of the California Birth Defects

Monitoring Program, publicly questioned the vitamin hypothesis: "It's not at all clear that Mexicans are deficient in folic acid because their diet—rice and beans—appears to be plentiful in folic acid."[162]

But the hypothesis had taken hold. Even as the medical literature emphasized that the etiology of anencephaly was multifactorial, the public emerged with a simplified understanding of the crisis as rooted in nutritional deficiency. In 1994, the *Houston Chronicle* reported that in a study of 19 mothers in the Valley affected by anencephalic births, only one had experienced a recurrence. The reporter callously blamed her, alleging that she "had refused to take the vitamin." He made no mention of a control group and no gesture toward statistical analysis. We know nothing about this woman's health status, living situation, or access to clean water and healthcare.[163]

Folic acid initiatives failed to eradicate NTDs at the border, but officials continued to rely on the quick fix. When the rate of anencephaly doubled in Cameron County in 1998, TDH epidemiologist Russell Larsen again blamed mothers by telling *The Monitor*, "Women are not protecting themselves." Texas First Lady Laura Bush responded to the increase by announcing the formation of the Texas Folic Acid Council, which would focus on health education about the vitamin.[164] For public health workers, the perceived problem shifted from anencephaly itself to the intractability of Valley women to reproductive education. Health campaigns sought to engage them through racially and linguistically inclusive marketing, including visits from health workers who went door to door.[165] Though well intentioned, these efforts were still underpinned by officials' blaming women who could not control the circumstances of their reproductive debility.

Seeking an explanation for folic acid's underwhelming efficacy in South Texas, some made the biologically essentialist suggestion that supplementation might be less effective in Hispanic women.[166] A research team at the California Birth Defects Monitoring Division pointed out that folic acid data in white women had been generalized to the border population in a race-blind manner. Their case-control study found that while white women in the state benefited from risk reduction due to folic acid, women of Mexican descent did not.[167] This was an important finding, but it again attributed biological difference to a population itself, while the external logic of nutritional supplementation remained intact.

The narratives of birth defect surveillance and folic acid distribution raise questions about the nexus of surveillance, care, and reproductive management. They illustrate the limited conditions under which a border population, unmanageable and undocumented, became visible to public health institutions. The year 1996 also offers an instructive contrast between two developments at the federal level, developments that mirrored the local response to anencephaly. First, under a new program, makers of grain products such as pastas and flours would begin fortifying their foods with folic acid for the general population, a practice made mandatory two years later by the US Food and Drug Administration. Second, a federal welfare law cut funding for virtually all services to undocumented immigrants, including prenatal care.[168] Government actors directed money and attention to public health solutions according to a paradigm of intrinsic defect, intensified by underlying assumptions about race and space. This institutional response to anencephaly prioritized technological expedience over long-term care and investment in border communities.

Conclusion

"For the parents and child, it is a nightmare beyond description. For the nation, it diminishes our most precious natural resource: the next generation of Americans in whose hands the future of our country lies." Thus, Lloyd Bentsen of Texas addressed his US Senate colleagues on July 1, 1992, in his remarks about the Texas Birth Defects Prevention Act.[169] One wonders how he reconciled calling children a "national resource" while ignoring one of the nation's more environmentally degraded regions, and while knowing that they were born to mothers on the periphery of citizenship.

The discovery of anencephalic births created an impetus for the state to catalogue nonnormative fetal bodies and to subject their mothers to an aspirational vision of reproductive surveillance. Previously neglected at the national margins, residents of the Valley also experienced increased intrusion by public health and media apparatuses. Despite these changes, the region remained fundamentally disenfranchised. All along, the epidemiologic puzzle of whether environmental hazards could be causally linked to anencephaly had obscured a more basic claim: the border community deserved access to clean air and water *regardless* of the public health crisis. Services that the ordinary citizen might take for granted as part of a contract with the nation-state were never extended to the Valley. To this day, numerous residents along the Texas border suffer conditions of debility due to persistent environmental degradation as well as fraught access to potable water and other basic needs.[170]

Anencephalic fetuses, and the social meanings attached to them, were shaped by the political, spatial, and historical contingencies of the borderlands. Racial otherness and biological vulnerability were not simply additive conditions; they worked together to intensify bodily impairment and difference. Mothers themselves were marked in relation to the pathological births they had produced. This chapter documents the range of their emotional responses, including ambivalence, care, and grief, that contradicted and complicated dominant portrayals. Affective resistance had its limitations, and these intimate ties should not be essentialized or expected to transcend the realities of political disenfranchisement or structural injustice. But they were all the more tangible and significant for the hostile conditions out of which they emerged. For this border community, expressions of love and care invoked a radical embrace of some of its most marginal bodies.

NOTES

1. David Grogan, "The Baby Killer," *People* Magazine, September 27, 1993.

2. Jerry Adler, "A Life and Death Puzzle," *Newsweek*, June 7, 1992.

3. Barry Schlacter, "Valley of Death: Mysterious Birth Defects Plague Brownsville," *Fort Worth Star-Telegram*, January 19, 1992; John M. McClintock, "Cluster of Babies in Texas Born Without Brains," *Baltimore Sun*, January 19, 1992; Adler, "Life and Death Puzzle."

4. Examples of the press reports include: "Feds Probe Mysterious Fetus Deformities in Border County," *Odessa (TX) American*, July 19, 1991; Schlacter, "Valley of Death"; "Mysterious Baby Deaths," *Battle Creek (MI) Enquirer*, February 19, 1992; James Pinkerton, "Cause of Border Birth Defects Remains a Mystery," *Houston Chronicle*, June 30, 1992; Dave Harmon, "Anencephaly Mystery Still Baffling to CDC, TDH," *The Monitor* (McAllen, TX), July 3, 1992.

5. Michael E. Young and Sandra Jacobs, "Reasons for Defect a Mystery," *South Florida Sun Sentinel* (Deerfield Beach), March 29, 1992.

6. "South Texas Stillborn Had Rare Disorder," *Houston Chronicle*, March 21, 1992; "State Briefs: Fifth Anencephalic Birth," *Houston Chronicle*, April 14, 1992.

7. Miriam Rich, "Monstrosity in Medical Science: Race-Making and Teratology in the Nineteenth-Century United States," *Isis* 114, no. 3 (2023): 513–36.

8. See Bianca Premo's chapter in this volume, pp. 27–56.

9. Gloria Anzaldúa, *Borderlands/La Frontera: The New Mestiza* (Aunt Lute Books, 1999), 25.

10. Leslie Reagan, *Dangerous Pregnancies: Mothers, Disabilities, and Abortion in Modern America* (University of California Press, 2010), 180. For additional scholarship that histor-

icizes deeply held assumptions about normative reproduction, see Janet Golden, *Message in a Bottle: The Making of Fetal Alcohol Syndrome* (Harvard University Press, 2005); Elizabeth Armstrong, *Conceiving Risk, Bearing Responsibility: Fetal Alcohol Syndrome and the Diagnosis of Moral Disorder* (Johns Hopkins University Press, 2005); Leslie Reagan, "Monstrous Births, Birth Defects, Unusual Anatomy, and Disability in Europe and North America," in *The Oxford Handbook of Disability History*, ed. Michael Rembis, Catherine Kudlick, and Kim Nielsen (Oxford University Press, 2018), 385–406; Miriam Rich, "Monstrous Births: Race, Gender, and Defective Reproduction in U.S. Medical Science, 1830–1930" (PhD diss., Harvard University, 2019).

11. The late 1980s and early 1990s witnessed bioethical debate about the personhood of anencephalic babies and its implications for organ transplantation. See, for example, Michael R. Harrison and Gilbert Meilaender, "Case Studies: The Anencephalic Newborn as Organ Donor," *Hastings Center Report* 16, no. 2 (1986): 21–23; Michael R. Harrison, "Organ Procurement for Children: The Anencephalic Fetus as Donor," *Lancet* 8520, no. 2 (1986): 1383–86.

12. Robert McRuer, *Crip Times: Disability, Globalization, and Resistance* (New York University Press, 2018): 20.

13. For one such study that takes this stance as its starting point, see Sharon Snyder and David Mitchell, *Cultural Locations of Disability* (University of Chicago Press, 2006).

14. Jasbir Puar, *The Right to Maim: Debility, Capacity, Disability* (Duke University Press, 2017).

15. Clare Barker and Stuart Murray, "Disabling Postcolonialism: Global Disability Cultures and Democratic Criticism," in *The Disability Studies Reader*, ed. Lennard J. Davis (Routledge, 2013); Mark Sherry, "(Post)colonising Disability," *Wagadu: A Journal of Transnational Women's and Gender Studies* 4 (2007): 10–22; Julie Livingston, *Debility and the Moral Imagination in Botswana* (Indiana University Press, 2005); Shaun Grech, *Disability and Poverty in the Global South: Renegotiating Development in Guatemala* (Palgrave Macmillan, 2015); Susan Reynolds Whyte and Benedicte Ingstad, "Introduction: Disability Connections," in *Disability in Local and Global Worlds*, ed. Susan Reynolds Whyte and Benedicte Ingstad (University of California Press, 2007); McRuer, *Crip Times*.

16. Alison Kafer, "Bodies of Nature: The Environmental Politics of Disability," in *Disability Studies and the Environmental Humanities: Toward an Eco-Crip Theory*, ed. Sarah Jaquette Ray and Jay Sibara (University of Nebraska Press, 2017), 201, 202.

17. Kelly Fritsch, "Toxic Pregnancies: Speculative Futures, Disabling Environments, and Neoliberal Biocapital," in *Disability Studies and the Environmental Humanities*, 365–66.

18. Fritsch, "Toxic Pregnancies," 368, 360, 375.

19. Eli Clare, "Notes on Natural Worlds, Disabled Bodies, and a Politics of Cure," in *Disability Studies and the Environmental Humanities*, 255.

20. Katherine Barrett and Richard Greene, "The Littlest Victims: An Ounce of Prevention," *Ladies' Home Journal* 102, no. 9 (September 1985).

21. Dorceta Taylor is one scholar who has traced the history of minority environmental activism, in *Toxic Communities: Environmental Racism, Industrial Pollution, and Residential Mobility* (New York University Press, 2014).

22. Veronica V. Chambers, "Self-Health Programs," *Essence* 22, no. 4 (August 1991): 14.

23. Barrett and Greene, "Littlest Victims," 187.

24. Dorothy Roberts, *Killing the Black Body: Race, Reproduction, and the Meaning of Liberty* (Vintage Books, 1997), 159.

25. Ruth Key, "Too Many Questions Remain," *The Monitor*, July 8, 1992.

26. Schlacter, "Valley of Death."

27. Adler, "Life and Death Puzzle."

28. J. Michael Kennedy, "Medicine Bordering on Crisis," *Los Angeles Times*, July 3, 1992.

29. Associated Press, "Study No Help in Texas Birth Defect Deaths," *Kerrville (TX) Times*, July 3, 1992.

30. Martha A. Slattery and Dwight T. Janerich, "The Epidemiology of Neural Tube Defects: A Review of Dietary Intake and Related Factors as Etiologic Agents," *American Journal of Epidemiology* 133, no 6 (1991): 526–40.

31. Dan Fagin, "Texas Birth Defect Mystery," *Newsday,* July 3, 1992.

32. Mark Feldstein and Steve Singer, "The Border Babies," *Time*, May 26, 1997.

33. Nancy Nusser, "Families Sue Maquiladoras over Links to Birth Defects," *Austin American-Statesman*, July 11, 1993.

34. Lina Maria-Murillo, "Birth Control on the Border: Race, Gender, Religion, and Class in the Making of the Birth Control Movement, El Paso, Texas, 1936–1973" (PhD diss., University of Texas at El Paso, 2016), 16, 98.

35. For example, Reagan examines how the rubella epidemic of the 1960s transformed abortion in the public eye, harnessing the privilege of white, middle-class status that eventually translated to greater access. Reagan, *Dangerous Pregnancies*, 5–6.

36. Rich, "Monstrous Births," 39; Reagan, *Dangerous Pregnancies*, 80.

37. Paula Adams Hillard, "Screening for Neural Tube Defects," *Parents* 62, no. 9 (September 1987): 194; D. M. Main and M. T. Mennuti, "Neural Tube Defects: Issues in Prenatal Diagnosis and Counselling," *Obstetric Gynecology* 67, no. 1 (January 1986): 1–16; Sue A. Meinke, "Anencephalic Infants as Potential Organ Sources: Ethical and Legal Issues," Bioethics Research Library, Joseph and Rose Kennedy Institute of Ethics, Georgetown University, Washington, DC, 1989.

38. Shlomo Shinnar and John Arras, "Ethical Issues in the Use of Anencephalic Infants as Organ Donors," *Neurologic Clinics* 7, no. 4 (November 1989): 729–43. A similar sentiment was expressed by James W. Walters, in "Anencephalic Infants as Organ Sources," *Bioethics* 5, no. 4 (October 1991): 326–41.

39. Ilana Löwy, *Imperfect Pregnancies: A History of Birth Defects and Prenatal Diagnosis* (Johns Hopkins University Press, 2017); Rayna Rapp, *Testing Women, Testing the Fetus: The Social Impact of Amniocentesis in America* (York: Routledge, 1999); Faye Ginsberg and Rayna Rapp, "Enabling Disability: Rewriting Kinship, Reimagining Citizenship," in *The Disability Studies Reader*, 237–53.

40. Tamar Stieber, "Hispanic Babies Born in '80s Hit Worst by Spinal Defect," *Albuquerque Journal*, July 10, 1992.

41. Mary J. Seller, "Unanswered Questions on Neural Tube Defects," *British Medical Journal* 294, no. 6563 (January 1987): 1–2.

42. R. D. Snyder, A. F. Fakadcj, and J. E. Riggs, "Anencephaly in the United States,

1968–1978: The Declining Incidence Among White Infants," *Journal of Child Neurology* 6, no. 4 (October 1991): 304–5.

43. Hector F. Garza-Trejo, "Genetic Testing for Peace of Mind," *Brownsville Herald*, June 9, 1992.

44. In the wake of *Planned Parenthood v. Casey*, reproductive rights evolved for different groups of women. For example, Dorothy Roberts has described how during this time New Jersey became the first state to obtain a federal waiver for a family cap provision, which openly discouraged welfare recipients from having additional children; women described being induced to undergo abortions they did not want. Roberts, *Killing the Black Body*, 212. On how genetic counseling sometimes encourages the elective termination of potentially disabled or disabled fetuses, see Alexandra Minna Stern, *Telling Genes: The Story of Genetic Counseling in America* (Johns Hopkins University Press, 2012).

45. Dan Meyers, "Babies of Brownsville Stir an Anguished Plea," *Philadelphia Inquirer*, August 29, 1993.

46. Fletcher quoted in James E. Garcia, "Brain Birth Defect Raises Ethical Questions," *Austin American-Statesman*, June 6, 1992.

47. Dave Harmon, "Mother's Love Keeps Anencephalic Baby Alive," *The Monitor*, September 22, 1992.

48. Grogan, "The Baby Killer"; Dan Fagin, "Border Town Mystery," *Newsday*, July 12, 1992; Sue Anne Pressley, "Years After Cluster of Birth Defects, Pain and Mystery Linger in Brownsville," *Washington Post*, September 17, 1995.

49. Perez quoted in Juanita Darling, "A River of Doubt: The Rio Grande's Pollution Is Part of the Debate over NAFTA," *Los Angeles Times*, August 31, 1993.

50. Elizabeth O'Brien, "The Many Meanings of *Aborto*: Pregnancy Termination and the Instability of a Medical Category over Time," *Women's History Review* 30, no. 6 (2021): 952–70.

51. "Medical Officials Puzzle over Cause of Rare Brain Disorder," *Odessa (TX) American*, February 9, 1992.

52. Associated Press, "Cause of Border Birth Defects Eluding Researchers," *North County Times* (Oceanside, CA), July 12, 1992.

53. James E. Garcia, "Family's Tragedy Puts State in Abortion Dispute," *Austin American-Statesman*, June 2, 1992.

54. James E. Garcia, "Senator Seeks a Change in Health Policy on Abortion," *Austin American-Statesman*, June 3, 1992.

55. Johanna Schoen, *Choice and Coercion: Birth Control, Sterilization, and Abortion in Public Health and Welfare* (University of North Carolina Press, 2005); Elena Gutiérrez, *Fertile Matters: The Politics of Mexican-Origin Women's Reproduction* (University of Texas Press, 2008); Roberts, *Killing the Black Body*; Elizabeth O'Brien, *Surgery and Salvation: The Roots of Reproductive Injustice in Mexico, 1770–1940* (University of North Carolina Press, 2023).

56. "Report: Baby Was Anencephalic," *The Monitor*, July 30, 1994.

57. Associated Press, "Baby Found near Grave 3 Years Later," *Fort Worth Star-Telegram*, August 4, 1994.

58. Josh Lemieux, "Dead Baby Discovered Frozen for 3 Years," *Austin American-Statesman*, August 5, 1994.

59. Patricia A. Gonzalez, "Anencephalic Baby Found in Cemetery 'Preserved,'" *The Monitor*, August 2, 1994.

60. Lynn Morgan, *Icons of Life: A Cultural History of Human Embryos* (University of California Press, 2009).

61. Rich, "Monstrous Births"; Livingston, *Debility and the Moral Imagination in Botswana*. I also look to David A. Ellison and Isabel Karpin's discussion of "grievability" in the context of cryopreserved embryos, as well as Mel Y. Chen's insights into affective politics. Ellison and Karpin, "Death Without Life: Grievability and IVF," *South Atlantic Quarterly* 110, no. 4 (2011): 795–811; Chen, *Animacies: Biopolitics, Racial Mattering, and Queer Affect* (Duke University Press, 2012): 125.

62. McClintock, "Cluster of Babies in Texas Born Without Brains."

63. Dave Harmon, "Funds, Study for Anencephaly Causes Sought," *The Monitor,* May 25, 1992; Schlacter, "Valley of Death."

64. For example, see Peggy Fikac, "Birth Defects Registry, Health Plan Becomes Law," *Fort Worth Star-Telegram,* June 16, 1993; Leigh Hopper, "A Mysterious Mix," *Austin American-Statesman,* January 20, 1997; Pressley, "Years After Cluster of Birth Defects, Pain and Mystery Linger in Brownsville"; Gillian Swanson, "Leaders Gather for Symposium," *The Monitor*, October 31, 1998.

65. Mark Feldstein, "Special Report on Rio Grande Valley," *CNN Evening News*, aired May 18, 1992.

66. "Texans Sue Mexican Factories for Birth Defects," *Morning Edition*, NPR, August 5, 1994.

67. Darling, "A River of Doubt."

68. Swanson, "Leaders Gather for Symposium."

69. Feldstein and Singer, "Border Babies"; "Medical Officials Puzzle Over Cause of Rare Brain Disorder."

70. Feldstein, "Special Report on Rio Grande Valley."

71. Megan K. Stack, "Birth Defect Research Hasn't Resolved Decade of Anguish," *Houston Chronicle*, January 21, 2001.

72. Feldstein and Singer, "Border Babies."

73. Meyers, "Babies of Brownsville Stir an Anguished Plea."

74. Feldstein, "Special Report on Rio Grande Valley."

75. Butler quoted in Ellison and Karpin, "Death Without Life," 800.

76. Feldstein, "Special Report on Rio Grande Valley."

77. Meyers, "Babies of Brownsville Stir an Anguished Plea."

78. It is necessary to acknowledge the tensions that arise from considering personhood in the fetus, with its practical implications for feminist and reproductive politics. Lynn Morgan reflects on these ethical stakes, and the need for dynamic and overlapping discourses, in "Fetal Relationality in Feminist Philosophy: An Anthropological Critique," *Hypatia* 11, no. 3 (1996): 47–70.

79. James Pinkerton, "No Links Found in Nine Born with Fatal Brain Defect," *Houston Chronicle*, July 20, 1991 (quote); Schlacter, "Valley of Death."

80. Pinkerton, "No Links Found in Nine Born with Fatal Brain Defect."

81. John M. McClintock, "Cluster of Babies in Texas Born Without Brains," *Baltimore*

Sun, January 19, 1992. Other examples can be found in Gaynell Terrell, "Tragic Puzzle Grips Families in the Border: Plant Pollution May Cause Brain Not to Develop," *Houston Post*, May 17, 1992; Fagin, "Border Town Mystery."

82. McClintock, "Cluster of Babies in Texas Born Without Brains."

83. McClintock.

84. Some journalists blamed Mexico for environmental degradation while ignoring the fact that many of the factories were based in the US. Jeff Silverstein, "Doctors Probe Anencephaly Outbreak," *Miami Herald*, April 19, 1992; Associated Press, "Health Officials Continue Checking Brain Abnormalities Along Border," *Tyler (TX) Courier-Times*, May 18, 1992.

85. Feldstein, "Special Report on Rio Grande Valley."

86. Meyers, "Babies of Brownsville Stir an Anguished Plea."

87. Fagin, "Border Town Mystery."

88. Fritsch, "Toxic Pregnancies," 361.

89. "Baby-Killing Disease Racks Texas Border City," *Dallas Times Herald*, February 18, 1992.

90. Mel Y. Chen, *Animacies: Biopolitics, Racial Mattering, and Queer Affect* (Duke University Press, 2012), 165; Associated Press, "Pollution Said to Cause Birth Defects in South Texas Babies, *Kilgore (TX) News Herald,* May 3, 1992.

91. Associated Press, "Emissions Checked for Link to Birth Defects," *El Paso Herald-Post*, May 18, 1992.

92. Silverstein, "Doctors Probe Anencephaly Outbreak"; Jean Brender and Lucina Suarez, "Paternal Occupation and Anencephaly," *American Journal of Epidemiology* 131 (1990): 517; "Rash of S. Texas Babies Born with Partial Brains Spurs Probe," *Houston Chronicle*, July 19, 1991.

93. Adler, "Life and Death Puzzle"; "Epidemiologic Investigation of a Cluster of Neural Tube Defects in Cameron County, Texas" (preliminary study report), June 24, 1992, Box 4, Folder 5, Amalia Rodriguez-Mendoza Papers, Austin History Center, Austin, TX (hereafter cited as Rodriguez-Mendoza Papers).

94. Cheek quoted in Gannett News Service, "Baby-Killing Disease Racks Texas Border City," *Times Herald*, February 18, 1992.

95. Roberto Suro, "Rash of Brain Defects in Newborns Disturbs Border City in Texas," *New York Times*, May 31, 1992; Schlacter, "Valley of Death."

96. At the 1992 South Texas Economic Development Conference, Texas state senator Eddie Lucio Jr. noted that the "issue of the anencephalic babies [would] definitely put a dent in the free trade negotiations." Lucio quoted in Tony Vindell, "NAFTA Dominates Conference," *Brownsville Herald*, May 24, 1992. See also Elizabeth A. Ellis, "Bordering on Disaster: A New Attempt to Control the Transboundary Effects of Maquiladora Pollution," *Valparaiso University Law Review* 30 (1996): 621–99.

97. McClintock, "Cluster of Babies in Texas Born Without Brains."

98. Kelly Reblin, "NAFTA and the Environment: Dealing with Abnormally High Birth Defect Rates Among Children of Texas-Mexico Border Towns," *St. Mary's Law Journal* 27 (1996): 929–65.

99. McClintock, "Cluster of Babies in Texas Born Without Brains"; Gannett News Service, "Baby-Killing Disease Racks Texas Border City."

100. Adler, "Life and Death Puzzle"; Laura Beil, "Rare Birth Defects Linked to Bad Corn," *Dallas Morning News*, February 5, 2005; Jeremy Bigwood, "Monsanto Weed Killer Blamed for Powerful Fungus," *Global Information Network*, August 21, 2003.

101. Hector F. Garza-Trejo, "Officials Start Study of Anencephaly Rate," *The Monitor*, May 19, 1992; Silverstein, "Doctors Probe Anencephaly Outbreak"; Associated Press, "Pollution Said to Cause Birth Defects in South Texas Babies"; Schlacter, "Valley of Death."

102. John MacCormack, "Activists Blast Not Designating Defects Epidemic," *San Antonio Express-News*, July 2, 1992.

103. R. Daniel Cavazos, "Maquilas Need to End Silence," *The Monitor*, July 5, 1992.

104. Bill Hethcock, "Activists List Points to Present to Panel," *Brownsville Herald*, May 22, 1992.

105. Dr. John A. Harris to Jennifer Howse, June 18, 1992, Box 4, Folder 5, Rodriguez-Mendoza Papers.

106. Amalia Rodriguez-Mendoza to Dr. David R. Smith, July 1, 1992, Box 4, Folder 6, Rodriguez-Mendoza Papers.

107. Pinkerton, "Cause of Border Birth Defects Remains a Mystery."

108. Smith quoted in Fagin, "Texas Birth Defect Mystery."

109. Perrotta quoted in Pinkerton, "Cause of Border Birth Defects Remains a Mystery"; "Rash of S. Texas Babies Born with Partial Brains Spurs Probe"; James Pinkerton, "10 Earlier Brain-Defect Victims Found," *Houston Chronicle*, May 30, 1992.

110. Dave Harmon, "Agencies' Anencephaly Findings Outrage Watchdog Group," *The Monitor*, July 2, 1992.

111. Fagin, "Texas Birth Defect Mystery."

112. Alexandra Minna Stern, "Buildings, Boundaries, and Blood: Medicalization and Nation-Building on the U.S.-Mexico Border, 1910–1930," *Hispanic American Historical Review* 79, no. 1 (1999): 41–81.

113. Miriam Alfie Cohen and Luis H. Méndez Berrueta, *Maquila y movimientos ambientalistas: Examen de un riesgo compartido* (Universidad Autónoma Metropolitana Azcapotzalco, 2000), 114.

114. Cohen and Méndez Berrueta, *Maquila y movimientos ambientalistas*, 247.

115. Cohen and Méndez Berrueta, 114.

116. Cohen and Méndez Berrueta, 125.

117. Diane Lindquist, "Environment Is Key Trade-Pact Issue; 'Wild Card' Issue Could Doom NAFTA," *San Diego Union-Tribune*, June 27, 1992, at Dl.

118. Lindquist, 126–27.

119. Ana María Ohem Ochoa, *Tendencias de localización de la industria maquiladora en México* (El Colegio de México, 1998), 76 (authors' translation).

120. *La Jornada* (Mexico City), June 2, 1992, 13.

121. *La Jornada*, March 28, 1993.

122. *Novedades* (Mexico City), June 7, 1997.

123. *La Jornada*, September 12, 1992.

124. *Excelsior* (Mexico City), Sección Financiera, August 27, 1995.

125. Gino Giacomini Filho, *Consumidor versus propaganda* (Summus Editorial, 1991).

126. James Garcia, "GM, Companies Settle Lawsuit over Brain Defects in Valley," *Austin American-Statesman*, August 26, 1995.

127. Quite literally so: As part of its research study, CDC-TDH administered a survey written in English. A Spanish-speaking person orally translated it but was unfamiliar with survey procedure. Kathi Lynn Groenendyk, "Covering the Story: A Rhetorical Analysis of Brownsville's Television News Coverage" (Master's thesis, Texas A&M University, 1994), 2.

128. Will Dunham, "U.S. Officials Grant Texas $1.6 Million to Fight Brain Defect," *The Monitor*, October 6, 1992; Dave Harmon, "Group's Plans Moving Ahead," *The Monitor*, December 8, 1992; Dave Harmon, "Rivalry Wastes Effort, Anencephaly Researchers Say," *The Monitor*, December 21, 1992.

129. Jim Morris, "Baby Tragedy Has No Bounds," *Houston Chronicle*, August 2, 1992.

130. Rodriguez-Mendoza's handwritten notes on Hector F. Garza-Trejo, "Anencephaly Investigations Inconclusive," *Brownsville Herald*, May 22, 1992, Box 4, Folder 5, Rodriguez-Mendoza Papers.

131. Jim Morris, "Birth Defect Sparks Concern: Data Scarce as Experts Probe Babies Born Without Brains," *Houston Chronicle*, September 22, 1991.

132. Laura E. Keaton, "Panel Urged to Authorize Birth Defects Registry," *Houston Chronicle*, February 5, 1993.

133. Colonias are largely impoverished housing developments that lack essential public services. "Brownsville Community Health Center," 1992, Box 95-019/920, Folder "Neural tube defects, 1992," Ann W. Richards Papers, Dolph Briscoe Center for American History, University of Texas at Austin (hereafter Ann W. Richards Papers).

134. Mary Ellen O'Brien, "Successful Birth Centers in the Rio Grande Valley," October 1989, Box 95-019/920, Folder "Neural tube defects, 1992," Ann W. Richards Papers; "Brownsville Community Health Center," 1992, Box 95-019/920, Folder "Neural tube defects, 1992," Ann W. Richards Papers.

135. Carolyn Poirot, "9 Babies with Brain Defect a Mystery to Texas Doctors," *Fort Worth Star-Telegram*, July 19, 1991.

136. Poirot, "9 Babies with Brain Defect a Mystery to Texas Doctors."

137. Elena Gutiérrez describes this stereotype and historical scrutiny of Mexican-origin women's reproductive lives, in *Fertile Matters*. See also Pinkerton, "No Links Found in Nine Born with Fatal Brain Defect."

138. Morris, "Birth Defect Sparks Concern."

139. Senator Carlos F. Truan to Acting Commissioner Robert MacLean, November 26, 1991, Box 4, Folder 5, Rodriguez-Mendoza Papers.

140. Pauline Arrillaga, "Senate OKs Birth Defect Listing," *Houston Chronicle*, March 12, 1993.

141. Fikac, "Birth Defects Registry, Health Plan Becomes Law"; "Birth Defect Statistic Project to Begin," *The Monitor*, November 25, 1993.

142. Carlos Truan, interview by David Todd, February 2, 2000, in Corpus Christi, Texas, Conservation History Association of Texas, Texas Legacy Project Records, Briscoe Center for American History, University of Texas at Austin.

143. "History of the Texas Birth Defects Registry," Texas Department of State Health

Services, accessed July 16, 2025, https://www.dshs.texas.gov/birthdefects/MotherStory
.aspx.

144. *Primary Care Services for the Underserved: Hearing Before the Subcommittee on Health and the Environment of the Committee on Energy and Commerce, House of Representatives*, 103rd Cong. (1993), 129.

145. Janet Bronstein delves into the role of risk categorization in reproductive governance and surveillance, in "The Cultural Construction of Preterm Birth in the United States," *Anthropology and Medicine* 27, no. 2 (2020): 234–41.

146. Todd Ackerman, "Health Group Foresees Threat in Texas," *Houston Chronicle*, February 21, 2002; Charlotte Huff, "State Cuts Back on Scope of Birth Defects Registry," *Austin American-Statesman*, March 13, 2002; "Proposed Health Agency Cuts Draw Fire," *Fort Worth Star-Telegram*, February 25, 2003.

147. See, for example, Samuel Roberts Jr., *Infectious Fear: Politics, Disease, and the Health Effects of Segregation* (University of North Carolina Press, 2009); Nayan Shah, *Contagious Divides: Epidemics and Race in San Francisco's Chinatown* (University of California Press, 2001).

148. Livingston, *Debility and the Moral Imagination in Botswana*, 161.

149. "Epidemiologic Investigation of a Cluster of Neural Tube Defects in Cameron County, Texas."

150. Associated Press, "Officials Battling Birth Defects with Vitamins," *Austin American-Statesman*, August 8, 1992; "Free Vitamins Offered," *Houston Chronicle*, October 7, 1992; Dave Harmon, "Folic Acid Vitamins Arrive in Droves," *The Monitor*, October 6, 1992; J. S. Simpson, "Neural Tube Defects: Surveillance, Epidemiologic and Folic Acid Activities in Texas," *Texas Preventable Disease News* 53, no. 1 (January 1993).

151. Dave Harmon, "Folic Acid Prescribed to Curb Birth Defects," *The Monitor*, August 4, 1992.

152. Folic acid supplementation is routinely recommended today as a standard of care to individuals who may become pregnant. Will Dunham, "Federal Plan to Fight Birth Defects Starts: Key Component Is Folic Acid," *The Monitor*, September 15, 1992.

153. "Prevention of Neural Tube Defects: Results of the Medical Research Council Vitamin Study," *The Lancet* 338, no. 8760 (July 1991): 131–37.

154. Andrew E. Czeizel and István Dudás, "Prevention of the First Occurrence of Neural-Tube Defects by Periconceptional Vitamin Supplementation," *New England Journal of Medicine* 327 (December 1992): 1832–35.

155. Centers for Disease Control, "Use of Folic Acid for Prevention of Spina Bifida and Other Neural Tube Defects—1983–1991," *Morbidity and Mortality Weekly Report* 40, no. 30 (August 1991): 513–16; W. C. Willett, "Folic Acid and Neural Tube Defect: Can't We Come to Closure?," *American Journal of Public Health* 82, no. 5 (May 1992): 666–68.

156. There was active debate about the efficacy of folic acid. Some in the medical community argued that the observational findings should be viewed as complementary and that they provided a "solid empirical basis" for generalizing randomized trial findings to women without a previous neural tube defect. Irene H. Yen, "The Changing Epidemiology of Neural Tube Defects," *American Journal of Diseases of Children* 147, no. 7 (July 1992): 857–61.

157. Will Dunham, "Federal Plan to Fight Birth Defects Starts."

158. Harold A. Nelson, "TDH's 'Sins of Omission,'" *The Monitor*, August 28, 1992.

159. Harmon, "Folic Acid Vitamins Arrive in Droves."

160. Dave Harmon, "Doctors Recommend Taking Folic Acid to Prevent Defects," *The Monitor*, August 7, 1992.

161. Lucina Suarez, Marilyn Felkner, Jean D. Brender, Mark Canfield, Huiping Zhu, and Katherine A. Hendricks, "Neural Tube Defects on the Texas-Mexico Border: What We've Learned in the 20 Years Since the Brownsville Cluster," *Birth Defects Research Part A: Clinical and Molecular Teratology* 94, no. 11 (November 2012): 882–92.

162. Hollace Weiner, "More Cities Report Neural Birth Defects," *Fort Worth Star-Telegram*, July 9, 1995.

163. Leslie Sowers, "MOD Asks Future Moms to Think Ahead," *Houston Chronicle*, June 6, 1994.

164. James Pinkerton, "Rise of Birth Defects Spurs Concern in Valley," *Houston Chronicle*, August 23, 1998; Allie Johnson, "Birth Defect of Brain Rises Again in Cameron County," *The Monitor*, May 4, 1999.

165. *Primary Care Services for the Underserved*, 129; Diane West, "Latina and Nutraceutical Trends Merge," *Pharmaceutical Executive* 30, no. 7 (2000): 118.

166. "Folic Acid's Pregnancy Benefits Reduced in Latinos, Study Finds," *Los Angeles Times*, April 17, 1995.

167. John A. Harris and Gary M. Shaw, "Commentary: Neural Tube Defects—Why Are Rates High Among Populations of Mexican Descent?" *Environmental Health Perspectives* 103, no. 6 (September 1995): 163–64.

168. Ruth SoRelle and James Pinkerton, "Battling Birth Defects: Grain Products to Get Folic Acid, Official Says," *Houston Chronicle*, March 1, 1996; Tim Golden, "Pregnant Immigrants Wait Out Policy Storm," *New York Times*, October 16, 1996; Roberts, *Killing the Black Body*, 202.

169. Statement by State Senator Lloyd Bentsen, July 1, 1992, Box 95-019/920, Folder "Anencephaly, 1979, 1987–1992," Ann W. Richards Papers.

170. Neena Satija and Alexa Ura, "Undrinkable: Many Along Texas Border Still Live Without Clean, Safe Water," *Texas Tribune* (Austin), March 8, 2015.

4

Debilitating Care

Mothers and Children in the Aftermath
of Zika in Brazil

K. Eliza Williamson

"I see how hard it is," said Bruna. "To wake up and have a child who needs your attention 24 hours a day."[1]

Bruna was sitting across a desk from me, under the fluorescent lights of a small exam room at Cepred, the state-run rehabilitation center in Salvador, Bahia, Brazil, in July 2017.[2] Her nearly two-year-old daughter, Naiara, dozed off in her arms as we talked after an effortful session of combined physical, occupational, and speech therapy. Naiara had been born in late 2015 with what is now known as congenital Zika syndrome (CZS), a condition caused by the Zika virus that affects the central nervous system and causes motor, sensory, and cognitive impairments in the children of infected pregnant women. Babies diagnosed with Zika-related malformations were funneled into "early intervention" therapy programs in the interest of cultivating their maximum potential development.[3] In addition to multiple weekly therapy appointments, these children were also expected to have frequent consultations with specialist physicians and undergo regular neurological, hearing, and vision testing. All these clinical commitments—collectively referred to as *atendimentos* (appointments)—involved a lot of moving around from place to place. Since most families did not own cars, this in turn meant a significant amount of waiting for and riding on public transportation, which left little time for parents and children to rest.

"You don't have time for anything," Bruna continued. "You wake up, you feed them, then you prepare the midday meal, you give *mingau* [porridge]. . . . Then before you know it, it's 11:00 and you have to rush to get ready [*se arrumar correndo*], because you leave, on the bus, and everything has a scheduled time, to take her to therapy . . ."

I had asked Bruna to describe a typical day with her daughter. Her narrative, like those of nearly all the Brazilian mothers I interviewed, revealed an exhausting daily routine of therapy sessions, doctor's appointments, and grueling travel to and from these atendimentos.

"Then, a lot of times," Bruna said, "you get stuck in traffic on the way here [to Cepred] and the way back, and you only get home at night. I'm so tired of leaving Cepred at 5:00 p.m. and arriving home at 8:00 at night. . . . Then the next day, you're in that [same] routine, that routine of doctor, physical therapist, doctor, physical therapist, just road and bus [só estrada e buzú]."

The busyness didn't abate at home. As Bruna and other moms told me, clinical occupational, physical, and speech therapists encouraged and expected them to "work" with their children between appointments, engaging in specific kinds of play that encouraged development of motor, sensory, and cognitive abilities. Home, too, became a quasi-clinical space.

Drawing on my ethnographic research with families raising children with congenital Zika syndrome in Bahia, this chapter foregrounds the ways care debilitates. Specifically, I attend to the ways mothers become debilitated through caring for their disabled children—what colleagues and I have elsewhere called *dis/abling care*.[4] Mothers' care work includes transporting children to multiple weekly appointments spaced out across the city, engaging in home-based therapeutic exercises and other forms of "chronic homework," tackling mountains of bureaucracy for paltry social assistance benefits, and doing all of this under formidable economic, social, and physical constraints, and it leaves mothers feeling worn down both physically and mentally. In plain terms, caregiving for disabled children debilitates mother-caregivers. I contend that mothers' debilitation through caregiving is augured by the paucity of social support for the manifold work of care, which itself reflects intersecting gender, racial, and class inequities in contemporary Brazil.[5] Dialoguing with my interlocutors' narratives of embodied struggles to care well in adversity, I show how mothers' debilitation underscores disability's political and relational aspects. Dis/abling care, I suggest, points to the need for a definition of disability justice capacious enough to include caregivers.

This chapter represents one facet of a larger ethnographic research project I am pursuing on disability and care in the aftermath of the 2015–16 Zika virus epidemic in Bahia. This ongoing longitudinal project asks how Bahian families living with Zika's embodied fallout are reconstituting their lives in the wake of the epidemic. My fieldwork has been both in-person and re-mote: I spent four years living in Bahia between 2015 and 2019 and doing ethnographic research on maternal and child health. In 2016 I began vol-unteering with the local parents' support group–turned-NGO, Associação Abraço a Microcefalia ("I Embrace Microcephaly" Association).[6] That work led me to Cepred, the state-run rehabilitation center that enrolled many of the Bahian children born with CZS into its early intervention program. There I conducted semistructured interviews with 15 parents and 3 therapists in addition to observing several children's therapy sessions. I also accompa-nied parents and children to informational sessions on cannabis oil for epi-lepsy; observed health worker training for caring for children with CZS in low-income households; joined parents in disability rights marches and other public protests; and participated in parents' WhatsApp message groups. Since returning to the US in 2019, I have stayed connected with my inter-locutors via WhatsApp and other social media, and I conducted five-year follow-up interviews with parents via Zoom in 2022 and 2025.

As I began to talk to parents—primarily mothers, who are the ones most involved in caring for children with CZS—I realized that their children were not the only ones who were disabled. Mothers themselves were becoming debilitated, or having existing chronic illness and disabilities exacerbated, through the intense care work they were doing day in and day out. To under-stand disability in the wake of Zika, I would have to take seriously mothers' debilitation. And to understand why mothers were becoming debilitated, I had to listen closely to their stories of intense care work under multiple forms of constraint.

Drawing on global health guidelines, the Brazilian Ministry of Health recommends intensive early-intervention therapy (*estimulação precoce*) for children born premature or with impairments, or both, during the period of zero to three years of age when brains are said to be at their most malleable.[7] While most of the children diagnosed with CZS, including Naiara, had pri-ority access to early intervention through Brazil's public healthcare system, the Sistema Único de Saúde (SUS), the tiring work of just getting to therapy sessions multiple times a week at Cepred, as well as the additional labor of doing regular stimulation exercises with children at home to maximize ther-apeutic benefits, fell squarely on mothers.[8] Therapists at the rehabilitation center exhorted mothers to be paratherapists, doing the kind of "chronic homework" without which, they warned, their children's developmental progress would ultimately be hindered.[9] Repetition of the kinds of sensory stimulation activities they did in the clinic was key to fomenting their abilities. Mothers' chronic homework also included administering medications, planning and preparing meals for children's specific dietary needs, and managing medical documentation. This specialized care work added to an already exhausting daily schedule of clinical care and domestic labors in which mothers engaged, most often with little or no help from others.[10] Maria, another mom, told me,

> I just ask God for strength, really, because sometimes it's very tiring. . . . We have to be out [*na rua*] all the time. There's an appointment in the morning, and since I live far from the city center, I have to stay out [*ficar pela rua*] to be able to go to the next appointment. And this is extremely tiring for him, and also for me. When we get home, I don't want to sit and stimulate [Bruno]. I don't want to do stimulation; I want to sleep. I want to rest, watch a movie. That's why I can't be a "therapist" at home, because of all this running around [*correria*].[11]

The remainder of this chapter dwells on what Maria glossed as *correria*—a constant, exhausting running around that wears mothers down. After contextualizing the Zika virus epidemic and its unequal impacts in Brazil, I turn back to my interlocutors' narratives about their labors of care for their disabled children. Drawing on my interlocutors' stories of intensified care routines in the virtual absence of social support, I show how care work debilitated mothers, creating or exacerbating their physical and mental health conditions. I conclude by underscoring the gender, race, and class inequalities that shape family care for disabled children in contemporary Bahia, Brazil.

Zika in Brazil

Zika is a flavivirus transmitted by mosquitoes, primarily *Aedes aegypti*, and through sexual contact. In pregnant people, Zika can pass through the placental barrier and infect the fetus, attacking the developing central nervous system and causing a range of neurological malformations now known as congenital Zika syndrome, which can include but is not limited to microcephaly (reduced cranial circumference). Babies born with CZS may have microcephaly, calcifications in the cerebral subcortex (the area of the brain responsible for motor control and skills learning), arthrogryposis (joint curvature), ocular damage (leading to low vision), and hypertonia (rigid muscles, causing mobility difficulties). They may also have cerebral palsy and epilepsy.[12] Most children diagnosed with CZS, therefore, have multiple impairments and rely on the care of others for eating, mobility, and toileting. The "others" doing this care work are, in most cases, the children's mothers.

Zika was identified in Bahia and reported to the Ministry of Health in early 2015.[13] In Northeast Brazil, the Zika virus found ample opportunity to spread quickly. *Aedes aegypti* mosquitoes can easily proliferate in even very small amounts of standing water, making densely populated urban areas like the *periferias* of cities like Salvador, with their irregular garbage collection, open sewage infrastructure, and pothole-ridden streets, prime breeding grounds for mosquitoes.[14] At the time of this writing, the state of Bahia had the second-highest number of confirmed cases of CZS in the country.[15] Residents of Salvador's poorly serviced periferias are majority Black—a product of environmental racism rooted in Brazil's long history of chattel slavery.[16] The human impacts of the Zika epidemic both reflected and exacerbated Brazil's socioeconomic and regional inequalities: low-income Black families in the Northeast were the most affected, and Zika's aftermath has further compounded economic precarity for many now living with its consequences.[17]

On its own, Zika was not initially considered much of an immediate threat to public health. Compared to other mosquito-borne diseases that were circulating at the time, such as dengue and chikungunya, Zika infections tended to occasion comparatively mild symptoms (quickly disappearing rashes and mild joint pain in many cases).[18] It wasn't until the latter part of 2015, when doctors in the Northeast reported a precipitous rise in cases of microcephaly in fetuses and babies, that alarm bells began to sound. Once a scientific consensus was reached that Zika was most likely causing microcephaly and other congenital anomalies, and as the virus spread to the rest of Latin America and beyond, Zika mushroomed into a national, then international, public health emergency. In other words, it wasn't the Zika virus itself, but its capacity to produce disability, that made it a public health priority.

The Zika virus outbreak emerged during a period of intensifying political and economic crisis in Brazil. A recession that had begun in the first half of the 2010s deepened, former Workers' Party president Dilma Rousseff was ousted by parliamentary coup, and her successor, centrist Michel Temer, proceeded to approve a series of severe austerity measures. One of the most drastic of these was Constitutional Amendment 95, which essentially froze public spending on healthcare, education, and social assistance programs for the following two decades.[19] Dubbed the "Constitutional Amendment of Death" (*PEC da morte*) by Temer's opposition, this amendment all but guaranteed that the three quarters of the population relying on these government-funded services—including those living with the consequences of Zika—would continue to fall deeper into economic precarity. For parents engaged in full-time care for disabled children, these retrograde policies tore at the threads of what little safety net they had.[20]

As if this turmoil weren't enough, the COVID-19 pandemic arrived in Brazil on the heels of Jair Bolsonaro's first year in office, which saw numerous human rights violations.[21] Faced with yet another global public health emergency, Brazil now had a president who flagrantly denied medical science: Bolsonaro refused to accept the predictions of national and international epidemiological experts, repeatedly minimized the gravity of the pandemic, and publicly promoted spurious COVID-19 treatments like hydroxychloroquine, all of which contributed to delays in lifesaving prevention and treatment measures and very likely contributed to the several hundreds of thousands of COVID-related deaths in Brazil.[22] During the pandemic, Brazil's economy plummeted deeper into recession with increasing inflation and unemployment rates. The meager emergency financial aid that Bolsonaro's administration approved in 2020 barely covered basic necessities for those who were hardest hit, and the poverty rate rose from 23 million before the pandemic to 28 million.[23]

Although the Zika epidemic was declared over almost a decade ago—in November 2016 by the World Health Organization and then in May 2017 by the Brazilian government—the Zika virus continues to circulate. Scientists have warned that Zika is one genetic mutation away from becoming even more contagious, thus putting the world at risk of another, possibly even graver, epidemic.[24] The long-term consequences of Zika also continue to reverberate in the lives of people across the country, especially those children born with congenital Zika syndrome and the families that care for them.[25]

Esgotadas e Debilitadas: The Weight of Care

Women bear the brunt of all kinds of care work in Brazil, remunerated and otherwise. This is also true of care for disabled children.[26] Mothers of children with CZS are the ones who attend to their families' basic needs, accompany their children to multiple weekly therapy sessions and doctors' appointments, and engage in therapeutic labors at home—such as administering medications, preparing ketogenic meals, and doing cognitive stimulation exercises.[27] Mothers also often take on the additional work of fighting for their children's rights to healthcare, food, and government assistance. They do all of these tasks while also attending to the needs of intimate partners, if they have them, and often other family members.[28] Over time, this intense, constant care work wears mothers down.

"It's that *correria*, that whole crazy thing," Leide said. Her words echoed Bruna's, featured at the beginning of this chapter. "Up and down, public transport, metro rail . . ."

Leide and I sat on a small couch in the living room of her family's auto-constructed home, accessible only by a steep flight of concrete stairs leading up from the small grocery store owned by her father-in-law. Diego, her son, lay belly-down on the floor next to us, watching Leide's cell phone as it played Galinha Pintadinha videos on YouTube a few inches from his face. I had taken three buses to get to Leide's home in the Subúrbio Ferroviário from my apartment across the city, about an hour and a half of travel, one-way. Two or three buses, plus a ride on the city's new light rail (*metrô*), were typical also for Leide and Diego on their daily journeys to and from Diego's *atendimentos*, which were spread out in different clinics across the city. "Up and down" wasn't just a metaphor; Salvador is laid out on hilly coastal terrain that takes substantial physical effort to navigate on foot, even when one isn't carrying a toddler or pushing a child's wheelchair. Telling me how she regularly navigated streets with few functional wheelchair ramps and poorly maintained sidewalks (where there were sidewalks at all), Leide described maneuvering her son's wheelchair up onto and off of curbs constantly. While pushing Diego's wheelchair was better than having to carry him, as she had done for the first few years of his life, it still hurt her back: "Just today I left the house with [Diego] in the wheelchair, the really heavy wheelchair, and me with back pain, *né*, going up and down stairs because accessibility here is awful. . . . When we arrive [home], we're destroyed [*arrasada*]!" she laughed bitterly. "Tired, hungry, and everything else."[29]

Both Bruna and Leide had left their jobs after their children were born, and nearly two years later, like all the other moms I knew, they hadn't been able to return despite their desire to do so. Caring for young children with congenital Zika syndrome was more than a full-time job, in large part because of the many hurdles involved in accessing medical care, vital social benefits, and even basic necessities. As a result, mothers' narratives of caregiving were also narratives of exhaustion (*cansaço*), of being worn out (*esgotada*).[30] From inaccessible urban landscapes and public transport to stigma and discrimination, from barriers to healthcare access to labyrinthine bureaucracies of social assistance programs, economic insecurity, lack of caregiving support from family, and the anxieties and restrictions of the COVID-19 pandemic, the weight of both social and bodily precarity, over time, wore mothers down.

Mothers' experiences of physical and mental wearing down are evident in their narratives of exhaustion, anxiety, and bodymind destruction, stories that index the results of gradual debilitation under conditions of considerable constraint.[31] Whereas their children are the ones officially recognized as disabled, their mothers—also their primary caregivers—experience a slow wearing down of their embodied capacities that largely elides the label of "disability." This wearing down is directly related to the care work they undertake: As they labor to provide their children with the therapeutic resources prescribed to cultivate their child's maximum developmental potential, in addition to taking care of other family members and the home—all while struggling with the chronic challenges of poverty, systemic ableism, and the COVID-19 pandemic—mothers themselves become debilitated. Their debilitation gestures toward the ways structural violence becomes embodied in the context of caregiving for disabled children and requires a capacious definition of disability justice.[32]

Sem Suporte

Despite all the initial media and political attention to Zika and microcephaly, mothers have found very little in the way of assistance with or support for their caregiving labors. This abandonment left mothers feeling they were "without support" (*sem suporte*). Securing and keeping children's various atendimentos, for example, posed a challenge all its own. Since health is defined as a right in Brazil's Constitution, all citizens have access to the SUS. There is also a thriving but poorly regulated private healthcare sector, and many Brazilians use a combination of both public and private services. While some mothers in my research have purchased low-cost private health plans (*planos de saúde*, akin to health insurance), most continue to rely primarily on the SUS for their children's medical needs, including early-intervention therapy, medications, and high-cost exams and procedures. Chronic underfunding, however, makes for long waitlists for some of these SUS services. Regular electroencephalograms (EEGs), for example, were used for measuring electric activity in children's brains to detect seizures and aid in the diagnosis of epilepsy, for which many of the children needed antiseizure medications. But EEGs in the SUS could often be scheduled only several months out, Bruna explained to me. "There are children who need electro-encephalograms who don't get them!" she said. "A child who has seizures might go four, five months on a [waiting] list to be able to get an electro-encephalogram."[33] Without regular EEGs, children couldn't get updated prescriptions, and their medication dosage might be too high or too low until they were able to get a new one. This had obvious negative consequences for children's well-being. For mothers, it also meant constant monitoring for seizures and more frequent trips to urgent care and the hospital, which in turn contributed to their exhaustion.

Then there were the restrictions clinical centers placed on access to the care they provided. Leide complained that both government-run and non-profit therapy clinics had "so many rules," including strict limits on how many appointments a child could miss before being cut from services and sent back to the end of the waitlist. Such rules, she added, were "inviable for a mother who is psychologically debilitated [*debilitada psicologicamente*]" like herself and so many others she knew. Just a couple of missed appointments could move their children to the back of the line, sending mothers once again in search of therapeutic care.[34] Being "psychologically debilitated" already, from all the other challenges of caring for multiply disabled children under intersecting constraints, made it more likely that mothers might miss their children's atendimentos, Leide suggested, and suffering the consequences of missing too many atendimentos could debilitate mothers even further.

If bureaucratic rules threatened children's access to therapies, they also complicated mothers' access to vital social benefits. Most families relied on government programs like the Benefício de Prestação Continuada (BPC) to make ends meet. The BPC is a government pension of one minimum monthly salary (*salário mínimo*) for disabled people whose family income is no higher than a quarter of the salário mínimo. When the disabled person is a child, the child's primary caregiver is the beneficiary. The BPC was a lifeline for mothers who had to stop working to take care of their children full time—which was most of them. Yet gaining access to these benefits often seemed to require Herculean effort and infinite patience. The first time Francisleia applied for her son Miguel's BPC, her application was denied because her former employer had failed to report to the social security system that she was no longer working at her factory job, which she had left to care for Miguel full time. Francisleia had to take her former employer to court, then present a document from the court proceedings to the INSS (Brazil's social security system) to prove that she was no longer working. Even after she had the document, getting an appointment to register for the BPC was no easy undertaking. Every INSS office she called in Salvador told her they had no available appointments. In our 2017 interview, she told me she had been calling since the previous year and was always told the same thing: no appointments available that year or the next year. Only by making the trip in person—which required multiple buses both ways with her son—to explain her situation to the INSS agents was she able to get an appointment to evaluate her case, after which she finally obtained the benefit.[35]

In all their care labors, mothers could count on little practical support from others, even close family members and coparents. Although Leide's husband, Danilo, was unemployed when we spoke in 2022, and therefore often at home, he participated only in certain aspects of Diego's care. Sometimes, Leide told me, he would give their son baths and watch him while Leide attended to other matters—"basic things," as she put it. But feeding and administering daily medications were usually left up to her, as well as the labor of planning and preparing meals, keeping track of medication times, and other necessary tasks. Danilo didn't "like" feeding Diego because it took a long time, Leide said, and he just didn't have the patience it required. "There are days when I feel so tired, so tired," she told me. "And I would like to go to bed earlier. But then I have to wait for the whole process of feeding, and after feeding, wait for [Diego] to digest, to then give him his medication, to put him in his bed, wait for him to fall asleep, to then go to bed myself."[36] In a brief conversation in October 2020, early in the COVID-19 pandemic, Leide lamented that it was nearly impossible to imagine a future for herself outside full-time dedication to her son's care. In one rare outing to run errands, she told me, she had left Diego with her husband, Diego's father. "It was hell!" she said. "He was calling me every five minutes to come back home. The boy only had lunch [much later] in the afternoon because he [his father] didn't want to feed the boy because of his eating difficulties. This routine is exhausting [*esgotante*] for me."[37]

During the COVID-19 pandemic, Leide contracted Chikungunya, an arbovirus transmitted by the same *Aedes aegypti* mosquito as Zika. The infection gave her "pain, fever, itching," and her body "begged for rest." She wanted to go to the hospital but felt she couldn't, with all the COVID patients and the risk of contracting that virus too. She preferred to stay home and self-medicate with over-the-counter analgesics. Not surprisingly, Leide found it nearly impossible to take care of Diego in this state, but she knew no one else would. It was only by chance, she said, that her sister called her and, when Leide told her about her situation, offered to take Diego for a few days while Leide recovered. This kind of help from siblings was not at all typical, though, she told me. She also fell and injured her knee and ankle on the irregular sidewalk outside their apartment building. After her X-ray at urgent care, she was told to stay off her ankle for several weeks—something she knew would be impossible with all the care work she was responsible for. The accumulation of these stresses, added to her feeling of being "trapped" and "a prisoner in [her] own home," led to a mental health crisis mid-pandemic. Leide said she became "very weakened" (*muito fragilizada*), having "anxiety attacks," "getting depressed," and discovering, through their exacerbation, "a series of psychological problems that I didn't even know I had."[38]

Even when mothers were surrounded by family, help with caregiving was not forthcoming. Maria's family often got together. Maria and Bruno lived in an apartment near the outskirts of Salvador, distant from most family members on the other side of the city and scattered around the metropolitan region, so these gatherings meant—ostensibly, at least—a reprieve from the grind and loneliness of their everyday routine. Other children in the family ran around playing with their cousins. Babies were passed from one set of auntie's arms to another in succession. Older cousins took care of younger ones. Other parents got a bit of a break, but not Maria: Even during these gatherings at her mother's home, she found little support with Bruno's care. While she enjoyed reconnecting with her family, she said, she often returned home feeling "worn out" (*esgotada*). "Because I get there and I have to do everything that I do at home, in an environment that isn't mine, and that isn't prepared [for a disabled child]. So I don't have a place to give him a bath. He's heavy, he's big. The place [physical space] isn't prepared, and I don't have much help. Actually, I *don't* have help." When I asked Maria why she thought her family members didn't help her with Bruno, she told me it was because "it's a lot of work. It's easier [for them] to say, 'I don't know how to do it,' or 'I'm afraid of what could happen.' Like, 'Ah, I'm afraid of him choking [if I feed him].' 'Ah, but I don't know what he eats.' You see?" Maria felt she couldn't relax on family visits because she still had to do "all the work," including simple things like changing Bruno's diaper, which, she reasoned, anyone could do. Whereas aunts, cousins, and grandmothers would often participate in caring for and playing with nondisabled kids in the family, Maria lamented that it was "very rare" for her to have this kind of practical support with Bruno even from close kin.[39] The lack of family engagement with their disabled children was a common experience among the mothers in my research, and this, too, contributed to their wearing down.

When I asked Bruna what came to mind when she thought about her future with her daughter Naiara, she expressed her worry that if she weren't around, no one else would be there to take care of Naiara. Bruna said she had recently experienced a flare-up of her own chronic illnesses, which had prevented her from taking Naiara to her atendimentos. She didn't elaborate on what illnesses these were, and I didn't press her on it, but she made it clear that they were bad enough that they affected her ability to leave the house and engage in childcare. Knowing Bruna lived with Naiara's father, I asked about him. Wouldn't the little girl's dad take over his daughter's care in her absence? "I don't think . . . he would know how to take care of her, you know, that he would have the patience that I have," she told me. When she was sick, no one, including her husband, stepped in to help with Naiara or even asked her if she needed assistance.[40]

The COVID pandemic further confounded mothers' caregiving struggles. Much like Leide, Maria described feeling "imprisoned" (*presa*) with her son in their small apartment and spoke of the "mental affliction" (*transtorno mental*) and "psychological pressure" around keeping Bruno safe from COVID infection—conditions also connected to insomnia that, as she put it, "dysregulated" her. Like other parents, Maria worried that in isolation her child would "lose" the developmental progress he'd made in his therapy sessions. At the same time, she feared taking him out of their home, even after lockdown measures had been lifted, because her son's weak immune response (*baixa imunidade*) meant that even mild respiratory infections could threaten his life.[41] And yet taking Bruno with her to buy groceries and run other errands was usually necessary, since she was a solo mom and no one else was usually available to watch Bruno while she went out. Besides the general panic regarding COVID, Maria had further reason to be on high alert: The year prior to the pandemic's onset, a respiratory infection had landed Bruno in the hospital for the third time in his short life. She was "really scared," she told me, and had doubts that her son would survive a COVID infection. "I got very neurotic," Maria said. "I wouldn't leave the house, and I didn't want to receive any visits."[42] "Neurotic" might have been hyperbole here, but Maria was quite literally sick with worry. "I . . . began to have anxiety attacks [*crises de ansiedade*]," she told me. "I had [anxiety] attacks where I called an ambulance because I had a blood pressure reading of 180/120 in the middle of the night, feeling really bad." Maria had hypertension and regularly used a home blood pressure monitor. As a way of coping with her anxiety and isolation, Maria often resorted to overeating, which left her feeling even more out of control. "I gained even more weight," she continued, "because [eating] was a way of compensating" for unmet emotional needs.

Disabling Care

In a 2023 report entitled "Esgotadas," based on a nationwide survey of care work and mental health among Brazilian women, the feminist organization Think Olga states: "Women arrived exhausted [esgotadas] in 2020, went through one of the worst crises of the century [the COVID-19 pandemic] and, even after its end, continue to be exhausted in 2023. Overload [*sobrecarga*] is one of the main reasons, if not *the* main reason, that women become ill and seek help and mental health care."[43]

Although the Think Olga report doesn't name them specifically, mothers of disabled children, and particularly those with limited access to support resources, financial and otherwise, fit squarely within the realities the report describes. Maria, Leide, Bruna, and Francisleia were overwhelmed and worn out both mentally and physically. For them, caring for their multiply disabled children is a full-time job. It requires constant presence and attention, as well as cultivation of expertise in specialized feeding practices, various healthcare technologies, and therapeutic stimulation exercises designed to maximize the development of their children's motor, sensory, and cognitive skills.[44]

These mothers are worn down by engaging in intense care work under multiple, interlocking forms of structural violence. Chronic economic precarity; stigma and discrimination; barriers to accessing public spaces, healthcare, and social assistance; exposure to illness and injury; government mishandling of viral pandemics; and the structural racism undergirding these—all have played a role in mother-caregivers' debilitation. That they faced these challenges virtually alone, with minimal support from family and government support, strained their bodyminds even further. The language mothers used to describe their experiences—exhaustion, anxiety, weakness, neurosis, mental affliction, dysregulation—foregrounds how caregiving under constraint debilitates.

Caregiving debilitates caregivers in part as a result of the same kinds of systemic ableism that constantly constrict disabled people formally recognized as such. While care routines for children with multiple disabilities tend to involve various forms of "chronic homework" that can in themselves be taxing, these were not the focus of my interlocutors' stories of debilitation. Rather, mothers underscored the laborious effort required to get even the most basic needs met: Inaccessible built environments, from broken sidewalks and nonexistent ramps to faulty wheelchair elevators on public buses, required extra time and energy spent planning routes and shuttling children to appointments. Some, like Leide, developed painful injuries from the strain of carrying children in their arms or pushing heavy wheelchairs up and down Salvador's hilly, unevenly paved streets. Accessing vital medical care and social benefits was practically a full-time job in itself and a significant source of mental and physical stress for mothers. With atendimentos spread out all over the city, they often spent entire days outside their homes with their children, navigating public transport to, from, and between clinics. Long wait times for important medical tests like EEGs sent mothers scrambling to find earlier appointments elsewhere—perhaps through informal channels if they had such recourse—and could leave them looking for stopgap measures to manage their children's frequent seizures in the absence of necessary medications. Clinics' often unforgiving missed-appointment policies failed to account for the myriad circumstances, including mothers' own illnesses, that prevented mothers from getting their children to all appointments on time, all the time. All of this resulted in constant stress that inevitably took its toll on mothers' bodyminds.

That the ones doing this care work were women, and specifically Black women, reveals how debilitation-through-caregiving is imbricated with deep social inequalities in contemporary Brazil. In Brazil as in many places of the world, care work is women's work. Brazilian women do twice the amount of unpaid domestic work that Brazilian men do.[45] The quantity and kinds of care work women do, however—and, by extension, the forms of caregiving-related debilitation they experience—depends on their racial identities and income levels. Black women are overrepresented in both unpaid and paid care work generally.[46] Whereas some middle-class mothers (who also tended to be white or lighter-skinned) could hire domestic help and purchase cars adapted for their children's wheelchairs, most others had to transport their children on foot and by public bus, resulting in more time and energy spent getting to and from appointments, and sometimes resulting in injuries. Many of the same socioeconomic factors that exposed these mothers to Zika infection in the first place—namely, being Black, poor, and northeastern—also augmented their debilitation through caregiving.

Finally, much of the care work that mothers were engaging in was geared toward habilitating their children's bodyminds in the hope of ameliorating impairment and avoiding or reducing their future disabilities. In laboring to cultivate their children's bodymind potential, guided by medical professionals and prescribed therapy regimens, mothers became (more) debilitated. This is why colleagues and I have framed such care as dis/abling: Carefully designed to cultivate capacity in others' bodyminds but poorly supported financially, socially, or infrastructurally, care can often simultaneously disable—debilitate, wear down—caregivers' own bodyminds.[47]

Scholars of disability in Latin America must take seriously how disability is produced through conditions of structural violence and social marginalization.[48] Doing so requires challenging the boundaries of disability as defined in much global north disability studies literature, beyond the confines of identity and into the more ambiguous territory of debilitation, taking seriously local categories of meaning and ways of indexing incapacitation. Accounting for the production of disability also necessitates careful consideration of how the many kinds of care work mobilized to sustain disabled and chronically ill bodyminds (one's own and others') may also produce or exacerbate disability and chronic illness in those doing the care work. It demands, too, critical assessment of how debilitation through care work manifests differently in specific gendered, racialized, and classed bodyminds. Disability justice is intimately entwined with caregiver justice. Continued engagement with the nexus of disability and caregiving in Brazil is vital to dreaming—and bringing forth—more just futures for disabled people and their loved ones.

NOTES

1. Bruna, interview with the author, July 17, 2017.

2. Cepred is the acronym for Centro Estadual de Prevenção e Reabilitação da Pessoa com Deficiência (State Center for Prevention and Rehabilitation of People with Disabilities).

3. Eliza Williamson, "Habilitating Bodyminds, Caring for Potential: Disability Therapeutics After Zika in Bahia, Brazil," *Cultural Anthropology* 39, no. 1 (February 22, 2024): 9–36.

4. K. Eliza Williamson, Cíntia Engel, and Helena Fietz, "The Chronicity of Home-Making: Women Caregivers in Dis/Abling Spaces," *Space and Culture* 26, no. 3 (August 1, 2023): 468–82.

5. My use of the term "debility" here draws on Jasbir K. Puar's work, particularly in *The Right to Maim: Debility, Capacity, Disability* (Duke University Press, 2017). For Puar, global arrangements of power and violence produce the debilitation and "slow death" of bodies in certain populations. Whereas "disability" has become a political identity and a category of classification for legal and social welfare purposes, debility often flies under the radar of recognition. Not all or even most of those who are debilitated would be officially recognized, or even identify themselves, as "disabled." I find the concept of debility useful for naming the various ways my interlocutors' embodied capacities are diminished, regardless of whether they might identify with the label "disabled" or qualify for such a status under any official definitions (and they usually do not).

6. At Abraço I made myself useful where I could: Among other things, I did clerical work for the NGO; helped organize regular gatherings and events; played with children while parents participated in these events; organized donated diapers, foodstuffs, and toys; and translated grant proposals to capture funds for the NGO.

7. Ministério da Saúde do Brasil, "Diretrizes de estimulação precoce: Crianças de zero a 3 anos com atraso no desenvolvimento neuropsicomotor decorrente de microcefalia" (Ministério da Saúde do Brasil, 2016), Biblioteca Virtual em Saúde, http://portalsaude .saude.gov.br/images/pdf/2016/janeiro/13/Diretrizes-de-Estimulacao-Precoce.pdf; UNICEF, "Early Childhood Development," United Nations Children's Fund, accessed March 23, 2022, https://www.unicef.org/early-childhood-development.

8. Several scholars have documented similar phenomena in the United States and elsewhere. See, for example, Laura Mauldin, *Made to Hear: Cochlear Implants and Raising Deaf Children* (University of Minnesota Press, 2016); Gail Landsman, *Reconstructing Motherhood and Disability in the Age of Perfect Babies* (Routledge, 2009); Brendan Gerard Hart, "Making an Autism World in Morocco: Parent Activism, Therapeutic Practice, and the Proliferation of a Diagnosis" (PhD diss., Columbia University, 2016); and Cheryl Mattingly, *The Paradox of Hope: Journeys Through a Clinical Borderland* (University of California Press, 2010).

9. Cheryl Mattingly, Lone Grøn, and Lotte Meinert, "Chronic Homework in Emerging Borderlands of Healthcare," *Culture, Medicine, and Psychiatry* 35, no. 3 (September 1, 2011): 347–75, https://doi.org/10.1007/s11013-011-9225-z.

10. Mattingly, Grøn, and Meinert, "Chronic Homework in Emerging Borderlands of Healthcare."

11. Maria, interview with the author, September 19, 2017. I translate *correria* here as "running around" because of the specific contexts in which my interlocutors use it. The word *correria* can also mean "busyness," "rushing," "hustle and bustle," and the like.

12. CDC (Centers for Disease Control and Prevention), "Zika Virus: Congenital Zika Syndrome and Other Birth Defects," January 31, 2025.

13. Debora Diniz, *Zika: From the Brazilian Backlands to Global Threat* (Zed Books, 2017); Gabriela Freitas and Soraya Fleischer, "A epidemia do vírus Zika nas Ciências Sociais no Brasil: Um estudo bibliográfico (2016–2018)," *Revista TOMO* 38 (January–June 2021): 309–38.

14. Alex M. Nading, *Mosquito Trails: Ecology, Health, and the Politics of Entanglement* (University of California Press, 2014).

15. Between 2015 and 2022, Brazil reported 1,857 confirmed cases of congenital Zika syndrome nationally. The state of Bahia's total, as of the latest available epidemiological report, was 335. These numbers come from *Epidemiological Bulletin* 55, no. 5 (March 5, 2024): 12.

16. Victor de Jesus, "Racializando o olhar (sociológico) sobre a saúde ambiental em saneamento da população negra: um continuum colonial chamado racismo ambiental," *Saúde e Sociedade* 29 (May 11, 2020): e180519.

17. Social and public health scientists highlight the way the Zika epidemic both exposed and exacerbated long-standing inequities in Brazil: lack of access to healthcare resources despite the existence of the SUS; unequal access to education; inadequate public transportation for parents who need to take children to medical appointments and therapy sessions, to pick up medications, nutritional supplements, and diapers, and to attend support group meetings; stigma and discrimination against disabled people; and the insufficiency of social assistance programs that are supposed to support them in caring for their children and themselves. Ilana G. Ambrogi, Luciana Brito, and Debora Diniz, "The Vulnerabilities of Lives: Zika, Women, and Children in Alagoas State, Brazil," *Cadernos de Saúde Pública* 36 (January 11, 2021); Adeolu Aromolaran et al., "Unequal Burden of Zika-Associated Microcephaly among Populations with Public and Private Healthcare in Salvador, Brazil," *International Journal of Infectious Diseases*, April 22, 2022; Diniz, *Zika*; Debora Diniz and Luciana Brito, "Epidemia Provocada Pelo Vírus Zika: Informação e Conhecimento," *Revista Eletrônica de Comunicação, Informação e Inovação Em Saúde* 10, no. 2 (June 2016); Amanda Estrela Gonçalves, Sibele Dayane Brazil Tenório, and Priscila Correia da Silva Ferraz, "Aspectos socioeconômicos dos genitores de crianças com microcefalia relacionada ao Zika vírus," *Revista Pesquisa em Fisioterapia* 8, no. 2 (April 17, 2018): 155–66; Ludmila Lobkowicz et al., "Neighbourhood-Level Income and Zika Virus Infection During Pregnancy in Recife, Pernambuco, Brazil: An Ecological Perspective, 2015–2017," *BMJ Global Health* 6, no. 12 (December 1, 2021).

18. For a brief time, Zika was even referred to as a "weak dengue fever" (*dengue fraca*). Raquel Aguiar and Inesita Soares Araujo, "A Mídia Em Meio Às 'Emergências' Do Vírus Zika: Questões Para o Campo Da Comunicação e Saúde, Aguiar, Revista Eletrônica de Comunicação, Informação e Inovação Em Saúde," *Revista Eletrônica de Comunicação, Informação e Inovação Em Saúde* 10, no. 1 (2016); Diniz, *Zika*.

19. The full text of Constitutional Amendment 95 can be found at Presidência da

República, accessed May 30, 2025, http://www.planalto.gov.br/ccivil_03/constituicao /emendas/emc/emc95.htm.

20. This assertion is based on my participant observation. See also "'PEC da morte' levou ao que vemos no sistema de saúde agora, diz Conselho," *CNN Brasil*, May 16, 2020.

21. Jurema Werneck and Erika Guevara Rosa, "1,000 Days of Bolsonaro and Brazil's Grave Human Rights Crisis," Amnesty International, October 20, 2021, https://www .amnesty.org/en/latest/news/2021/10/mil-dias-bolsonaro-grave-crisis-derechos-humanos -brasil/.

22. Francisco Ortega and Michael Orsini, "Governing COVID-19 Without Government in Brazil: Ignorance, Neoliberal Authoritarianism, and the Collapse of Public Health Leadership," *Global Public Health* 15, no. 9 (September 1, 2020): 1257–77.

23. Nathalia Garcia and Pedro Ladeira, "Fome, inflação e informalidade desafiam discurso de Bolsonaro sobre 'economia pujante,'" *Folha de São Paulo*, September 10, 2022, sec. Mercado; Raquel Landim, "Quase 28 milhões de pessoas vivem abaixo da linha da pobreza no Brasil," *CNN Brasil*, July 10, 2021, https://www.cnnbrasil.com.br/business /quase-28-milhoes-de-pessoas-vivem-abaixo-da-linha-da-pobreza-no-brasil/. While this chapter was in copyediting, there was a major development in Brazil. On July 1, 2025, after years of dogged activist efforts by parents of children with CZS across Brazil who formed a national front, Brazil passed a law (Lei No. 15.156) offering reparations to Zika-affected families. Under this law, each family will receive a one-time reparations payment of R$50,000 in addition to a lifetime monthly pension of several thousand reais—about six times the minimum salary. (Presidência da República, Lei No. 15.156 de 01, de julho de 2025, https://www.planalto.gov.br/ccivil_03/_ato2023-2026/2025/lei/l15156.htm.) Law 15.156 stands to eliminate many of the financial struggles I have documented here. It remains to be seen how mother-caregivers' experiences will change in the wake of this much deserved victory.

24. Jose Angel Regla-Nava et al., "A Zika Virus Mutation Enhances Transmission Potential and Confers Escape from Protective Dengue Virus Immunity," *Cell Reports* 39, no. 2 (April 12, 2022); Laith Yakob, "Zika Virus After the Public Health Emergency of International Concern Period, Brazil," *Emerging Infectious Diseases* 28, no. 4 (April 1, 2022): 837–40.

25. Erica Charters and Kristin Heitman, "How Epidemics End," *Centaurus* 63, no. 1 (2021): 210–24.

26. Helena Moura Fietz, "Construindo futuros, provocando o presente: cuidado familiar, moradias assistidas e temporalidades na gestão cotidiana da deficiência intelectual no Brasil" (PhD diss., Porto Alegre, Universidade Federal do Rio Grande do Sul, 2020); Helena Hirata, "Comparando relações de cuidado: Brasil, França, Japão," *Estudos Avançados* 34 (May 8, 2020): 25–40; Bila Sorj and Adriana Fontes, "O care como um regime estratificado: implicações de gênero e classe social," in *Cuidado e cuidadoras: As várias faces do trabalho do care*, ed. Helena Hirata and Nadya Araujo Guimarães (Editora Atlas, 2012), 103–16.

27. Soraya Fleischer, "Segurar, caminhar e falar: notas etnográficas sobre a experiência de uma 'mãe de micro' no Recife/PE," *Cadernos de Gênero e Diversidade* 3, no. 2 (July 30, 2017), https://doi.org/10.9771/cgd.v3i2.21983; Raquel Lustosa da Costa Alves and Yazmin

Bheringcer dos Reis e Safatle, "'Mães de Micro': Perspectivas e desdobramentos sobre cuidado no contexto da síndrome congênita do zika vírus (SCZV) em Recife/PE,," *Áltera Revista de Antropologia* 1, no. 8 (2019): 115–45, https://doi.org/10.22478/ufpb.2447-9837 .2019v1n8.42464; K. Eliza Williamson, "Care in the Time of Zika: Notes on the 'Afterlife' of the Epidemic in Salvador (Bahia), Brazil," *Interface—Comunicação, Saúde, Educação* 22 (September 2018): 685–96.

28. Fleischer, "Segurar, caminhar e falar"; Rosamaria Carneiro and Soraya Resende Fleischer, "'I Never Expected This, It Was a Big Shock': Conception, Pregnancy and Birth in Times of Zika Through the Eyes of Women in Recife, PE, Brazil," *Interface—Comunicação, Saúde, Educação* 22, no. 66 (September 2018): 709–19; Diego Alano de Jesus Pereira Pinheiro and Marcia Reis Longhi, "Maternidade como missão! A trajetória militante de uma mãe de bebê com microcefalia em PE," *Cadernos de Gênero e Diversidade* 3, no. 2 (July 30, 2017): 113–33; Russell Parry Scott et al., "A Epidemia de Zika e as Articulações das Mães num Campo Tensionado entre Feminismo, Deficiência e Cuidados," *Cadernos de Gênero e Diversidade* 3, no. 2 (July 30, 2017): 73–92; Russell Parry Scott et al., "Itinerários terapêuticos, cuidados e atendimento na construção de ideias sobre maternidade e infância no contexto da Zika," *Interface—Comunicação, Saúde, Educação* 22, no. 66 (September 2018): 673–84.

29. Leide, interview with the author, February 16, 2022.

30. The theme of *cansaço* in mothers' narratives has also been explored by Raquel Lustosa da Costa Alves and colleagues. See Raquel Lustosa da Costa Alves, "Um dia com Josi: uma fotoetnografia do cuidado e do cansaço," *Interface—Comunicação, Saúde, Educação* 22 (September 2018): 975–80; Raquel Lustosa da Costa Alves and Soraya Resende Fleischer, "'O que adianta conhecer muita gente e no fim das contas estar sempre só?': O desafio da maternidade em tempos de Síndrome Congênita do Zika Vírus," *Revista AntHropológicas* 29, no. 2 (2018); Raquel Lustosa da Costa Alves and Yazmin Bheringcer dos Reis e Safatle, "'Mães de Micro': Perspectivas e desdobramentos sobre cuidado no contexto da síndrome congênita do zika vírus (SCZV) em Recife/PE," *Áltera Revista de Antropologia* 1, no. 8 (2019): 115–45.

31. My use of the term "bodymind" here is inspired by disability studies scholarship that takes body and mind as intimately entwined rather than separate, and that calls us to acknowledge the embodied impacts of structural forms of oppression and marginalization intersecting with disability that can manifest both physically and mentally. See Margaret Price, "The Bodymind Problem and the Possibilities of Pain," *Hypatia* 30, no. 1 (2015): 268–84; Sami Schalk, *Bodyminds Reimagined: (Dis)Ability, Race, and Gender in Black Women's Speculative Fiction* (Duke University Press, 2018).

32. By "structural violence," I mean the ways in which structural conditions—such as global capitalism, anti-Blackness, and ableism as well as the social, spatial, and health inequities they produce—impede survival and thriving for marginalized people. This definition comes from sociologist Johan Galtung, in "Violence, Peace, and Peace Research," *Journal of Peace Research* 6, no. 3 (1969): 167–91. It has been further developed by anthropologists such as Paul Farmer. See Farmer, "An Anthropology of Structural Violence," *Current Anthropology* 45, no. 3 (June 2004): 305–25.

33. Bruna, interview with the author, July 17, 2017.

34. Leide, interview with author, February 16, 2022.

35. Francisleia, interview with the author, July 18, 2017.

36. Leide, interview with author.

37. Leide, WhatsApp message exchange with the author, October 2020.

38. Leide, interview with author.

39. Maria, interview with the author, February 8, 2022.

40. Bruna, interview with author.

41. Many mothers insisted that their children with CZS had weakened immune responses and often fell ill.

42. Maria, interview with author, February 8, 2022.

43. Psychologist Juliane Callegaro Borsa quoted in Think Olga, "Esgotadas," accessed November 24, 2023, https://lab.thinkolga.com/esgotadas/, 29 (emphasis added).

44. Williamson, "Habilitating Bodyminds."

45. World Bank, "Brazil," World Bank Gender Data Portal, accessed November 27, 2024, https://genderdata.worldbank.org/en/economies/brazil.

46. "Em 2022, Mulheres Dedicaram 9,6 Horas Por Semana a Mais Do Que Os Homens Aos Afazeres Domésticos Ou Ao Cuidado de Pessoas," Agência de Notícias—Instituto Brasileiro de Geografia e Estatísticas, August 11, 2023.

47. Williamson, Engel, and Fietz, "Chronicity of Home-Making."

48. N. Erevelles, *Disability and Difference in Global Contexts: Enabling a Transformative Body Politic* (Palgrave Macmillan US, 2011); Laura Jordan Jaffee, "Disrupting Global Disability Frameworks: Settler-Colonialism and the Geopolitics of Disability in Palestine/Israel," *Disability and Society* 31, no. 1 (January 2, 2016): 116–30; Puar, *Right to Maim*; Helen Meekosha, "Decolonising Disability: Thinking and Acting Globally," *Disability and Society* 26, no. 6 (October 1, 2011): 667–82; Shaun Grech and Karen Soldatic, eds. *Disability in the Global South: The Critical Handbook*, International Perspectives on Social Policy, Administration, and Practice (Springer International, 2016); Rosamund Greiner, "Towards *Critical Studies of Disabilities*: Engaging Latin American Theoretical Perspectives on Congenital Zika Syndrome," *Horizontes Antropológicos* 28 (October 2022): 143–72, https://doi.org/10.1590/S0104-71832022000300006.

5

Slavery, Litigation, and the Construction of Disability in Late Colonial Lima, Peru

Adam Warren

In 1803 Esteban Tirado, an enslaved man in Lima, the capital of the Spanish Viceroyalty of Peru, invoked his disability, poor health, and status as a *miserable*, or wretch, in a civil suit he initiated against his owner, Francisco Tirado. Working most likely through a notary and eventually a procurator, or legal advocate, with the goal of improving his circumstances as an enslaved person, Esteban Tirado alleged that Francisco Tirado had sent him to work in a *panadería*, or bakery, "with the punishment of the stock that has been placed on me," after he failed to find a new owner to purchase him at a specified price. Panaderías and supply houses (or warehouses) known as *casas de abasto* typically served as sites of incarceration, punishment, and work for enslaved people deemed rebellious or unruly in colonial Lima. Noting that Francisco Tirado was willing to sell him only for a price greater than what he believed himself to be worth, Esteban Tirado asked the courts not just to have himself removed from the panadería, but also to have him appraised by an expert, perhaps a physician or surgeon, and be permitted to seek a new owner who would purchase him at a lower price. Claiming that "I'm not worth the 300 pesos he asks for me" and that he became "herniated in the groin" before entering the panadería, his overall condition worsened after his owner disobeyed the court's previous ruling and sent him there. Having become "herniated in two places," he described himself as suffering multiple illnesses; those drafting his petition emphasized "the imminent danger in which he finds himself." Esteban Tirado's dire condition, his petition pointedly argued, was a direct consequence of the harsh treatment to which he was subjected in the panadería, which rendered him "broken and crippled in two places." Having found a new buyer and using an emerging legal language of disability rooted in traditional legal principles, Esteban Tirado sought to draw on the opinion of experts to attain the court's mercy and protection.[1]

Tirado's story is not unlike those of the many urban enslaved people who toiled on their owners' behalf in the streets, bakeries, supply houses, and homes of eighteenth- and early-nineteenth-century Lima while suffering from ill health and various forms of disability. Rather than just dwell on the quotidian violence of slavery that Tirado's testimony conveys, this chapter asks what court cases about the purchase and sale of enslaved people and court cases initiated by enslaved people and their kin can tell us about the history of disability in late colonial Peru. How did residents of Lima— including the enslaved, the notaries and procurators who recorded their petitions and advocated for them, family members, owners, and the healers who provided expert testimony—understand, construct, and navigate what we would call disability? How did ideas about disability circulate, and how did they come about in relation to slavery? How were claims of disability, and of the related violence of slavery, strategically deployed to transform the fates of individual slaves, many of whom sought what Michelle McKinley describes as "fractional freedoms"?[2]

To address these questions, this chapter engages two types of civil cases. The first type of case, which I discuss only briefly, took place between owners who engaged each other in litigation to contest the value, health, and ability to labor of the enslaved adults and children they purchased and sold. Known as redhibitory cases, they are not unlike lawsuits between buyers and sellers in the US antebellum South over the "soundness" of enslaved people who had been transacted; Jenifer Barclay has examined these lawsuits in depth.[3] Dozens, if not hundreds, of redhibitory cases are archived in Peru's National Archives and Lima's Archbishopric Archive, and they provide insights into how owners navigated the relationship between ability, disability, and commodification, seeking always to maximize the return on their investment in human property. Esteban Tirado's lawsuit against Francisco Tirado, on the other hand, illustrates the second kind of case, examples of which sit alongside the first kind in the archives and merit greater attention. Rooted in a different legal culture from that of the British colonies and the United States, the justice system in the Iberian world provided enslaved people greater levels of legal personhood and allowed them to initiate civil cases. Increasingly, they and their kin took owners to court with the help of notaries and procurators to make accusations and press for demands, among them the provision of treatment for their injuries and ailments, protection from violence and abuse, removal from specific labor sites, transfer to different owners, and exercise of the right to self-purchase. In these cases, enslaved people constructed their own understandings of disability by engaging discourses of value and commodification, by challenging their positions within slavery, and by drawing on the protections that Spanish colonial law afforded.

Court cases of these two kinds prompt questions about how disability operated in the social world and economic relations of both urban and rural slavery in colonial Peru. Focusing largely on civil cases from Lima from the eighteenth and early nineteenth centuries, a period that witnessed a surge in civil litigation initiated by enslaved people, this chapter not only reconstructs how the violence of slavery created actual disability and exacerbated existing disabilities among the city's enslaved, but also analyzes how enslaved people and others invoked that violence in constructing understandings of what we would call ability and disability, deploying such allegations strategically for specific ends.[4] It juxtaposes the testimony of the enslaved as recorded by their notaries and procurators with that of family members, slaveholders, and the city's surgeons and physicians, who often testified as experts on the health of enslaved people and their suitability for work. In doing so, it provides a social and cultural history of disability on Peru's coast and the obligations that free and enslaved members of colonial society believed they had to each other.

In pursuing these goals, this chapter benefits not just from Michelle McKinley's and Linda Newson and Susie Minchin's research using redhibitory cases and other litigation involving enslaved people from Lima,[5] but also from Frank Trey Proctor III's research on Lima's enslaved litigants and their accusations against their owners.[6] It takes broader inspiration from Bianca Premo's comparative analysis of civil cases involving the enslaved in Lima and other parts of the Spanish Empire. Premo demonstrates how enslaved people transformed Iberian law and concepts of freedom through litigation in the eighteenth century, arguing that they brought a "process of becoming into the Spanish American courts" and posited, "through their petitions and legal initiatives, that they were becoming free."[7] This chapter asks how enslaved people's claims of what we would call disability and debility, often supported by family members' and healers' testimony, and demands of protection and care fit into these processes of navigating and transforming legal channels and pursuing greater forms of freedom. How did placing obligations on slaveholders to provide treatment, limit their exploitation, or allow sale to a new owner, for example, shape ideas about the rights of the disabled enslaved? How did these obligations, along with practices of protection and care among enslaved people and their kin, shape ideas about disabled enslaved personhood? Notably, by focusing not just on slaveholders but also on enslaved litigants, notaries, procurators, family members, and healers, this chapter argues that civil cases gave rise to an idea of disability based not on the liberal notion of universal rights that informs our modern understanding, but rather on enslaved people's claims to centuries-old legal principles that recognized forms of corporate status based on vulnerability, exclusion, and suffering that under Spanish law could warrant and require protection. Rooted in medieval and early modern Iberian law and its gradual evolution, this emerging concept of disability preceded the rise of definitions of disability linked to nineteenth-century industrial workplace legislation and workers' protections and rights, which dominate the historiography today.[8] Its earlier emergence is a consequence of the mobilization of law by enslaved people with disabilities against their masters.[9]

A Note About the Term "Disability" and the Violence of Slavery

To engage these civil cases, it is important to consider broadly what would count as "disability" in the late colonial period. While terms like *lisiado* and *imposibilitado*, which we would now consider potentially offensive and would translate as "disabled" or "incapacitated," appear occasionally in litigation from eighteenth- and early-nineteenth-century Lima, they did not have the same power and connotations as stable legal categories that "disability" has today, nor did they serve as the dominant terms by which enslaved litigants and their kin made claims about themselves and their suffering; for their part, owners, physicians, and surgeons employed the terms inconsistently. My work is thus attentive to the varied lexicon through which historical actors described the "complex embodiment"[10] of disability and communicated forms of both disability and disablement, with the latter term referring to the processes of overwork, deprivation, and violence by which one was rendered disabled, sometimes intentionally.[11] Through my own grappling with archival sources, I concur with Dea Boster, Stefanie Hunt-Kennedy,

Barclay, and others that one must think expansively about what constituted disability in specific historical contexts during the early modern period and the nineteenth century, rather than simply projecting narrower understandings from the present onto the past.[12] Disability could include physical injuries and congenital traits, but it could also include behaviors like flight and drunkenness. Incurable maladies, including diseases of poverty, malnutrition, and sexual contact that were common in eighteenth-century Lima and elsewhere, also counted.[13] In some cases, enslaved peoples' bodies were simply described as worn out due to the effects of a hard life. For their part, enslaved people claimed such conditions in order to make demands of their owners in court, petition for the provision of care for themselves and their loved ones, and secure greater forms of freedom. By rejecting the "commonplaceness of disability" and drawing on the medical knowledge of physicians and surgeons as well as the testimony of their neighbors and fellow enslaved people,[14] they collaborated with notaries and procurators to shape how disability would operate within late colonial Spanish law.[15]

About the depictions of violence that appear in civil litigation involving enslaved people who were sick or disabled: In recent years, scholars have rightly questioned the ethics, purpose, and consequences of reproducing in academic writing the violence found in the archives of slavery, arguing that to do so reinscribes that violence while doing little to capture the world-making of the enslaved themselves or to reconstruct or foreground their own voices. Several scholars have problematized this issue of depiction and narration in relation to the broader silences of the archive.[16] I take these cautions seriously, but ultimately have decided to include depictions of violence in my analysis. I do so because enslaved litigants and their kin deliberately drew attention to such violence as part of a strategy to change their circumstances by making their suffering known and visible. In vivid descriptions and evidence of abuse and neglect, they found tools to secure greater freedoms and, they hoped, bring their processes of world-making to fruition. In this sense, I do not narrate violence inflicted on enslaved people whom the archive has silenced or rendered voiceless. Rather, I reconstruct how enslaved people used their own voices, though filtered by notaries, procurators, and scribes who recorded and modified their testimony, to emphasize how the violence inflicted on them created and exacerbated disabilities and ultimately constituted cause for judicial intervention on their behalf. Enslaved people made the violence carried out against them productive in ways that contravened its original purpose, narrating it and exhibiting its physical consequences on their bodies in order to place limits on their owners' power.[17]

Slaveholders, Disability, and Value in Cases of Redhibition

How did slaveholders think about and contest disability in eighteenth- and early-nineteenth-century Lima? To answer this question, it should be noted that Spanish colonial law was far from static. While largely based on the Siete Partidas, a medieval legal code dating back to the thirteenth century, the system itself was malleable and adaptable, and legal reasoning changed in response to the circumstances of Spanish colonization and the development of colonial societies in the Americas after 1492.[18] In this context, concepts like Blackness and slavery came to occupy meanings and legal space that went beyond what was established in the Siete Partidas. New concepts like "Indian" (for Indigenous peoples of the Americas), which did not exist at the time of the Siete Partidas' drafting, also changed over the colonial period, signifying a race in addition to a status. Terms like *lisiado* or *imposibilitado* also shifted meanings and in usage in Spanish colonial law, especially during the eighteenth century. Owners of enslaved peoples participated in this process of change through their lawsuits with one another, which focused on questions of value and productivity.

In redhibitory cases, the purchaser of an enslaved person typically sought to annul a transaction or secure the partial return of a payment already made for an enslaved person, reasoning that the seller and previous owner had failed to disclose the person's *tachas y defectos*, or "blemishes and defects," as required. The buyer alleged that by failing to make clear the enslaved person's limitations prior to completing the transaction, the seller had deceived the purchaser, charging a price that exceeded the enslaved person's actual value based on their ability to labor productively. According to this reasoning, the enslaved could not provide a reasonable return on the investment the owner had made. Owners sometimes invested in treatments when there was hope of maintaining or improving the enslaved workers' ability to labor; these treatments then served as evidence. That said, some owners went so far as to claim that the enslaved person was unable to work at all, constituting a financial burden and a responsibility that the previous owner had shirked. In this sense, they occupied a position similar to that of a "chargeable" in the US antebellum South; the cost of maintaining them exceeded any profit to be gained from them.[19] Sellers, on the other hand, denied the existence of physical or behavioral impediments to work, at least at the time of sale. In this sense, ability and disability became fundamentally linked to labor, and disability became a problem in that it disrupted the commodification and exploitation of enslaved people's bodies.[20]

The 1712 case of Luisa de Chávez illustrates how slaveholders contested the transaction of their property and questions of value. Representing his sister, doña María de Aguiar, Friar Nicolás de Aguiar took Chávez's former owner, Luis de Zegarra, to court to demand that he return the 500 pesos doña María had paid for her. Friar Nicolás alleged that about two months after the purchase had been completed, Chávez suffered "a great shedding of blood, and since it appeared to said woman, my sister, that it was the menses [*costumbre*] that ordinarily flows from women, she did not provide care. But the persistence of said affliction [*accidente*] obliged her to examine the origin from which it came, and it was found that she had in her belly an old and dangerous mass [*bulto*], according to the medics who examined her." The origin of this bulto, or tumor, was unclear but "all of them assured us that it presented a risk." This led Friar Nicolás to assert that "don Luis concealed the vice and defect from which said black woman suffered." He demanded that the contract be annulled.[21]

Friar Nicolás pushed for the annulment because, he reasoned, given the presence of the tumor, Chávez, at forty-five years old, was not even worth 40 percent of what had been paid to purchase her. In this way, his central concern was whether Chávez's condition impeded her ability to work and thus prevented her commodification. He argued that she "was not worth 200 pesos, not any half-wit [*hombre de mediano juicio*] would give that amount." He would not even have paid 100 pesos, "since one purchases the slave so that she can serve in domestic tasks, and she is unable to do so due to said affliction." For these reasons, he suggested, "one [thus] sees that [doña María] was most enormously harmed in having given such an exorbitant sum for her, given that she is not useful." Friar Nicolás asserted, furthermore, that Luisa's former owner had deliberately deceived doña María. Knowing of her illness, he "sold [Luisa] to [doña María] assuring her that she was one of the best slaves that there was in said city."[22]

Such ways of thinking about health, disability, value, and commodification persisted across the eighteenth century among slaveholders, as the 1781 redhibitory case of Rosa Ramona demonstrates. Doña Bernardina Losada took to court the executor of doña María Dávila's estate, don Agustín de los

Ríos, after having purchased Ramona from the estate for 350 pesos. Losada claimed to have been assured that "the slave mentioned was capable of being used for her service, and was well and healthy and free of the vices and defects that have [since] been discovered." Ramona, however, allegedly sought to continue working in the streets earning *jornal*, or wages, "so that her vices would not be discovered." Particularly in urban slavery in Peru, this arrangement, in which masters allowed enslaved people to work as *jornaleros* (journeymen), laboring for others on the condition that they hand over a large portion of their earnings, was common. Having searched for her after she failed to provide payments, Losada found her "sick, afflicted throughout [*traspasado*] with syphilis [*gálico*], the effects of which have been allowed to persist on an arm that is crippled." Hoping to secure treatment for her, Losada placed her "in the Hospital of San Bartolomé, where today she is found, almost without remedy, due to the painfulness of the injury."[23]

Ramona, however, not only suffered from a disabling physical condition but also exhibited behaviors that allegedly further reduced her productivity. Losada saw these, too, as impediments to her commodification, claiming that "the black woman mentioned suffers from the vices of being a drunk and a runaway [*cimarrona*], and all in all there is no blemish or defect that she does not have." For these reasons, Losada went back to Ramona's previous owner's executor, de los Ríos, but he claimed to no longer have the money. She nevertheless pleaded in her petition that the contract of sale be annulled and the money returned, emphasizing that "I am an unhappy poor woman weighed down with jobs, who had to sell the few assets I had in order to pull that amount of money together."[24]

In her own testimony, however, Ramona sought to influence the outcome by confirming the allegations that diminished her value. In doing so, she demonstrated that while redhibitory cases sought to reduce enslaved people to commodified bodies, the enslaved could participate in them in ways that reflected their strategies for navigating and shaping the terms of their subjugation. Ramona confirmed via the scribe that before Losada purchased her, she was already suffering "from the pain in her hand while under the authority of her previous owner, doña María Dávila." Once her sale to Losada had been completed, however, she sought to conceal her health problems "with the motive of not being in doña Bernardina's house, but rather in the street." This changed, however, about seven months later when Losada summoned her to pay *jornales*. Since Ramona could not pay them in full, her scribe wrote, "they put her at a trough [*batea*] to do washing. The pain in her hand came to be discovered because the declarant could no longer hide it." Once the injury was discovered, Losada sent her to the Hospital of San Bartolomé, "where she has been attended to carefully, without having been able to achieve her health." Moreover, while Ramona claimed to have fled multiple times during the period she was owned by Losada, and while she admitted to drinking, she denied engaging in excess. Her scribe noted that "with regard to the vice of drunkenness, she claims that although she has had her drinks of *aguardiente*, she has never done so to the point of losing her senses." In this sense, Ramona invoked and confirmed her physical and behavioral traits with the hope of being freed from her current owner, potentially resulting in better circumstances for her as an enslaved person.[25]

Enslaved Litigants, Disability, and Masters' Obligations

As can be seen in the previous section, enslaved people found ways in redhibitory cases to shape perceptions of their "tachas y defectos." In doing so, they sought to move beyond slaveholders' concerns about commodification and productivity and impress on authorities their owners' failure to take seriously their needs and disabilities. Litigation initiated by the enslaved, however, provided more favorable opportunities for making such demands than redhibitory cases did. Mentioned at the start of this chapter, Tirado provides one example, but he was far from alone in claiming what we would call disability and litigating against his owner in pursuit of fractional freedoms. He built on a long tradition of enslaved people contesting their subjugation over the course of the previous century as well as earlier.

The legal strategies that enslaved people employed resulted in the articulation of concepts of disability that built on, but also diverged from, those that slaveholders invoked in redhibitory cases. Rather than speak of disability only in terms of commodification, enslaved people built on such frameworks but also characterized their physical characteristics, infirmities, behaviors, and suffering in ways that highlighted their need for protection under early modern legal principles. Likewise, they sought to reinforce the obligations of their owners, emphasizing disability as a state that required the provision of care, and they in some cases sought the testimony of expert healers to bolster their claims.

This section analyzes the legal arguments of enslaved people and their notaries and procurators that instantiated disability as a category in Spanish colonial law. As a legal strategy, enslaved litigants with disabilities often claimed to have been rendered *miserables* (wretches), those whose vulnerability and destitution necessitated the intervention of the Spanish Crown. *Miseria* (wretchedness) was a long-standing category in medieval and early modern Spanish law, and its use over the course of the colonial period expanded to encompass various populations, including people with disabilities. Claims to miseria were often grounded in accusations that masters had practiced *sevicia* (cruelty) against their enslaved property. Sevicia could take the form of inappropriate labor demands, violence, or abuse, but it could also take the form of neglect, the refusal to provide for the enslaved person's basic needs.[26] In both cases, enslaved litigants linked *sevicia* to resulting disabilities. Fearing their master's wrath, some also sought *amparo*, the Crown's protection in the form of separation and placement in a location the master could not reach.[27] In doing so, they made the case that the Crown had distinct obligations toward those living with disabilities.

This section highlights the actions of three enslaved litigants, Francisco de Rojas, Plácida Laines, and María Josefa Lavalle, in order to explore those legal strategies. In addition, it examines how these litigants and their advocates utilized themes of piety and obligation and sought healers' expertise to further their claims.

Francisco de Rojas

Among the many who appear in Peru's National Archives, Francisco de Rojas exemplifies the practice of seeking the protection of the courts especially well. A creole enslaved man from Lambayeque in the Corregimiento of Zaña, on Peru's north coast, Francisco was nicknamed "el Tullido," or "the Lame," at a young age because, according to the recorder of his initial request, he "was born from the belly of his mother lame and he can barely walk, as one sees, with his backside." In legal correspondence that began in 1774, Francisco claimed and invoked this very identity, describing himself as "crippled in both feet without being able to use them for any exercise or bodily work." When Francisco reached age sixteen, his owner, don Pedro de Rojas, nevertheless required that Francisco begin paying him a jornal, or a portion of his wages, amounting to two reales per day, or eight pesos per month. Since Francisco could not work, he gathered the money for these payments by begging and seeking alms, "which piety allows me [to attain], since if I do not do so [don Pedro] punishes me until causing me to bleed."[28]

Don Pedro was a priest, but his behavior was far from Christian. Indeed, Francisco's strategy and that of those involved in his legal case was to characterize don Pedro as straying from the values of a cleric in his treatment of his disabled property. He alleged that don Pedro neglected his obligations as a master, lacked pity, made excessive demands, and acted abusively in ways that amounted to sevicia. He even refused to make exceptions for religious holidays when calculating jornal obligations, and he punished Francisco severely for failing to make payments for those days. According to his petition, after Francisco refused to provide the corresponding jornal, don Pedro "took him to the *tira* [place of punishment], which belongs to Licenciado don José Manuel de Ripalda, and there they put him in the stocks and punished him, giving him fifty lashes from the hand of another *moreno* [Black man]." In this way, the petition accused don Pedro of brutally punishing Francisco, determined to profit from his investment despite the enslaved man's inability to work.[29]

Beyond the owner's use of violence, Francisco and his legal advocates portrayed don Pedro as failing to fulfill his obligations as a master and a Christian in other ways as well. Among other accusations, they alleged that don Pedro refused to provide for Francisco's most basic necessities. Don Pedro would not feed him or supply him with clothing "as all the neighbors of the village can report, likewise there are witnesses here [in Trujillo] who can declare it." This was the case even though Francisco had helped amass funds for this purpose. While Francisco had gathered money "in the crowds with the intention of buying myself things to wear," he claimed that once handed over to don Pedro, the priest "never ended up verifying that with this money he would buy me a shirt, or a coat, since it was necessary, that I ask for them [from others] out of charity."[30]

Francisco, however, was not the only person who observed don Pedro's un-Christian behavior and cited it to further the enslaved man's journey toward freedom and protection. The scale of sevicia inflicted on Francisco in the form of punishments ultimately led another priest, don Matías de Soto, to take pity on Francisco and seek to transform his circumstances. According to Francisco's petition, having brought Francisco to his own home to provide refuge, don Matías allegedly offered to pay don Pedro 50 pesos "to give [Francisco] freedom out of God's charity." Don Pedro initially agreed but later changed his mind, capturing Francisco when he left don Matías's home and returning him to the tira. There, the scale of abuse allegedly escalated, with don Pedro determined to dissuade Francisco from seeking a new owner. According to Francisco's petition, "They put him in the stocks and punished him, giving him fifty lashes even though the supplicant had welts on his rear. The welts burst open from the lashes, and upon seeing this, the major-domo said to [don Pedro], 'look at the blood flowing.'" Don Pedro, however, rejected the majordomo's concerns and exhibited little more than disdain, allegedly saying, "Leave him there to die, for having been a friend of seeking freedom."[31]

Working most likely with his procurator in developing this account, Francisco positioned don Matías as a model of piety while characterizing don Pedro as dismissing Francisco's life as worthless and ordering punishment inflicted on the specific part of his body that had been the locus of his disability since birth. Since Francisco was disabled and sought freedom, don Pedro's reasoning went, he deserved punishment. According to the scribe, don Pedro then sought to further hinder Francisco's mobility to prevent his escape, writing that "they put a *corma* [wooden clamp] so heavy on the supplicant that it barely let him move." Francisco, however, broke the lock on the corma and fled from Lambayeque to Trujillo, where he appealed to the bishop's compassion for help. Noting that "my master is a priest and the ecclesiastical judge in Lambayeque is his friend," Francisco declared that he had traveled to Trujillo "so that in attending to the evidence of cruelty that I have exposed, your Illustriousness might oblige [don Pedro] to receive the money corresponding to my value." The bishop, however, claimed he lacked the authority to force Francisco's owner to receive the money and approve the sale. Francisco therefore proceeded on to Lima and appealed to the Real Audiencia, asking for protection and assistance as a "miserable" in light of "the circumstances of oppression from which I suffer."[32]

For his part, Don Pedro's legal representative in the case, don Bernardo Durán y Meza, adopted a strategy common in such cases. Rather than defend don Pedro's piety, he sought to malign Francisco's character and insist on his ability to work in spite of his disability. He depicted Francisco as being "of perverse inclinations" and noted that "had he not found himself impeded by nature, he would have been the most villainous bandit of that province." Moreover, Durán y Meza claimed that "despite his bodily defect, [Francisco] has frequent quarrels with all classes of people, and he has been accused before the law various times of blows and wounds, which he has inflicted with his legs and other instruments on diverse people." Durán y Meza reasoned that Francisco could in fact work, declaring that "when he flees, he applies himself to earning jornal by grinding sugar and cacao, grinding corn for chicha, cooking, and whatever other exercise it may be, because he has no other impediment than being unable to walk straight with his feet." In this sense, Durán y Meza alleged that Francisco could be made productive.[33]

Speaking on don Pedro's behalf, Durán y Meza also complained of Francisco's tendency to flee, arguing that this was a greater hindrance to fulfilling his value as a slave than his physical disability. In this sense, from the master's perspective flight was the true disability, not the physical traits with which he was born and that prevented him from working. He argued that simply declaring the absence of abuse and returning Francisco to don Pedro's custody "would have no effect, because said Francisco would frustrate me by fleeing, to which he is accustomed, in the same way that he did to come here from Lambayeque, and he would proceed on, to where they have no news of him." He feared that Francisco would end up so far away "that the cost of his return would be greater than what he is worth." He argued that, as it was not just that he litigate while Francisco "lives in abandonment, at risk of committing crime atrociously in accordance with his evil propensity, and of getting lost," the authorities should "return him to me to put him back, under the guarantee that I offer of not offending him, and of feeding him, as always." If it was not immediately possible to return Francisco to don Pedro, Durán y Meza requested that "for now, may he be placed in the hospital where he is subject to the majordomo, and detained, serving the poor sick, until the case is resolved."[34]

An initial ruling came from the *oidores* (judges) of the Real Audiencia on June 1, 1774. In it, Francisco's wishes were not granted, but neither were don Pedro's *sevicia*, abuse, and impious behavior dismissed. Rather, Francisco was ordered to be returned to his owner, but "under the guarantee that [don Pedro] offers of his good treatment, and of not punishing him." In addition, Francisco could not be removed from Lima, and "in case he becomes sick, he will be put in the Hospital of San Bartolomé for his recovery, without loss of the protection put before the referenced slave." The oidores ordered don Pedro to treat Francisco well, "not removing him from this city, and leaving him free so that he may make use of his right, as it is more widely known." In contesting this decision, however, Francisco requested a new procurator to represent him, who then asked that "considering (and attending to) the disease on which my client is found to be sick, and lame, and inept for all service, he be granted freedom." This request was based on Francisco's vulnerability and need of protection, and it resulted in a final decision issued on September 2, 1774. While the terms of the decision remained the same, it furthered the construction of an idea of the disabled as worthy of the audiencia's consideration and intervention.[35]

Plácida Laines

Whereas Francisco de Rojas's legal strategies in pursuit of fractional freedoms centered on his owner's sevicia in the form of inappropriate labor demands, violence, abuse, and absence of piety, and while his petitions took the form of appeals for compassion and protection, Plácida Laines's strategies rested on her owner's sevicia in the form of neglect and his obligations in light of her perilous state of health. Laines initiated a case against her owner, don José Inclán, in November 1799. She claimed urgently that, "finding myself gravely injured and with ongoing diseases, the aforementioned my master has disregarded [*descascarado*] the causes, abandoning [not treating] them principally to avoid their costs, which is why I have not achieved the health I so longed for." She added that while Inclán had granted her permission to find a new owner, he had also threatened, should she fail to find one, to send her to the highlands, "where I understand my death will be certain." Fearing his indignation, she sought to shield herself from him by hiding while asking that he be made to fulfill his duties. Describing herself as a "defenseless person," and noting that "my state of fugitivity increases the dangers to my life during the peak of my illnesses," she appealed "to the compassion of Your Honor so that my master might be reduced to what dominion obliges him out of charity."[36]

As part of a legal strategy, Laines and those assisting her boldly asserted that, given her grave condition and in accordance with what the law provided, she could in fact put forth a request that she be declared free. She could then document her condition and seek treatment in the hospital that corresponded to her status. Instead, however, she opted to work strategically within the system of slavery, claiming that "I aspire only to the relief of my health right away, and to a robust recovery in order to please my master in what he orders of me." She asked the ecclesiastical judge to prevent her owner from selling her outside Lima and to order him to provide her with "the radical treatment that I need, continuing it until I am fully recovered, without him demanding service of me in the meantime when I am not in full health." In this sense, she worked to seek the Crown's protection, building on the concept of amparo.[37]

Laines's demands, however, expanded over the remaining weeks of 1799, building on earlier actions taken. In early December, she and those advocating for her submitted a second petition, in which she referred to asking for a "reduction in price, considering my notorious and ongoing illness in my person." In this sense, Laines played against Inclán's and other slaveowners' considerations of value and productivity in relation to worsening illness, emphasizing the disabling effects of the maladies from which she suffered. Noting that Inclán had already been informed of her request, she asked that he be notified again, lamenting that "each day, sir, I deteriorate further, given that my ongoing illnesses are putting me in the most deplorable state one can imagine, and there is nobody who would pay 100 pesos for me."[38]

In his response and drawing on others' testimony, Inclán sought to prove that Laines was not stating her motives truthfully and that she had long denied him revenue to which he was entitled. Working through his own legal representative, he rested his defense on downplaying Laines's debilities and claiming that she engaged in inappropriate conduct as an enslaved person, making him, as her owner, the true victim. He argued that she sought "food, treatments, or better said—libertinage," and he summoned witnesses to confirm this. Manuel Pacheco, for example, testified that "libertinage, embezzlement, and willfulness" characterized her behavior, and he asserted that during the period in which she had been Inclán's property, "she has not satisfied jornal payments, and to the contrary has caused her master, *licenciado* Ynclán [*sic*], infinite losses." On the question of embezzlement, Pacheco added that at a *masamorrería* (food shop), where she worked, Laines "rebelled with the principal and the earnings, for which it was still necessary to pay for her for the consecutive months in the shop." Following this episode, he alleged, jornales became "a drug for her, and she has lived as if she were free." Similarly, Joaquín Marcelo described her as being "of a vagabond and dissolute life" and as "of bad skill and conduct: [one] who has not satisfied her jornales for her master, and for whom everything has been a drug." Manuel Muñoz added that "from what has been presented, he has believed that her perditions are worthy of the greatest punishment."[39]

Together, these witnesses suggested that rebelliousness was Laines's true disability, in that it prevented her commodification. Additional documentation from previous years indicated that Laines had indeed lived independently of Inclán for some time and that she had claimed to be married, when she was in fact single, to prevent being sold outside Lima. Claiming that Laines "lives according to her whim and spontaneous willfulness" and that due to her malice Inclán "lacks her service and the jornal payments she should contribute to me," Inclán's legal representative submitted an additional petition in February 1800 to impose limits on her mobility. Through him, Inclán asked that "you might order that the aforementioned slave be placed in a casa de abasto, until her sale is brought about, and avoid in this way the losses that can result for me in relation to her value." The legal representative then submitted an additional petition in mid-February 1800, responding to Laines's actions "regarding demanding treatments from me" for her infirmities. Casting doubt on her behavior and invoking his own sense of piety, Inclán asked, "What slave doesn't recognize subordination to their master? Plácida, who has never once given me jornal payments, who has lived extravagantly [*exóticamente*] without acknowledging her servitude. My kindness has kept me from capturing her, using the corresponding leniency so that forgetting the feelings of a priest, I try to secure my money and avoid infinite guilt before God, which cannot be allowed."[40]

Laines responded to her owner's criticisms by citing and emphasizing his obligations. She asserted that while she had indeed misbehaved, it was nevertheless his responsibility to offer assistance to cure her once she became sick and debilitated. Describing herself as suffering "the totality of ongoing maladies that draw me closer to the grave," and noting that her owner had defamed her character in previous testimony, Laines argued:

> All my master has alleged in order to make use of his power, is that I am bad, prone to vice, and licentious. I concur that it is all true, but if I was once bad, now I am a valetudinarian sick woman. Back then I deserved correction, and now, with as much as I have suffered, I need curing and attending to, and for my master to cover the cost. This was not the time to prove that I was bad, but rather that I was good and healthy. He has said nothing about my health, and his silence is the confession of what impedes me.

Pushing for either the improvement of her health or her own freedom, Laines added:

> The sick slave should be cured, and to not do so matters as a form of abandonment which the law compensates with freedom. A radical cure or freedom is the

choice of the day. I press and clamor for or one or the other, because having hidden for so long for fear of being apprehended and sold in the highlands, I neither go outside for fresh air, nor exercise, which worsens my dropsy and obstruction, nor do I hear mass, nor do anything other than be consumed with hypochondria.[41]

Laines, however, did not reject the system of slavery itself, even as her demands escalated and she doubled down on accusations of neglect. She argued that the ecclesiastical judge should protect her by refusing, for now, "to allow the exercise of dominion that I confess, I recognize." At the same time, she suggested, using the language of medicine and cures, that since it was "the master's duty to attend to and treat the diseases of the slave," the ecclesiastical judge should "order that I be examined with a summons to my master, and via the experts that you name, so that they may report, and certify, my sick state, and with what results from my grave affliction." Once completed, her master should be "notified to either place me under treatment in the hospitals of this city or leave me free to seek my own assistance, and travel [*haser exercicio*] on foot, and on horseback [*a bestia*], which is the medicine that will benefit me most." Reversing the typical obligations between enslaved person and master, she argued that this arrangement should take place "with the mere charge of giving me a daily real and continuing it until I am healthy, and strong, and can serve my master and give him jornal payments if it suits him more." Laines warned, moreover, that if Inclán were to provide for her in terms of treatments and time, and "wait for me to recover and convalesce, [then] he will see his money; should he not do so, prepare for my burial and entrust me to God. For I have expressed all of this and other favorable things here, negating and contradicting the harmful."[42] In this way, describing herself as debilitated by illness and a victim of sevicia in the form of neglect, Laines sought, in essence, to exert her own will over her master, conveying in vivid terms the stakes involved in either fulfilling his obligations toward her or granting her greater forms of freedom.

María Josefa Lavalle

Like Rojas and Laines, María Josefa Lavalle strategically navigated the courts to push for the improvement of her condition based on claims of disability resulting from illness, violence, and neglect. To an even greater extent than her fellow litigants, however, Lavalle centered the language of medicine and succeeded in her efforts to secure the testimony of an expert healer to further her case. The resulting records thus provide insight into how both enslaved people and healers negotiated emerging concepts of disability in late colonial Lima.

Lavalle, an enslaved woman described as a *"mulata achinada clara,"* or lighter-skinned woman of African and Spanish descent, litigated against her owner, doña Teresa Pacheco between December 3, 1803, and September 9, 1805. Having claimed for years to be too weak to work on her behalf, Lavalle accused Pacheco, the wife of the colony's *protomédico* (chief medical examiner), Juan José de Aguirre, of mistreating her and inflicting harm, further disabling her in the process. Refusing to acknowledge Lavalle's ill health, Pacheco denied that she had done anything wrong and countered that she was in fact herself the victim, having suffered the misfortune of owning a disobedient, dishonest, and unproductive slave. For this reason, and finding herself unable to sell Lavalle for a sufficient price, Pacheco claimed she had no other choice but to use bodily violence and confinement to enforce her will.[43]

According to the person who recorded Lavalle's initial petition and who was likely a notary, Lavalle claimed that she resembled a *"cadáver animado,"* or living corpse, and, in her accusation, suggested that Pacheco's use of punishment was excessive. He wrote that on one occasion Pacheco "cut, scratched, and mistreated her gravely as [Lavalle] is showing with the scratches on her arms, giving her cruel blows with the reasoning that [Lavalle] had asked for one real for firewood." Perhaps more important, however, the scribe framed such violence ironically using the language of cures. He wrote, for example, that when Lavalle initially asked Pacheco to seek treatments for her diminished eyesight and her prolapsed uterus, which along with other problems left her weak and made it difficult to stand and walk, "the cure she gave her was to put her in the kitchen for the first time, where the effort and work is quite difficult to do [even] for the good and healthy. . . . This was one of the medicines she applied."[44] The "second cure" was to lock Lavalle in a panadería named La Acequia Alta for one year, followed by three years in another panadería known as Los Pericotes. After eventually negotiating with Lavalle to release her on the condition that she find a new owner to purchase her— something she was unable to do given her physical condition—Pacheco beat her cruelly. In this way, neglect to provide treatment turned into revenge and led to the infliction of disability, as Lavalle proved unable to "cure" herself through the principal duty of slaves: work.[45]

In her petition, Lavalle requested that the judge hearing her case order "that the said owner neither bother her for jornales, nor bother her person due to the incapacitated state [*imposibilidad*] in which she finds herself."[46] Eventually, she also asked to be inspected by a healer. Emphasizing her own suffering and seeking to further substantiate her claims of disability and discredit Pacheco, she strategically requested that José Manuel Valdés, a notable Latin surgeon in the city, examine her "and certify the state in which he finds me," believing his testimony would work in her favor.[47]

To a considerable degree, Valdés's diagnosis of Lavalle reflected a different understanding of disability and a different valuing of the enslaved woman's body and her capacity to work than those that her owner articulated, though he, like many other physicians and surgeons of the period, did not outright reject ideas about the commodification of enslaved peoples' bodies. There is little evidence to suggest that Valdés, a highly respected Afro-descendant surgeon in Lima, saw himself as an ally of enslaved people. Rather, he took such cases to further his status as a professional and an expert. He began by noting that he could not confirm allegations that Lavalle had consistently coughed up blood, since "that required a more extensive and repeated observation." However, he did note that she exhibited "a prolapse of the uterus so considerable that she has the womb outside the vulva." Furthermore, he found that she had a cataract forming in her left eye, which like the prolapsed uterus was absolutely incurable "not just due to its nature, but also due to [Lavalle's] age and reduced strength." He believed she would eventually go blind in both eyes. Given both of these conditions, he judged her "incapable of any kind of work," thus engaging Pacheco's focus on labor while refuting her view that Lavalle could still be productive. His diagnoses led the judge hearing the case to acknowledge Lavalle's condition and grant her request that she be freed from the panadería.[48]

In making his diagnosis, Valdés furthered Lavalle's journey toward greater forms of fractional freedom through her claims of disability and disablement, responding to her own demands in her petitions that she be granted protection. While Pacheco largely disregarded Lavalle's suffering and refused to address her bodily debilities seriously, Valdés spoke of the severity of her conditions and the inability of medicine to restore her health fully. While Pacheco spoke of a lost investment and the need to confine Lavalle to panaderías to ensure her productivity, Valdés spoke of Lavalle's well-being and incapacity for work without taking a clear position regarding sevicia, the cruelty, neglect, and mistreatment she suffered. In doing so, and at Lavalle's urging, Valdés evaluated the enslaved woman's body and testified about its disabilities using Pacheco's, and other slaveholders', own language of labor and usefulness. He furthered Lavalle's efforts to seek protection from her owner but did so by drawing on frameworks employed by Pacheco and other slave owners, who viewed enslaved people as lacking any value beyond their ability to generate revenue. While Teresa Pacheco provided testimony to reinforce her power to make use of Lavalle's body for her own gain, she ultimately failed to have her way. Instead, Lavalle crafted a successful claim of disability, most likely with the help of a procurator, and solicited the medical expertise of a respected healer to support it.[49]

Family Litigants, Disability, and Care

The aforementioned cases form part of a late colonial surge in litigation by enslaved individuals who advocated on their own behalf with the help of notaries and procurators and sought the courts' intervention to place limits on their masters. In many cases, however, litigation involved larger kin networks. As Barclay notes for the US antebellum South, "The presence of disability produced distinct social relations and power dynamics that played out in [enslaved people's] families, communities, and interactions with whites."[50] In Peru, the justice system recognized family relations and allowed family members to petition on behalf of enslaved kin who had been disabled, had fallen sick, or were otherwise rendered unable to work. In many of these cases, parents, spouses, and others pursued fractional freedoms by following strategies similar to those that individual enslaved litigants employed, emphasizing miseria, sevicia, and amparo.

Manuel de Aguirre's petition to the courts in 1795 on behalf of his wife, Petronila Rosa Gutiérrez, exemplifies this pattern. Gutiérrez had suffered for five years from problems "in her eyes, in which she has two large clouds and is completely blind in one and almost blind in the other, since she only sees shapes." Accusing Petronila's owner, María del Carmen Gutiérrez, of neglect, Aguirre complained that she "has not spent even a real in treating her, and has had the conscience to receive eight pesos of jornal during all of this lengthy time." Aguirre further claimed that even though he made his wife's jornal payments, "for I love and esteem my wife so much," María del Carmen

Gutiérrez had decided to separate them and confine him "with the goal that I would not see my wife." This cruelty, he asserted, would cause "most grave harm, both due to not being able to console my wife and because the unhappy woman has no other refuge than my protection and my personal labor." Seeking to prevent this separation, he argued that "it is of supreme hatred and great tyranny for this woman [her owner] to behave with extreme cruelty, wishing to divorce us as if she had the powers that reside in your honor."[51]

The case of an enslaved woman named Quitería in 1785 further illustrates how kin used the courts, basing their claims on notions of suffering, neglect, and obligation. Quitería's husband, Ramón Rivera, sought to have a physician sent to the panadería where Quitería was confined and had become ill. He requested that "once my wife, Quitería, is examined by a professor of medicine in the panadería where she is found, and once her illness is confirmed, may she be released from that imprisonment so that she can be given medicine." He found it difficult, however, to secure help for her, because neither her new owner nor her former owner would acknowledge her as their property; one claimed the sale had been annulled, while the other considered it valid. Rivera complained that "in the meantime my wife is blamed and suffers, and at the same time the illness causing her to cough up blood worsens."[52]

Hermenegilda Morales, on the other hand, provides an example of how enslaved people used accusations of deliberate cruelty to advocate for their kin. Morales litigated against Josefa Estacio, the owner of her husband, José de Jesús, to prevent her from selling him outside Lima, "separating him from the conjugal union, which we have maintained with such bondedness for so many years." Noting that "the separation is of the greatest severity," she requested that Miguel Cavello, the owner of the panadería in which José was confined, under "no title nor pretext place him at the disposition of his mistress without her first justifying before your honor the reasons that require of him such a painful separation." In other words, and perhaps counterintuitively, Morales actually sought to keep her husband imprisoned in the panadería so that he could not be taken away from her.[53]

Family members also used claims of suffering to force the purchase and sale of their disabled kin. For example, an enslaved woman named María de la Natividad was described in a *boleta de venta* (sales ticket) from 1764 as being offered for purchase "without guaranteeing that she is without any vices or illnesses, [and] with the declaration that she has suffered from marks [*manchas*] all over her body." For these reasons, "a redhibitory case may not be brought," but Natividad was nevertheless sold for 300 pesos. According to her owner, María Josefa Negreiros, María de la Natividad suffered from "syphilitic rashes" (*manchas galicosas*). Moreover, according to an accompanying petition, "after the affliction [*accidente*] is examined, those who want to purchase her refuse, and they only offer the 300 pesos referenced that her mistress excuses herself from receiving." For Natividad, these visual disfigurements and her failure to generate an adequate price had prompted "the revenge of said masters," who treated her cruelly. In response, Natividad's mother, Juana María Ibáñez, sought in 1765 to force Negreiros to sell the enslaved woman on the grounds that she had been mistreated. In this way, kin coordinated with their enslaved family members to push for the fractional freedoms to which they believed they were entitled.[54]

Conclusion

Civil cases involving enslaved people as litigants and as objects of litigation shed light on the complex ways in which ideas about what we would call disability operated in late colonial Lima. As other scholars have shown, slavery itself produced disability in the bodies of the enslaved, and slaveowners and others normalized disablement and disability in many ways. At the same time, the enslaved themselves, slave owners, notaries, procurators, healers, kin, and ordinary residents of Lima constructed variegated ideas about disability and used legal channels to transform their positions within and in relation to the system of slavery. While slaveowners negotiated disability through the language of commodification, value, and productivity, enslaved people found opportunities by emphasizing their suffering, mistreatment, neglect, and debility. Invoking sevicia in this way afforded them protections in the courts through early modern legal principles of miseria and amparo, which centered questions of vulnerability, exclusion, difference, and the Crown's obligation to protect. Through this strategy and by soliciting the testimony of respected healers on whom slaveholders also relied, enslaved people placed limits on their owners, transformed their own lives, gained fractional freedoms, and rendered disability a condition that did not always result in exclusion or a lower social position but sometimes secured protections. Civil cases involving enslaved people and disability thus contributed to the construction of disability as a malleable legal category that was rooted in centuries-old legal principles and existed outside liberal notions of universal rights. It was one through which enslaved people could gradually move closer to freedom.

NOTES

1. Archivo Arzobispal de Lima (hereafter cited as AAL), Causas de Negros XXXV: 23, 1803.

2. "Fractional freedoms" refers to the specific and incremental forms of autonomy that enslaved people could attain through various strategies. Noting that most of the enslaved subjects and former slaves in her research lived in "a state of quasi-emancipation or conditional liberty," McKinley emphasizes the idea that all states of being fell along a spectrum between free and unfree. She argues that "contingent liberty (or fractional freedom) was the reality that all—whether enslaved, freed, or free—accepted and to which they accommodated their lives. Neither total bodily autonomy nor absolute bondage was the norm for most enslaved peoples in Lima during this period." Michelle McKinley, *Fractional Freedoms: Slavery, Intimacy, and Legal Mobilization in Colonial Lima, 1600–1700* (Cambridge University Press, 2016), 11.

3. Jenifer L. Barclay, *The Mark of Slavery: Disability, Race, and Gender in Antebellum America* (University of Illinois Press, 2021), ch. 3.

4. For explanation of this surge in litigation, see Bianca Premo, *The Enlightenment on Trial: Ordinary Litigants and Colonialism in the Spanish Empire* (Oxford University Press, 2017).

5. McKinley, *Fractional Freedoms*; Linda Newson and Susie Minchin, *From Capture to Sale: The Portuguese Slave Trade to Spanish South America in the Early Seventeenth Century* (Brill, 2007).

6. Frank Trey Proctor III, "'Alien to My Sex': Enslaved Women and Their Gendered Notions of Abuse in Eighteenth-Century Peru," *Journal of Women's History* 31, no. 2 (2019): 57–79; Proctor, "An 'Imponderable Servitude': Slave Versus Master Litigation for Cruelty (*Maltratamiento* or *Sevicia*) in Late-Eighteenth-Century Lima, Peru," *Journal of Social History* 48, no. 3 (2015): 662–84.

7. Premo, *Enlightenment on Trial*, p. 223.

8. Stefanie Hunt-Kennedy similarly argues for the existence of a notion of disability in the British Empire that preceded nineteenth-century understandings and was rooted in slavery. See Hunt-Kennedy, *Between Fitness and Death: Disability and Slavery in the Caribbean* (University of Illinois Press, 2020).

9. Here I take inspiration from Catherine Kudlick's description of US disability history's focus on "a need to challenge the prevailing assumptions about disability, and the importance of granting people with disabilities historical agency"; Kudlick, "Comment: On the Borderland of Medical and Disability History," *Bulletin of the History of Medicine* 87, no. 4 (2013): 551.

10. On the concept of complex embodiment, Barclay writes that "[the array of conditions] show that disabling environments produced and affected 'people's lived experience of the body' while simultaneously acknowledging that 'some factors affecting

disability, such as pain, secondary health effects, and aging, derive[d] *from* the body.' For some enslaved people, the disabling conditions they experienced derived from their bodies and deeply affected their lived experiences under slavery, while for others the conditions of slavery impaired their bodies and gave rise to new and sometimes chronic experiences of disability." Barclay, *Mark of Slavery*, 16.

11. Here I use the term "disablement" as the act or experience of becoming disabled, in this context through the violence and overwork of slavery. I note that other scholars use this term to refer to the deliberate inflicting of disability in individuals, drawing on Neloufer de Mel's definition. Linking disablement to behavior in war zones, de Mel defines the term as "the deliberate, willful maiming of abled, physically strong" individuals. Applying the term outside war zones, I draw on Hunt-Kennedy's call to recognize "the violence inherent in slave societies." In doing so, I recognize a certain amount of ambiguity in slaveholders' intentions while noting that the structures and expectations of slavery were designed to inflict injury and wear down the bodies of the enslaved. Hunt-Kennedy, *Between Fitness and Death*, 9 (quoting De Mel).

12. Barclay, *Mark of Slavery*; Dea H. Boster, *African American Slavery and Disability: Bodies, Property, and Power in the Antebellum South, 1800–1860* (Routledge, 2013); Hunt-Kennedy, *Between Fitness and Death*.

13. Here I engage Beth Linker's call for scholarly attention to the "unhealthy disabled" in disability history. See Linker, "On the Borderlands of Medical and Disability History: A Survey of the Fields," *Bulletin of the History of Medicine* 87, no. 4 (2013): 526. Kudlick suggests that such studies might "take special note of the complex, porous boundaries between disease and disability to understand places where they overlap and where they conflict, not just in terms of diagnoses and definitions, but also in terms of how they play out experientially." Kudlick adds that when considering the role of chronic illness from a disability history perspective, "the issue has less to do with whether someone is 'healthy' or 'unhealthy' than with how discussions of health, pain, illness, and disability are framed in larger social, economic, political, and medical contexts. And of course we must always ask who is doing the framing, in which contexts, and why." Kudlick, "Comment," 554.

14. On the "commonplaceness of disability," Barclay notes that in the US South, "the institution of slavery produced unsound, impaired bodies, and an estimated 9 percent of the enslaved population . . . experienced their daily lives through these bodies." Barclay, *Mark of Slavery*, 9.

15. Drawing on Alison Kafer's argument that "seeing disability as political, and therefore contested and contestable, entails departing from the social model's assumption that 'disabled' and 'nondisabled' are discrete, self-evident categories," my work follows her call to "explore the creation of such categories and the moments in which they failed to hold. Recognizing such moments of excess or failure is key to imagining disability, and disability futures, differently." Kafer understands "the very meanings of 'disability,' 'impairment,' and 'disabled' as contested terrain." Kafer argues, moreover, that we should think about disability "not as a category inherent in certain minds and bodies but as what historian Joan W. Scott calls a 'collective affinity.'" For Scott (quoted here by Kafer), collective affinities "play on identifications that have been attributed to individuals by their societies,

and that have served to exclude them or subordinate them." This definition enables Kafer to consider "disability" and "disabled person" as terms for which the parameters are "always open to debate." Kafer, *Feminist, Queer, Crip* (Indiana University Press, 2013), 10, 11.

16. Many scholars have contributed to these debates. See, for example, Saidiya Hartman, *Scenes of Subjection: Terror, Slavery, and Self-Making in Nineteenth-Century America* (Oxford University Press, 2007); Hartman, "Venus in Two Acts," *Small Axe: A Journal of Criticism* 12, no. 2 (2008): 1–14; Marisa Fuentes, *Dispossessed Lives: Enslaved Women, Violence, and the Archive* (University of Pennsylvania Press, 2016); Michel-Rolph Trouillot, *Silencing the Past: Power and the Production of History* (Beacon Press, 2015).

17. For theorizing of violence in this manner, see Nicole Guidotti-Hernández, *Unspeakable Violence: Remapping U.S. and Mexican National Imaginaries* (Duke University Press, 2011).

18. Brian Owensby, *Empire of Law and Indian Justice in Colonial Mexico* (Stanford University Press, 2018); Premo, *Enlightenment on Trial*.

19. In the South, as Barclay explains, slaveholders considered enslaved people with disabilities "financially worthless and sometimes even 'chargeable'—meaning that the cost of their care was a financial liability." Barclay, "Mothering the 'Useless': Black Motherhood, Disability, and Slavery," *Women, Gender, and Families of Color* 2, no. 2 (2014): 117. For another discussion of the category "chargeable," see Barclay, *Mark of Slavery*, 22.

20. This discussion builds on Tobin Siebers focus on the "ideology of ability" and asks what that ideology looked like and how it functioned in a very different time and place. Siebers writes: "The ideology of ability is at its simplest the preference for able-bodiedness. At its most radical, it defines the baseline by which humanness is determined, setting the measure of body and mind that gives or denies human status to individual persons." Disability identity, Siebers argues, "stands in uneasy relationship to the ideology of ability, presenting a critical framework that disturbs and critiques it." Siebers, "Disability and the Theory of Complex Embodiment—For Identity Politics in a New Register," in *The Disability Studies Reader*, ed. Lennard J. Davis (Routledge, 2013), 273. Drawing on Siebers's definition, Barclay argues that "employing disability as a critical category of analysis provides a unique vantage point to consider the lives and experiences of enslaved people. It also challenges scholars to be cognizant of gaps in historical knowledge that exist because of the 'ideology of ability.'" Barclay, "Bad Breeders and Monstrosities: Racializing Childlessness and Congenital Disabilities in Slavery and Freedom," *Slavery and Abolition* 38, no. 2 (2017): 298.

21. AAL, Causas de Negros XXVI: 60, 1713.

22. AAL, Causas de Negros XXVI: 60, 1713.

23. AAL, Causas de Negros XXXI: 5, 1781.

24. AAL, Causas de Negros XXVI: 5, 1781.

25. AAL, Causas de Negros XXVI: 5, 1781.

26. Frank Trey Proctor III has studied enslaved women's shifting use of *sevicia* as an accusation against their owners in late colonial Lima, arguing that the term's meaning varied according to gender. See Proctor, "'Alien to My Sex.'"

27. Evelyne Laurent-Perrault, "Esclavizadas, cimarronaje, y la ley en Venezuela,

1770–1809," in *Demando mi libertad: Mujeres negras y sus estrategias de resistencia en la Nueva Granada, Venezuela, y Cuba, 1700–1800*, ed. Aurora Vergara Figueroa and Carmen Luz Cosme Puntiel (Universidad ICESI, 2018). 165–96.

28. Archivo General de la Nación, Lima (hereafter AGN) (3009), XVIII, 189, 159, 10, 1774.

29. AGN (3009), XVIII, 189, 159, 10, 1774.

30. AGN (3009), XVIII, 189, 159, 10, 1774.

31. AGN (3009), XVIII, 189, 159, 10, 1774.

32. AGN (3009), XVIII, 189, 159, 10, 1774.

33. AGN (3009), XVIII, 189, 159, 10, 1774.

34. AGN (3009), XVIII, 189, 159, 10, 1774.

35. AGN (3009), XVIII, 189, 159, 10, 1774.

36. AAL, Causas de Negros XXXV: 4, 1799.

37. AAL, Causas de Negros XXXV: 4, 1799.

38. AAL, Causas de Negros XXXV: 4, 1799.

39. AAL, Causas de Negros XXXV: 4, 1799.

40. AAL, Causas de Negros XXXV: 4, 1799.

41. AAL, Causas de Negros XXXV: 4, 1799.

42. AAL, Causas de Negros XXXV: 4, 1799.

43. Instituto Riva-Agüero (hereafter IRA), Colección Maldonado, A-I-80.

44. IRA, Colección Maldonado, A-I-80. Lavalle also suffered from blood in her sputum, an injured foot, and trembles.

45. IRA, Colección Maldonado, A-I-80.

46. IRA, Colección Maldonado, A-I-80.

47. Lima's surgeons fell into two types: romance surgeons, who spoke Spanish in their training and work and possessed a less formal education based on apprenticeship, and Latin surgeons, who studied and were proficient in Latin, received more formal training, and were eligible for the title of *bachiller*. Latin surgeons were assumed to possess more extensive knowledge of the body than romance surgeons.

48. IRA, Colección Maldonado, A-I-80.

49. IRA, Colección Maldonado, A-I-80.

50. Barclay, *Mark of Slavery*, p. 3.

51. AAL, Causas de Negros XXXIII: 25, 1795.

52. AAL, Causas de Negros XXXI: 31, 1785.

53. AAL, Causas de Negros XXXI: 31, 1785.

54. AGN (2691), XVIII, 153, 1283, 44, 1765.

6

Madness in Ecuador, 1900–1943

Indigenous People and Intellectual Impairment

David Carey Jr.

After two years during which her Indigenous husband Juan Guano was in "a complete state of insanity," María Natividad Mesabanda was in the "difficult" position of having to put him in the Ecuadorian *manicomio* (madhouse), where he would live "without any hope of getting better."[1] As an illiterate mother of seven children who had to "work to maintain the most constant and resilient manner [from] a tiny little piece of land" in order to feed and clothe her young children, Mesabanda could not afford to do the same for her husband. "[It] is extremely difficult to do so as a poor widowed mother with so many children," she explained, because of the "lack of supplies [and] life's difficulties." That description captured the struggles of many poor and working-class women in Ecuador. In 1943, Mesabanda asked the president of the Junta Central de *Beneficencia* (Central Board of Benefits) to provide for her husband, concluding that "an act of humanism toward the impotent will be prized."[2] Although the director's response is lost, based on the scarce resources at such institutions, one may infer that even this small concession was far from assured.

By identifying herself as a widow, Mesabanda highlighted her vulner-

I want to thank our editor Ahmed Ragab, my coeditor Heather Vrana, participants and volume contributors at the workshop sponsored by the Center for Black, Brown, and Queer Studies, and three anonymous reviewers for critical comments and suggestions that sharpened this essay. Stefanie Hunt-Kennedy, Julie Minich, Matt Mulcahy, Bianca Premo, Michael Rembis, Sara Scalenghe, and Allen Wells, also offered insightful critiques that strengthened this chapter. The multitalented Maeve Hill assisted with references and footnote revisions.

ability in gendered ways. In a patriarchal society where husbands were expected to provide for their family, Guano's inability to do so, which Mesabanda attributed to his "*demencia*" (madness or insanity) compelled her (like many of her female contemporaries) to be the sole provider for her family.[3] Like race and class, gender intersected with ableism and sanism to ensure that unproductive Ecuadorians were counted among the disabled. As mutually constituting practices, ableism and sanism are systems of power and ideologies that privilege people based on different notions of fitness (ability and sanity) and systematically oppress and discriminate against people with physical or mental impairments, or both.[4] Unable to afford at-home care, Mesabanda had little choice but to institutionalize her husband, which compelled her to reimagine and recalibrate her family unit as female-centered.[5] Common throughout Latin America, female-headed households challenged ableist and sanist patriarchal discourse that portrayed masculinity as powerful and femininity as fragile.

Alongside patriarchy and misogyny, the intersecting forces of sanism, ableism, and racism regularly marginalized people of color and women.[6] Deploying what she calls a "politics of curiosity," Therí Alyce Pickens shows how Blackness and madness are in dialogue with gender and other "slippery" identities and notions in a "complex constellation of relationships."[7] In turn, scholars have exhibited how elites and authorities deployed ableism and anti-Indigenous racism to exploit and discount Indigenous people.[8] To undergird their claims of superiority and prejudicial practices embedded in eugenics, elites and officials invoked ableist and sanist logics.

More apparent among Hispanic than among Indigenous Latin Americans, sanism shaped how colonialism and imperialism structured power. As far back as the colonial era, Spanish authorities and officials developed "discourses and practices surrounding the inferior intellectual abilities of the natives," notes historian Christina Ramos.[9] She further suggests that judicial officials (and by extension the Spanish Crown) deployed "discourses regarding the protected legal status of the mad and Indians . . . to delegitimize" political adversaries and squelch Indigenous uprisings.[10] Such conflation of discourses and diagnoses continued to serve those in power in postcolonial Latin America where psychiatrists often assumed poor, Indigenous, Afrodescendant, or female individuals were mad, which reinforced social hierarchies that marginalized those groups.[11] Psychiatry emerged from physicians who, in underfunded fits and starts, medicalized "pathologies of the mind" and thereby delivered more power to medical professionals and authorities than therapy to mad people.[12]

Whereas historians of scientific medicine and historians of institutions might depict patients benefiting from psychiatric care, rehabilitation, and occupational therapy, disability and mad historians see inmates conscripted to work as part of efforts to control their socially deviant behavior.[13] Alison Kafer's "political/relational model of disability" interrogates, rather than opposing or valorizing, scientific medical intervention and locates disability "in built environments and social patterns that exclude or stigmatize particular kinds of bodies, minds, and ways of being."[14] Informed by her model, I argue that Ecuadorian elites, authorities, and scientific medical professionals in the first half of the twentieth century deployed anti-Indigenous racism and sanism to undermine Indigenous people's claims to equality and citizenship.

Rather than recognize *indígenas* (Indigenous people) as innovative and resourceful citizens who did not conform to Western notions of individuality, materialism, or comportment, Latin American officials and elites labeled them ignorant, lazy (and sometimes deranged) drunks.[15] People who existed outside elite cultural mores or who allegedly threatened modernization frequently found themselves labeled mad.[16] In her study of the Manicomio Pacheco in Bolivia during the 1940s, historian Ann Zulawski discovered that elites labeled behavior in indígenas that exceeded their station as madness.[17] Such pathological taxonomies facilitated scapegoating indígenas for national shortcomings and excluding them from modernization's benefits. By marginalizing those who did not conform to their notions of sanity and cognitive competence, officials and medical professionals used sanism to reinforce restrictive citizenship that excluded indígenas and privileged non-Indigenous Latin Americans.

This essay adapts the "revised social model" of disability that distinguishes between disability and impairment. As explained in this volume's introduction, this model argues that disability is a product of restrictive built environments and social policies that either do not account for or actively discriminate against people with impairments, and that impairment is simply part of human variation rather than a deficit in need of cure or eradication.[18] In Ecuador (and Latin America more broadly), Indigenous and non-Indigenous peoples held unique social and cultural values regarding impairments and thus often accommodated them distinctly. Since impairment and disability are socially constructed and historically contingent, they must be studied in their historical and social contexts. A nuanced approach is critical to moving beyond simplistic and reductive notions of the social model. With its origins in the twentieth-century disability rights movement in the United Kingdom, the revised social model cannot be mapped easily onto other times and places. Centering madness as a focal point, this essay traces connections between mental impairments and people's material conditions and identities such as poverty, ethnicity, race, class, and gender to demonstrate how sanism, ableism, and (particularly anti-Indigenous) racism intersected in ways that reified those systems of power and increasingly marginalized those who fell outside those socially constructed norms.

As is true in much archival evidence from Ecuador, the person labeled disabled or mad—Juan Guano in this case—has no voice in the documents that survive. Disability and mad historians read against the grain of such archival sources and through the filters of the medical professionals, officials, and assistants who penned them to search for what disability and madness meant to those identified by others as such. Although the field of mad history in the United States and Europe is increasingly recognized as distinct from disability history and disability studies,[19] in Latin America and the Caribbean scholars and activists generally consider madness as part of a larger pantheon of impairments.[20] In my analysis of madness, I follow the lead in the Ecuadorian archives whereby neither scientific medical professionals, authorities, elites, nor *indígenas* considered cognitive impairments (and the many meanings and manifestations thereof) to be distinct from what they considered physical or sensory impairments.

Reading against the grain of Ecuadorian archival materials reveals how ableism, sanism, and anti-Indigenous racism intersected to inform disability categories in medicine and culture.[21] That intersectionality shaped and was shaped by broader political and economic changes. In ways akin to historian Stefanie Hunt-Kennedy's insights about the relationship between disability and Blackness in the colonial British Caribbean, Indigeneity and insanity in Ecuador were "inextricably intertwined and mutually constitutive forces that worked to further entrench the connections between racism . . . ableism," and, I would add, sanism.[22] In a related pattern identified by Hunt-Kennedy, like the British who perceived enslaved Africans as intellectually disabled, Ecuadorian officials and elites portrayed indígenas as mentally deficient to justify their inferior social status.[23] If indígenas were mad, then non-Indigenous authorities and economic powerbrokers could deny them full citizenship and denigrate them as good for little else than manual labor, on which the extractive economic system (and elites' wealth) depended.

Evidently familiar with such denigration, Mesabanda cast a wide net in her petition to the president of the Board of Benefits, who was first and foremost a government authority but also a quasi-medical authority and (to a lesser extent) a quasi-religious authority. Amid its religious overtones, her petition suggests knowledge of how scientific medicine framed intellectual impairments. Acutely aware of her husband's (and perhaps her own) Indigeneity, Mesabanda advanced notions of sanism and ableism to highlight the urgency of her plight, which (in her framing) dovetailed with her husband's urgent need for care. We never hear from her husband, but Mesabanda reveals the challenges that mothers (and other family members) faced when trying to care for mad relatives and their children. Like many of her contemporaries, Mesabanda apparently approached scientific medicine as a possible solution, if not a cure, for her husband's insanity.[24] Her petition also suggests that she adopted values associated with scientific medicine and modernity more broadly. As she strategically communicated and navigated the racist, sexist, ableist, and sanist categories that often discriminated against her (and particularly her husband) and undermined her ability to eke out a living for her family, Mesabanda asserted her and her husband's humanity.

Madness's Many Meanings in
the Ecuadorian Historical Context

Tacking between describing her husband as insane, mad, incurable, and impotent, Mesabanda reveals the many pliable descriptions of disability and madness in multilingual, multicultural, hybrid healthcare contexts where medical professionals increasingly imposed their nomenclature, diagnoses, and "treatments" for impaired bodies and minds. Understandings of disability were unsettled, unstable, and pluralized.[25] As Ramos observes, "The very ambiguity and malleability of the term ["madness"] . . . underscores the historicity of mental disorders."[26] With shifting diagnoses and descriptions of the delusions, hallucinations, and paranoia recorded in the archives, embodied madness evoked distinct responses across time, place, culture, race, gender, and class.[27] From doctors and authorities to family members and individuals with impairments, people conceptualized, categorized, and experienced disability and particularly neurological diversity differently.

In the first half of the twentieth century, Ecuador generally isolated and stigmatized people with mental disabilities. Although Mesabanda concluded that "an act of humanism toward the impotent will be prized," if the archival record is any indication, few of her contemporaries would have agreed. Set against longer histories of vulnerability and disability in Latin America, Mesabanda's portrayal of incapacity—her husband's lack of productivity rendered him dead to her—suggests poor and working-class people shaped and comprehended the middle area between elite notions of capacity and disability. As is true in other parts of the Americas, Ecuadorian narratives of the past obscure histories of madness.[28]

The various terms for madness and disability across Latin America's rich linguistic and ethnic diversity speaks to the multiple understandings of these conditions.[29] They also highlight the problem of translating terms such as "disability" and "madness" across languages (Spanish, Indigenous, English), epistemologies (Indigenous, folk, Western, biomedical), historical periods, and ontologies. For the *hank'akuna* (disabled people) in the Inka Empire (1400–1533), which included present Ecuador, atypical body configuration could be a source of power. Respected and powerful figures in Inka society, hank'akuna served as governors and judges. Bodily difference facilitated their authority.[30] The Inka nobleman Guaman Poma's writings and drawings reveal more specific Quechua words for disabled people such as *k'umukuna* (people with kyphosis), *t'inrikuna* (people with dwarfism), *ñawsakuna* (people with blindness), and *upakuna* (people who are nonverbal). Informed by those meanings and conceptions, Quechua speakers did not assume those with physical, sensory, or mental impairments to be deficient or impaired. On the contrary, they often afforded them great influence and power. But few Quechua terms for mental or physical impairments aligned fully with the colonial (pseudo-)scientific medical notions or terms for disability that Spaniards brought after they invaded the Inka Empire in 1534.[31]

Deeply conflicted, the meanings of madness in colonial Latin America were seldom evident. In revealing a number of different Spanish words and phrases to describe neurodiversity in colonial archives, Ramos observes that madness was imprecise.[32] Historian Irina Metzler agrees that madness was a "notoriously ambiguous conceptual category."[33] Since the boundaries between the sane and insane were more porous than firm and categorical, "definitions of madness could shift according to context and intention," Ramos concludes. "While medical theory had parsed madness into several distinct varieties—mania, melancholy, furor, or frenzy—diagnosing a particular disorder was never straightforward."[34]

Conflation of and confusion around the meanings of madness continued into the postcolonial era. Recall that Mesabanda described her husband as being mad, insane, incurable, unproductive, and impotent. In her 2010 essay, "El triunfo de la locura," María Tausiet catalogs more than 30 Spanish words for madness.[35] The Ecuadorian archives are similarly fecund with descriptions of *locura* (insanity). "If insanity includes all types of anomalies and extreme thoughts and emotions," Tausiet asks, ". . . how can one decide where it started and where it ended?"

Early-twentieth-century Ecuadorian authorities and allopathic medical professionals did not claim to know those parameters, but they readily criticized the state for exacerbating madness. They also recognized the state's failure to provide adequate care. In 1910 city council president Pedro Traversari visited the San Lazaro *hospicio* (extended care facility), which he considered "a refuge of misery and something of a 'pandora's box' in which are crammed all miserable and ill-fated humans . . . [including] the unhappy *loco* [lunatic]."[36] Intent on improving institutional health care, Traversari drafted a report to the Asistencia Pública (Public Assistance) board. Read today, his observations resonate with Michel Foucault's argument about bureaucratic states classifying the poor and working classes as mad or criminal to control them.[37] At a time when other nations were classifying criminals as mad, Traversari distinguished between the two. In so doing, he advocated for mad people's rights and care rather than simply their confinement or incarceration.[38] Traversari intimated that the government had failed its citizens: "We do not vacillate in our belief that the government should reflect public philanthropy and yearn for what a notable hygienist said 'To conserve the health of the nation and facilitate this in general and with its denizens in particular, the means to recuperate when they have lost it.'"[39] Some hospital officials were as critical of non-Indigenous authorities as they were of Indigenous patients. A unified scientific "medical state" never completely coalesced in Ecuador. Focusing on Indigenous people and rural mental health care offers a unique perspective on institution- and urban-focused histories of psychology.

Even as authorities and capitalists (particularly cacao and other agro-export landowners) relied on their physical labor, they described indígenas as being physically, mentally, and emotionally impaired. Nineteenth-century Ecuadorian historian Pedro Fermín Cevallos lauded indígenas' ability to carry heavy loads over long distances but otherwise considered them "weak and lazy" and an "absolutely negative" factor "in the civilization of the country."[40] Such (often cognitively dissonant) perspectives were typical of most late-nineteenth-century and early-twentieth-century Ecuadorian elites, who framed indígenas as problematic and sought to disrupt their cultural, economic, and social systems.[41] Despite such denigration, capitalists depended on able-bodied indígenas for their profits even as they employed them on *fincas* and plantations in ways that impaired their bodies.

Although they seldom considered indígenas their equals, Ecuadorian elites understood that indígenas' well-being was essential to national development. By the 1920s, Ecuadorian indígenas organized and collaborated with other rural laborers to demand the recognition of their rights and to improve rural working and living conditions.[42] Indígenas increasingly positioned themselves at the center of national discourse and identity as a military coup led to the 1925 Revolución Juliana (Julian Revolution), which promised more humane government. Although it restricted citizenship to literate men and women (thereby excluding most indígenas even though it was the first Latin American constitution to grant female suffrage), the 1929 Constitution created a Senate seat to represent, guide, and defend indígenas. In that sense, Ecuador's authoritarian rule had a semblance of representative governance. Yet archival traces of Indigenous laborers' and activists' protests suggest relationships between indígenas and *hacendados* (hacienda owners) were marked by contention. Early-twentieth-century Indigenous leaders and entrepreneurs who carved out spaces of autonomy and wealth were the exception; the majority of indígenas struggled to thrive amid marginalized living, working, and health conditions in a nation characterized by unequal land distribution.[43]

Political instability that manifested in fifteen different administrations in the 1930s resulted in a decade-long power vacuum that facilitated indígenas' integration into Ecuador's economy and politics on their own terms.[44] In November 1935, the first Conferencia de Cabecillas Indígenas (Indigenous Leaders Conference) was held in Quito, and the Comité Central de Defensa Indígena (Indigenous Defense Committee) was founded the following year.

In turn, the 1937 Ley de Comunas (Community Law) helped indígenas establish their freedom from haciendas and position themselves more centrally in Ecuador's nation formation process.[45] As an economic crisis lasted into the 1940s, Indigenous and other popular groups enjoyed increasing influence.[46]

Those openings notwithstanding, Ecuadorian Indigenous populations generally had little access to resources, education, or authority. By 1940, Ecuador had a population of about 3 million people. Although 39 percent of Ecuadorians were identified as Indigenous, that estimate likely undercounted indígenas.[47] The nation's racial order—shaped by conquest, colonization, and slavery—varied over time, but its broad contours remained consistent: A few entrepreneurial and professional indígenas and Afro-Ecuadorians notwithstanding, lighter-skinned citizens enjoyed more social, economic, and political privileges than their darker-skinned counterparts.[48] Forced labor systems restricted Indigenous mobility, autonomy, and wealth well into the twentieth century.[49]

Eugenic Madness

For Hispanic elites and authorities who deployed eugenics and other scientific racisms to marginalize indígenas, sanism (like ableism) contributed to that goal. With citizenship in nineteenth- and early-twentieth-century Latin America reserved for those elites deemed capable of participating in civic life—namely, urban, cosmopolitan, able-bodied and -minded Hispanic citizens—eugenicists often relegated indígenas and locos to society's margins.[50] Perceived competency was a form of governmentality and citizenship. Some Latin American eugenicists associated locos with indígenas. In a condemnation resonant with disparaging discourse about ignorant, lazy indígenas, some officials and medical professionals suggested locos impeded national progress. Such conflated disenfranchisement demonstrates how medical science and racism combined to discount indígenas and mad people.

Throughout Latin America, eugenicists contrasted clean, healthy, light-skinned citizens with filthy, diseased people of color.[51] Discourse advancing the confluence of race and disability particularly marked nations with large Indigenous and Afro-descendant populations. Hispanic, *blanco-mestizo* (white mixed-race Ecuadorian), and other elites portrayed indígenas and Afro-Latin Americans as, by their nature, ignorant and susceptible to disabling diseases.[52] Targeting indígenas, Latin American leaders adopted a eugenic lexicon that framed national inclusion in terms of proper hygiene and good health and national exclusion in terms of foulness and pestilence.[53] That lexicon mapped nicely on to discourse that framed indígenas as unhygienic incubators of disease.[54] Concerned about "pathological *patrias*," many Latin American authorities deemed those regularly or incurably ill, impaired, or mad devoid of citizenship.[55] Ecuador followed eugenicist thinking but sometimes framed its efforts as attempts to improve a national (rather than solely Indigenous) race.

Regional differences distinguished Kichwa speakers in the Andes mountains, various Amazonian tribes, and a few Indigenous groups along the coast. Most Ecuadorian indígenas lived in the mountains. Those who shed their Indigenous markers, such as language and clothing, could adopt a blanco-mestizo identity and hope for the spoils that came with it. But many indígenas remained steadfast in their claims of ethnicity and citizenship.

In the first half of the twentieth century, the governments of Ecuador sought to spread scientific medicine among the population. These efforts were more robust in cities, with their clinics, hospitals, and Spanish-speaking populace, than in the rural highlands populated primarily by indígenas who had distinct languages, cultures, and healing epistemologies and practices. Ethnicity distinctly shaped perceptions of and care for madness. Even though Ecuadorian allopathic medical professionals and authorities did not generally identify indígenas as inherently insane, Ecuadorian elites and officials racialized mental health to further marginalize indígenas.

Disparaging Indigenous intellect facilitated conflating disease with Indigeneity. By the 1920s, eugenicists who targeted indígenas and locos were particularly passionate about conditions such as *bocio* (goiter or thyroid tumor) that they considered to be at the intersection of madness and Indigeneity. In February 1930, the Ecuadorian health delegation of Tungurahua in Ambato reported frequent incidences of bocio among "the indigenous race . . . the inhabitants of the white race or a little mixed . . . almost do not suffer from the disease[;] in contrast the Indians affected are very numerous."[56] By framing a physical impairment among indígenas as an indication (and consequence) of their cognitive incompetency, authorities and scientific medical professionals expanded the ways sanism excluded indígenas in Ecuador.[57] Dating to the colonial period, goiter was associated with mental disability.[58] According to the Tungurahua health delegation, *indígenas*' stunted intellect propelled their propensity for *bocio*: "Almost everyone who suffers from the disease is mentally degenerate[;] they do not have any interest in curing themselves much less doing so with their children." Informed by eugenics, Tungurahua officials proposed prohibiting "*bocios*" from marrying "because heredity is inevitable and for the degeneration of the race and the precarious situation in which those unhappy people live."[59] This assertion reflected the opinion of Ecuadorian officials who, by the early twentieth century, had embraced the French theory of degeneracy that claimed mental and physical diseases were passed from one generation to the next in ever more destructive doses.[60] In the 1920s and 1930s, authorities who advanced eugenics applied the term "degenerate" to those they considered intellectually inferior and thus unfit to reproduce.[61] Conflating race and mental deficiencies and attributing them to *bocio* distinguished those Ecuadorian eugenicists from their compatriots who framed eugenics along national rather than ethnic lines. That officials felt compelled to prohibit marriage indicates that "bocios" enjoyed and acted on the right to do so. In another manifestation of resistance to sanism and racism, indígenas with goiter also apparently reared and raised their children according to their own values and practices.

Disability and madness became tools for eugenic policies. Eugenicists framed Indigenous and poor people as disabled to justify marginalizing them. Presumptions that indígenas were cognitively deficient and irrational made them susceptible to diagnoses of psychological disabilities or madness. Even though archival and oral records are replete with evidence of indígenas embracing modernity, many allopathic medical professionals insisted insane indígenas were "fundamentally unfit for modernity."[62]

Discounting Indigenous intelligence was not uncommon. In his 1939 description of the community of Tocachi, where the "population . . . is almost completely Indigenous," health inspector Dr. Rogelio Yañez claimed, "At each step one finds idiots, morons and the majority with mental deficiency that forces one to despair."[63] By claiming that ignorance marked Indigeneity, Yañez revealed the intersection of sanism and racism. He deployed eugenic terms such as "idiot," "moron," and "mental deficiency" in his report, which signaled that people with mental illness were not only intellectually inferior but unfit to be citizens or to reproduce.[64] Like nineteenth-century US antebellum enslavers and twentieth-century U.S. immigration officials who portrayed Black people and Mexican immigrants respectively as disabled, Yañez suggested indígenas were mentally and cognitively impaired and thus incapable of caring for themselves let alone contributing to the nation. In crafting a discourse of defective indígenas, Yañez and his contemporaries conflated ethnicity and madness to "constitute and maintain social hierarchies" and advance eugenics.[65] Yet the broader Ecuadorian archival record suggests a more nuanced understanding of Indigenous intellect than racist portrayals in the press and public discourse betrayed.

In some cases, madness countervailed discourses of Indigenous ignorance. Appreciation for what readers today might recognize as "neurodiversity" among Indigenous populations is most obvious in diagnoses of madness. Without assuming intellectual inferiority, some doctors and nurses respected Indigenous patients in hospitals enough to correct other officials' misdiagnoses of madness. Although such actions were unusual, some scientific medical professionals resisted the pervasive medicalization of impairments.

Mad Care and Indigeneity

Mesabanda's initial efforts to care for her Indigenous husband despite the permanence of his disability—she framed it as an innate characteristic rather than a phase or condition—and subsequent appeal for humanitarian institutionalization provide evidence of ranges, alternatives, and pluralism in the ways that cultures, societies, and nations approached racially pathologized disabilities and particularly madness. Historically, mad people have had many collaborators, ranging from family and community members to allopathic medical professionals and traditional healers. With families having long served as the first custodial and therapeutic options in Latin America and elsewhere, only as societies increasingly embraced the Enlightenment and later modernization did institutionalization—being confined in a residential facility—become a strategy for marginalizing the insane.[66] Even when groups preferred communal and familial care, authorities and allopathic medical professionals framed madness as a disability that necessitated institutionalization.

A process that countervailed Indigenous culture, ethics, relationships, and worldviews, sanist institutionalization violated the self-determination of many "unhappy *indios*."[67] Like many Latin American *indígenas*, Kichwas in Ecuador rooted their ethnic belonging to shared local cultural understandings. Characterized by dynamic holistic approaches that took into account individuals' psychological, emotional, and physical well-being, Ecuadorian Indigenous health practices sought to maintain a balance between corporeal, community (society), natural, and supernatural forces.[68] In addition to the physical and psychological privations in asylums, *indígenas* while confined lost those vital connections to their culture, community, and families. That Mesabanda sought to institutionalize her husband speaks to the effects of the desperate poverty that marked her family's life.

With a tendency to incorporate rather than institutionalize people with impairments, Indigenous communities could be welcoming places for people with physical or mental impairments. A willingness to integrate community members with impairments was not unique to Indigenous communities or the modern era, but it sharply contrasted with non-Indigenous Ecuadorian (and many other Latin American) approaches to intellectual, physical, and sensory disability informed by scientific medicine.

Since few poor rural Indigenous families were equipped to care for mad family members, many poor indígenas like Guano were committed to insane asylums that, according to city council president Pedro Traversi, "would make the whole world cry."[69] Scientific medical professionals, particularly psychiatrists, who defined normal versus abnormal human behavior contributed to nation formation.[70] Those who racialized mental health in nations with large Indigenous populations like Ecuador further marginalized indígenas.

As Mesabanda's choice to identify herself as a widow suggests, families that remanded loved ones to mental health care and other scientific medical institutions understood they might never see them again—particularly if, as her husband's surname suggests, they were indígenas. In Ecuador, Indigeneity could hinder access to and the provision of health care.[71] Buttressed by eugenics, anti-Indigenous racism shaped mental healthcare processes, outcomes, nosology, and diagnoses.

In Ecuador, allopathic medical professionals tended to conflate cognitive disability with mental illness, though few explicitly said so. Deployed by doctors, the term *ebrio y lisiado* (drunk and disabled by alcohol) suggests a hinge between intellectual disability and madness in that inebriated individuals regularly received diagnoses of both.[72] An ebrio y lisiado diagnosis positioned both types of disability in a single frame. Assumptions about Indigenous tendencies toward inebriation facilitated their association with intellectual deficiencies and madness. Some nineteenth-century elites considered drunkenness "innate" in indígenas.[73] By suggesting that normally timid, cowardly indígenas became violent savages with alcohol, Conservative president Gabriel García Moreno (1860–75) associated Indigeneity with inebriation and portrayed indígenas as wards rather than citizens of the state.[74]

Grappling with categories and diagnoses reveals the socially constructed, spurious, and entwined nature of mental health and racial classifications. Tracing the forces that informed the creation of such categories exposes how elites and authorities portrayed marginalized people in ways that justified their institutionalization, incarceration, and sterilization.[75]

Associations of *indígenas* and alcohol continued into the twentieth century. In 1940, the minister of health warned, "*Guarapo* is causing disastrous effects on the health of *indígenas*, because of the toxicity of the drink that is not prepared properly[;] the alcohol grade that undoubtedly is added produces a psychological disorder." To address this "dangerous and bleak [development] for the unhappy *indio*," health commissioner Amable Viteri visited *chicherías* (taverns serving chicha) where he found "innumerable *indígenas* hanging out in the patios, encircled by flies and in obscene postures, men as well as women, a truly disturbing situation."[76] Like Viteri, the Tungurahua *intendente de carabineros* (police chief), Mayor Gustavo A. Torres, considered chicherías "dens of corruption and vice where *la raza india* degenerates."[77] To Torres's mind, chicherías and other drinking establishments exacerbated indígenas' intellectual inferiority, which made them unfit to reproduce or otherwise contribute to the nation.[78] Worse still, he thought them dangerous. When "the true poisons called *chicha* are ingested, they awaken in those that consume them primitive, criminal, and wild instincts."[79]

Institutions and Manifestations of Madness

In late-nineteenth- and early-twentieth-century Latin America, authorities and medical professionals hotly debated germ theory, sanitation, hygiene, disease containment, and other issues related to mental health and the ability of scientific medicine to address disruptions thereof. Public health and other officials often attributed disease to some mix of Indigenous, African-descendant, poor, rural, and other marginalized populations' allegedly unhealthy behaviors, practices, and customs. By portraying Indigenous people as backward, ignorant, lazy, and prone to inebriation, Ecuadorian elites co-constituted indigeneity with disability and madness at a time when psychology was shifting from religious and carceral approaches to mental health and medical approaches that involved expanding institutions, secularizing mental health care, and moving away from guardianship toward cure.[80]

Prior to establishing the first insane asylum Manicomio Velez in 1881, where only the most publicly or violently people experiencing mental troubles and distress were admitted (and categorized as having *trastornos mentales* or mental disturbances), Ecuadorian authorities housed mad people in jails or hospitals. Throughout Latin America, municipalities that oversaw those institutions had paltry budgets but significant legislative power to regulate personal behavior considered threatening to public health. Madness often fell into that category.[81] As confinement (a practice inconceivable in much of colonial Latin America) and care transferred to centralized asylums in the late nineteenth and early twentieth century, some inmates became more vulnerable. Insane asylums often served as isolation wards for contagious patients, which increased asylum death rates.[82]

By the turn of the century, allopathic medical professionals were increasingly convinced that madness was rooted in the nervous system and could be treated accordingly, which undergirded the medicalization and institutionalization of mental impairments and such labels as *enfermedades nerviosas* (nervous system illnesses).[83] According to the Ecuadorian minister of the interior in 1910, "All of the sources of human misery find their remedy in the altruistic action of the Juntas [government assemblies]: the orphan and the aged have their shelter, the leper and the madman have their refuge, and the ill recover their health in the hospital."[84] As part of modernization, the state deployed ableism and sanism by separating allegedly weak, incompetent, or less abled and minded people from their normalized counterparts.

Asylums and hospitals were sites of negotiation, conflict, and healing. While national officials were convinced "locos" were adequately and appropriately served, public health inspections shed a harsher light on Ecuadorian institutional care, particularly in rural areas. The hospice or orphanage and *lazareto* (quarantine hospital for infectious diseases; isolation hospital) in Latacunga—a region so remote and dispersed that health inspectors regularly exhausted (sometimes fatally) their horses in getting there—offer counterexamples to urban institutions.[85] Long considered destinations of death, hospitals and asylums were dangerous and foreign spaces for many rural indígenas.

The problematic nature of scientific medical professionals' ableist and sanist assumptions and incarceration of people notwithstanding, wretched health care could induce madness. When the aforementioned city council president Pedro Traversari visited the San Lazaro lazareto and hospicio in 1910, he exclaimed: "I never imagined that an establishment assigned the wretched who suffer from the terrible disease elephantiasis would be found in such deplorable conditions." He continued, "The establishment is crowded, dirty, humid, dark, anti-hygienic; after a few days in that pigsty, an individual who has the misfortune of landing there even in good mental and physical health would undoubtedly lose their mind and health[;] each and every one of the departments in that house are frightening and repugnant."[86] His observations reflected the prevailing dialectical relationship between reason and unreason.[87] Given that contemporary scientific medical professionals considered clean, ample spaces crucial to mental health improvement, the Latagunga lazareto was particularly problematic.[88] Like prison sentences, hospital stays could drive patients insane.[89] To counteract that possibility, Traversari recommended an "immediate . . . serious disinfection of the Lazareto" and that orphans and the elderly be moved to any other institution of the Asistencia Pública, since "leaving them where they are is an inhuman and even cruel act."[90] If institutions of scientific medical care could cause madness, they would seem counterproductive venues in which to address neurological diversity.

In his report to the Asistencia Pública, Traversari deployed insanity to incite interest in reform. Similar to the way Mesabanda portrayed her husband's madness as his death to her, Traversari rendered institutionalization as a fate worse than death to provoke his superiors to reform those institutions. After recommending a crematorium oven be constructed to incinerate lepers' "rags," Traversari insisted lepers not "leave to the street with [their] grave threat to public health."[91] Like many of his contemporaries, he sought to exclude lepers and their impairments from broader society rather than reform society in ways that could accommodate lepers.

Informed by the doctors who accompanied him, Traversari had a keen sense of how one's environment shaped convalescence. "The sick," he predicted, "with pure air, with spacious areas, with gardens and meadows where to entertain themselves and obligated to [perform] certain manual labor appropriate to the state of their sickness, would be cured of their mental derangement and at the same time would . . . help maintain the home." Claiming that work could cure insanity was particularly convenient in a nation dependent on the labor of indígenas portrayed as cognitively deficient. "Since colonial times," he observed, "we have had the *lazareto* in the heart of a city like Quito where there was no pure air where one lived in true overcrowding without precautions . . . or hygiene."[92] With 20,000 pesos, he claimed, they could secure a better place for a new lazaretto and "finish this work of vital importance."[93] "With patriotism and good will," he insisted, "anything is possible, but it is necessary to go step by step if we do not want to fail."

Critical of hospitals, Traversari was shocked by asylums. In a February 16, 1910, critique of staff who disregarded insane inmates, he denounced the "inhumane places" he toured in Pifo, with "closed, dark, small cells . . . without ventilation or release . . . and even without light . . . [where] the sane become insane and the insane are auctioned off."[94] The council president suggested that sane and insane were not absolute categories or innate characteristics. Rather, environments could make people insane or facilitate their recuperation. "With nothing to entertain their despondent spirits and distract their lost minds," he lamented, "their ghosts of terror and fear twirl around and come only in Dante's circles of hell."[95] Indigenous families that cared for the mentally impaired in their communities and homes offered a stark contrast to these institutions of medical science. The Asistencia Pública board "applauded" Traversari's report and his focus on care and rehabilitation rather than custodialism—marking a shift in the early twentieth century.[96] Evident among medical professionals who sought to incorporate indígenas into public health initiatives, and among indígenas who embraced medical science and adhered to public health mandates, indígenas were sufficiently central to the nation's identity and modernization that such institutional abuse was denounced in Ecuador.[97]

Across the Americas, insane asylums resembled decrepit confinement centers.[98] Some authorities deployed asylums as weapons whereby "inconvenient" family or community members could be deemed "dangerous" and institutionalized to isolate them from society.[99] So ill-equipped were doctors to diagnose symptoms that some inmates diagnosed themselves.[100] Regardless of conditions, insane asylums almost invariably assessed and treated individuals based on scientific medicine, which also was deeply flawed. As Kichwa conceptions that consider well-being as rooted in the dynamic interdependency and delicate balance of psychological, emotional, and physical health suggest, Indigenous notions of mental health did not necessarily resonate with scientific medical conceptions of madness.[101] As a result, scientific medicine practiced in asylums often alienated Indigenous inmates.

Ecuadorian inmates were subjects of scientific research and voyeurism, though not to the extent that Peruvian Lina Medina experienced, as Bianca Premo documents in this volume (chapter 1). In his March 2, 1911, report about the lazaretto in Pifo, a Dr. Villavicencio complained that persons confined there became sources of entertainment and fascination. "I understand that the *Lazareto* is a house of reclusion and isolation, but with outrage I have known and even witnessed that equal access is given to anyone who tries to inspect this new curiosity, as if the wretched *elefanciacos* were rare animals," he explained.[102] He wanted to "absolutely prohibit" anyone who was not an employee or did not have an order from the president from visiting the lazaretto. The Junta Central de Beneficencia (Central Board of Benefits) endorsed Villavicencio's prohibition.[103]

Once an individual had been admitted and diagnosed with mental impairment, it was often difficult to discharge them, even for a day. Eloisa C. de Betancourt wanted to take her husband Enrique Betancourt out to the *campo* (country) to convalesce on a June day in 1943. While the Junta Central de Beneficencia director approved Betancourt's leave, his doctor advised against it, claiming that Betancourt was a "danger to public order and the people's safety."[104] Enrique Betancourt is silenced in the archival record even as he was denied what would seem a basic human right to convalesce in public.

Under such conditions, it is not surprising that inmates fled asylums. Although he was quickly captured, the November 10, 1911, escape of the "lunatic M. Bedoya" sufficiently frightened the local population to warrant forming a tribunal to investigate the scandal and punish those found at fault.[105] Like Enrique Betancourt and so many of his counterparts in other asylums, Bedoya had no voice in the archival records that documented his incarceration and flight. We do not even learn his first name. His self-emancipation suggests how vehemently he disagreed with the scientific medical diagnoses and treatment he received. When the Ecuadorian president visited that hospicio in response to the escape, he was "convinced it lacked the most indispensable medicine to attend to the sick."[106] Bedoya may not have disagreed with him.

Conclusion

Ethnicity and race shaped changing conceptions of mental health when officials and medical professionals portrayed indígenas as mentally and intellectually deficient by their nature. In turn, race and racism are historically contingent social constructions that shaped and were shaped by notions of physical and mental disability. Those intersecting processes make racism, ableism, and sanism particularly valuable analytics with which to examine mental health, cognitive competence, neurodiversity, and perceptions thereof. Tracing the historically intersecting constructions of ableism, sanism, and racism reveals how those systems of power changed and took different forms in distinct places and times.[107] To exclude indígenas from citizenship and access to the many resources that came with it, Ecuadorian scientific medical and political authorities layered anti-Indigenous racism with sanism to maximize the marginalization of Indigenous people.

Ethnicity cut many ways. In Ecuador where social medicine had a long history, mental health care languished throughout the first half of the twentieth century. Mad people struggled to receive scientific medical services and social acceptance. The push to isolate mad individuals that accompanied modernization contravened Indigenous approaches to mental health and healing. Sanism and racism, in combination with ethnicity and class, compelled some poor indígenas to institutionalize mad loved ones because they lacked the resources to care for them. In that sense, sanism further facilitated racist denigration and marginalization of indígenas.

Certain scientific medical conditions such as bocio became tropes particularly for eugenicists who associated Indigeneity with mental deficits to justify marginalizing indígenas. According to Ecuadorian public health officials and authorities, those conditions were more pronounced and more dire among indígenas than among non-Indigenous people. Yet hospital records in Ecuador suggest that fewer Indigenous people than non-Indigenous people were confined. Even in Ecuador, where indígenas enjoyed significant autonomy and mobility, public health responses to bocio reinforced social hierarchies that disadvantaged indígenas.[108] Like other heavily Indigenous Latin American countries, Ecuador pathologized neurodiversity to buttress sanism and eugenics and solidify the privileges that non-Indigenous people enjoyed over indígenas.

NOTES

1. Museo de Medicina, Quito, Ecuador (hereafter MM), Asistencia Pública (hereafter AP) 0251, Hospicio, Director de Junta Beneficencia de María Natividad Mesabanda, 1943. Originating in the Kichwa (Quechua) language, Guano was a common surname among Indigenous peoples in Ecuador. See Gregory T. Cushman, *Guano and the Opening of the Pacific World: a Global Ecological History* (Cambridge: Cambridge University Press, 2013), 3; Kim Clark, email correspondence with the author, November 20, 2023.

2. MM, AP 0251, Hospicio, Director de Junta Beneficencia de María Natividad Mesabanda, 1943.

3. Since they identified individuals as mad or insane, *demencia* and *demente* were powerful terms to use when seeking state intervention. When a major general in the military asked the city *hospicio* to assume care for José Pavon, he referred to the artillery man as a "demente." See MM, AP 1101, Major General del ejército a Director de Junta Beneficiencia, April 18, 1925.

4. Jessica Cowing, "Occupied Land Is an Access Issue: Interventions in Feminist Disability Studies and Narratives of Indigenous Activism," *Journal of Feminist Scholarship* 17 (Fall 2020): 9–25; Susan Burch, *Committed: Remembering Native Kinship in and beyond Institutions* (University of North Carolina Press, 2021), 9; Lennard Davis *Enforcing Normalcy: Disability, Deafness, and the Body* (Penguin Random House, 1995). Manifested through discrimination, stereotypes, restricted access, and violence, ableism regulates the bodies and minds of those deemed disabled *and* normal. In late nineteenth- and twentieth-century Latin American nations obsessed with progress and order, people with impairments were diagnosed with a range of disorders and considered obstacles to modernization, whether they were labeled disabled or not.

5. Historians of disability have demonstrated how medical institutionalization, by denaturalizing the family unit, reconfigures families (often violently). See Alexandra Minna Stern, *Eugenic Nation: Faults and Frontiers of Better Breeding in Modern America* (University of California Press, 2015); Jay Dolmage, *Disabled upon Arrival: Eugenics, Immigration, and the Construction of Race and Disability* (Ohio State University Press, 2018); Regina Kunzel, "Queer History, Mad History, and the Politics of Health," *American Quarterly* 69, no. 2 (June 2017): 315–19, https://doi.org/10.1353/aq.2017.0026; Burch, *Committed*.

6. Catherine J. Kudlick, "Disability History: Why We Need Another 'Other,'" *American Historical Review* 108, no. 3 (June 2003): 763–93; Alexis Padilla "Cross-Coalitional Anti-Racist and Anti-Ableist Movements? Building on Maroon/Fugitive Knowledges and Global South Epistemologies," *Disability Studies Quarterly*, 43, no. 1 (2023); Kimberlé Williams Crenshaw, "Mapping the Margins: Intersectionality, Identity Politics, and Violence Against Women of Color," *Stanford Law Review* 43, no. 6 (1991): 1241–99; Anna Stubblefield, "'Beyond the Pale': Tainted Whiteness, Cognitive Disability, and Eugenic Sterilization," *Hypatia* 22, no. 2 (2007): 162, 179; Susan Burch and Michael Rembis, "Re-Membering the Past: Reflections on Disability Histories," in *Disability Histories*, ed. Susan Burch and Michael Rembis (University of Illinois Press, 2014), 1; Douglas Baynton, "Disability and the Justification of Inequality in American History: The Uses of Disability in Citizenship Debates," *PMLA* 120, no. 2 (March 2005): 33–57.

7. Therí Alyce Pickens, *Black Madness, Mad Blackness* (Duke University Press, 2019). See also La Marr Jurelle Bruce, *How to Go Mad Without Losing Your Mind: Madness and Black Radical Creativity* (Duke University Press, 2021), esp. ch. 4.

8. Ryan Scott Hechler, "The Fourth Lifeway: Recognizing the Legacy of Bodily Difference and Disability within the Inka Empire," *Disability Studies Quarterly* 41, no. 4 (Fall 2021); Scott Thomas Gibson, Sara Newman, and Antonia Carcelen-Estrada, "Indigeneity and Disabilities in the Ecuadorian Oral History Archives," *Disability Studies Quarterly* 41,

no. 4 (Fall 2021); Alexander Yarza de los Ríos, "Abya Yala's Disability: Weaving with the Thread and Breath of the Ancestors," *Disability Studies Quarterly* 41, no. 4 (Fall 2021); Siobhan Senier, "Blind Indians: Káteri Tekakwí:tha and Joseph Amos's Visions of Indigenous Resurgence," in *Disability Studies and the Environmental Humanities: Toward an Eco-Crip Theory*, ed. Sarah Jaquette Ray and Jay Sibara (University of Nebraska Press, 2018), 269–89.

9. Christina Ramos, *Bedlam in the New World: A Mexican Madhouse in the Age of Enlightenment* (University of North Carolina Press, 2022), 154.

10. Ramos, *Bedlam in the New World*, 150–51. Historians and scholars of other regions, including Europe, have noted the political nature of institutionalization. See Michel Foucault, *Madness and Civilization: A History of Insanity in the Age of Reason*, trans. Richard Howard (Vintage Books, 1988); Erwin H. Ackerknecht, "Political Prisoners in French Mental Institutions before 1789, during the Revolution, and under Napoleon I," *Medical History* 19 (1975): 250–55; Jonathan Andrews, Asa Briggs, Roy Porter, Penny Tucker, and Keir Waddington, *The History of Bethlem* (Routledge, 1997).

11. Manuella Meyer, "Madness and Psychiatry in Latin America's Long Nineteenth Century," in *The Routledge History of Madness and Mental Health*, ed. Greg Eghigian (Routledge, 2017), 204.

12. Cristina Rivera Garza, "Dangerous Minds: Changing Psychiatric Views of the Mentally Ill in Porfirian Mexico, 1876–1911," *Journal of the History of Medicine* 56 (2001): 42, 43; Andrew Scull, *The Insanity of Place, the Place of Insanity: Essays on the History of Psychiatry* (Routledge, 2006); Susan Cahn, "Border Disorders: Mental Illness, Feminist Metaphor, and the Disordered Female Psyche," in *Disability Histories*, ed. Susan Burch and Michael Rembis (University of Illinois Press, 2014), 258–83.

13. Michael Rembis, Catherine Kudlick, and Kim E. Nielsen, "Introduction," in *The Oxford Handbook of Disability History*, ed. Michael Rembis, Catherine Kudlick, and Kim E. Nielsen, (Oxford University Press, 2018), 9; Burch, *Committed*, 4; Adria L. Imada, *Archive of Skin, Archive of Kin: Disability and Life Making During Medical Incarceration* (University of California Press, 2022); Allison C. Carey, Liat Ben-Moshe, and Chris Chapman, *Disability Incarcerated: Imprisonment and Disability in the United States and Canada* (Palgrave McMillan, 2014); Cristina Rivera-Garza, "'She Neither Respected nor Obeyed Anyone': Inmates and Psychiatrists Debate Gender and Class at the General Insane Asylum La Castañeda, Mexico, 1910–1930," *Hispanic American Historical Review* 81, nos. 3–4 (2001): 676; Antonia Hylton, *Madness: Race and Insanity in a Jim Crow Asylum* (Legacy Lit, 2024). For explorations of the debates between historians of medicine and of disability, see *Bulletin of the History of Medicine* 87, no. 4 (Winter 2013).

14. Alison Kafer, *Feminist, Queer, Crip* (Indiana University Press, 2013), 6. Kafer's model also calls for problems of disability to be solved through social change and political transformation rather than medical intervention or surgical normalization.

15. David Carey Jr., *I Ask for Justice: Maya Women, Dictators, and Crime in Guatemala, 1898–1944* (University of Texas Press, 2013); Burch, *Committed*, 9–10.

16. Meyer, "Madness and Psychiatry."

17. Ann Zulawski, *Unequal Cures: Public Health and Political Change in Bolivia, 1900–1950* (Duke University Press, 2007), 157–89.

18. Michael Rembis, "Challenging the Impairment/Disability Divide: Disability History and the Social Model of Disability," *The Routledge Handbook of Disability Studies* (Routledge, 2019), 380–81, 383, 387.

19. Geoffrey Reaume, "How Is Mad Studies Different from Anti-Psychiatry and Critical Psychiatry?," in *The Routledge International Handbook of Mad Studies*, ed. Peter Beresford and Jasna Russo (Routledge, 2021); Alex Gillis, "The Rise of Mad Studies," *University Affairs / Affaires universitaires* (November 2015), https://www.universityaffairs .ca/features/feature-article/mad-studies/.

20. Rivera Garza, "Dangerous Minds"; Mariano Plotkin, *Freud in the Pampas: The Emergence and Development of a Psychoanalytic Culture in Argentina* (Stanford University Press, 2001), 16; Julia Rodriguez, "The Argentine Hysteric: A Turn-of-the-Century Psychiatric Type," in *Argentina on the Couch: Psychiatry, State, and Society, 1880 to the Present*, ed. Mariano Plotkin (University of New Mexico Press, 2003), 31; Jonathan Ablard, *Madness in Buenos Aires: Patients, Psychiatrists, and the Argentine State, 1880–1983* (University of Calgary Press; Ohio University Press, 2008); Stefanie Hunt-Kennedy, personal communication with the author, February 1, 2024.

21. Intersections of disability and indigeneity are also evident in other historical (and related) studies, including archaeology, art history, oral history, and oral traditions. See, for example, Hechler, "Fourth Lifeway"; Christian Prager, "Enanismo y gibosidad: las personas afectadas y su identidad en la sociedad Maya del tiempo prehispánico," in *La organización social entre los Maya prehispánicos, coloniales, y modernos*, ed. V. Tielser Blos, R. Cobos, and M. Greene Robertson (Instituto Nacional de Antropología e Historia, 35–67); William Gassaway, "Divining Disability: Criticism as Diagnosis in Mesoamerican Art History," in *Disability and Art History*, ed. A. Millet-Gallant and E. Howie (Routledge, 2017), 60–81; Scott Thomas Gibson, Sara Newman, and Antonia Carcelen-Estrada, "Indigeneity and Disabilities in the Ecuadorian Oral History Archives," *Disability Studies Quarterly* 41, no. 4 (Fall 2021), https://doi.org/10.18061/dsq.v41i4.8454; Alexander Yarza de los Ríos, "Abya Yala's Disability: Weaving with the Thread and Breath of the Ancestors," *Disability Studies Quarterly* 41, no. 4 (Fall 2021); Siobhan Senier, "Blind Indians: Káteri Tekakwí:tha and Joseph Amos's Visions of Indigenous Resurgence," in *Disability Studies and the Environmental Humanities: Toward an Eco-Crip Theory*, ed. Sarah Jaquette Ray and Jay Sibara (University of Nebraska Press, 2018), 269–89.

22. Stefanie Hunt-Kennedy, *Between Fitness and Death: Disability and Slavery in the Caribbean* (University of Illinois Press, 2020), 124.

23. Hunt-Kennedy, *Between Fitness and Death*, 80–81, 149–54, 159.

24. David Carey Jr., *Health in the Highlands: Indigenous Healing and Scientific Medicine in Guatemala and Ecuador* (University of California Press, 2023).

25. Kafer, *Feminist, Queer, Crip*, 7, 15–17.

26. Ramos, *Bedlam in the New World*, 20.

27. Sander L. Gilman, "Madness as Disability," *History of Psychiatry* 25 (2014): 441–49; H. C. Erik Midelfort, *A History of Madness in Sixteenth-Century Germany* (Stanford University Press, 1999); Charles E. Rosenberg, "Framing Disease: Illness, Society, and History," in *Framing Disease: Studies in Cultural History*, ed. Charles Rosenberg and Janet Golden (Rutgers University Press, 1992).

200 David Carey Jr.

28. Jennifer Lambe, *Madhouse: Psychiatry and Politics in Cuban History* (University of North Carolina Press, 2017), 6.

29. Kafer, *Feminist, Queer, Crip*, 4.

30. Hechler, "Fourth Lifeway."

31. Sophie Kasonde-Ng'andu, "Bio-Medical versus Indigenous Approaches to Disability," in *Disability in Different Cultures: Reflections on Local Concepts*, ed. Brigitte Holzer, Arthur Vreede, and Gabriele Weigt (Transcript Verlag, 1999), 114–21; Hechler, "Fourth Lifeway."

32. Meyer, "Madness and Psychiatry," 197; Ramos, *Bedlam in the New World*, 20–22, 40, 76, 120.

33. Irina Metzler, *Fools and Idiots? Intellectual Disability in the Middle Ages* (Manchester University Press, 2016), 1.

34. Ramos, *Bedlam in the New World*, 181, 122.

35. María Tausiet, "El triunfo de la locura: discurso moral y alegría en España Moderna," *Bulletin of Spanish Studies* 87, no. 8 (2010): 33–55.

36. MM, AP1120, Informe cerca del predio La Concepción de Pifo, February 16, 1910.

37. MM, AP1120, Informe cerca del predio La Concepción de Pifo, February 16, 1910; Foucault, *Madness and Civilization*.

38. Julia Rodriguez, *Civilizing Argentina: Science, Medicine, and the Modern State* (University of North Carolina Press, 2006); Marcos Cueto, *The Return of Epidemics: Health and Society in Peru During the Twentieth Century* (Routledge, 2017), 55.

39. MM, AP1120, Informe cerca del predio La Concepción de Pifo, February 16, 1910.

40. Pedro Fermín Cevallos, *Resumen de la historia del Ecuador* (Lima, 1870), 13–14.

41. Diego C. Iturralde, "Nacionalidades Indígenas y estado nacional en Ecuador," in *Nueva historia del Ecuador*, Vol. 12: *Ensayos generales II: Nación, estado y sistema político*, ed. Enrique Ayala Mora (Editorial Grijalbo Ecuatoriana / Corporación Editora Nacional, 1995), 12; Carey, *Health in the Highlands*.

42. Confederación de Nacionalidades Indígenas del Ecuador (CNIE), *Las nacionalidades indígenas en el Ecuador: nuestro proceso organizativo* (Ediciones Tinicui-Abya Yala, 1989).

43. Pablo Ospina Peralta, *La aleación inestable: origen y consolidación de un Estado transformista: Ecuador, 1920–1960* (Editorial Teseo / Universidad Andina Simón Bolívar, Sede Ecuador, 2020), 26, 429; Guillermo Bustos Lozano, *El culto a la nación: escritura de la historia y rituales de la memoria en Ecuador, 1870–1950* (Fondo de Cultural Económica / Universidad Andina Simón Bolívar, 2017); Tribunal Supremo Electoral de Ecuador, *Elecciones y democracia en el Ecuador* (1989), 56, accessed March 9, 2021, https://repositories.lib.utexas.edu/bitstream/handle/2152/17573/libro_18.pdf?sequence=2; Marc Becker, *Indians and Leftists in the Making of Ecuador's Modern Indigenous Movements* (Duke University Press, 2008), 18–22; George Stuart McCook, *States of Nature: Science, Agriculture, and Environment in the Spanish Caribbean, 1760–1940* (University of Texas Press, 2002), 10.

44. Kim A. Clark, "Race, 'Culture,' and Mestizaje: The Statistical Construction of the Ecuadorian Nation, 1930–1950," *Journal of Historical Sociology* 11, no. 2 (June 1998): 193, 208n26; Ospina Peralta, *Aleación inestable*, 21–22, 430.

45. José Antonio Lucero, "Locating the 'Indian Problem': Community, Nationality,

and Contradiction in Ecuadorian Indigenous Politics," *Latin American Perspectives* 30, no. 1 (2003): 27–29; Becker, *Indians and Leftists*, xvi, 72, 78–80.

46. Juan Maiguascha and Liisa North, "Orígenes y significado del velasquismo: lucha de clases y participación política en el Ecuador, 1920–1972," in *La cuestión regional y el poder*, ed. Rafael Quintero, 89–159 (Corporación Editora Nacional, 1991); Juan Maiguascha, "Los sectores subalternos en los años 30 y el aparecimiento del velasquismo," in *Las crisis en el Ecuador: los treinta y ochenta*, ed. Rosemary Thorpe (Corporación Editora Nacional, 1991), 79–94; Carlos Marchán Romero, "La crisis de los años treinta: diferenciación social de sus efectos económicos," in *Las crisis en el Ecuador*, 31–60; Kim A. Clark, "Racial Ideologies and the Quest for National Development: Debating the Agrarian Problem in Ecuador," *Journal of Latin American Studies* 30 (1998): 375–76, 381.

47. John Saunders, *The People of Ecuador: A Demographic Analysis* (University of Florida Press, 1961); Dirección Nacional de Estadísticas, *Ecuador en Cifras* (Quito, 1944), 55; Marc Becker, *¡Pachakutik! Indigenous Movements and Electoral Politics in Ecuador* (Rowman and Littlefield, 2010).

48. Rodrigo Chávez, *El mestizaje y su influencia social en América* (Imprenta Municipal, 1937), 77–79; Becker, *¡Pachakutik!*, 3–5; A. Kim Clark and Marc Becker, "Indigenous Peoples and State Formation in Modern Ecuador," in *Highland Indians and the State in Modern Ecuador*, ed. A. Kim Clark and Marc Becker (University of Pittsburgh Press, 2007), 12.

49. MM, AP 1188, Correspondencia recibida de Moyurco, cartas de Anibal Maldonado, Hacienda Moyurco, October 10 and 15, 1946; MM, AP 1188, Correspondencia recibida de Moyurco, carta de Anibal Maldonado, Hacienda Moyurco, October 10, 1946; CNIE, *Nacionalidades indígenas*; Andrés Guerrero, "Una imagen ventrílocua: el discurso liberal de la 'desgraciada raza indígena' a fines del siglo XIX," in *Imágenes e imagineros: representaciones de los indígenas ecuatorianos, siglos XIX y XX*, ed. Blanca Muratorio (FLACSO-Ecuador, 1994), 197–253; Andrés Guerrero, "La desintegración de la administración étnica en el Ecuador" in *Sismo étnico en el Ecuador*, ed. José Almeida et al. (Quito: DEDIME, 1993), 91–112; A. Kim Clark, *The Redemptive Work: Railway and Nation in Ecuador, 1895–1930* (Scholarly Resources, 1998), 76–83; Clark and Becker, "Indigenous Peoples and State Formation."

50. Rebecca Earle, *The Return of the Native: Indians and Myth-Making in Spanish America, 1810–1910* (Duke University Press, 2007), 163.

51. Nancy Stepan, *"The Hour of Eugenics": Race, Gender, and Nation in Latin America* (Cornell University Press, 1996); Alexandra Minna Stern, "Responsible Mothers and Normal Children: Eugenics, Nationalism, and Welfare in Postrevolutionary Mexico, 1920–1940," *Journal of Historical Sociology* 12, no. 4 (1999): 369–97; Patience Schell, "Eugenics Policy and Practice in Cuba, Puerto Rico, and Mexico," in *Oxford Handbook of Global Eugenics*, ed. Alison Bashford and Philippa Levine, 485–87 (Oxford University Press, 2011); Elizabeth O'Brien, "Pelvimetry and the Persistence of Racial Sciences in Obstetrics," *Endeavor*, 37, no 1 (2012): 21, 23, 24, 26–28; Stefan Pohl-Valero, "'La raza entra por la boca': Energy, Diet, and Eugenics in Colombia, 1890–1940," *Hispanic American Historical Review* 94, no. 3 (2014): 457–58, 474–75; Carlos Ernesto Noguera, *Medicina y política: discurso médico y prácticas higiénicas durante la primera mitad del siglo XX en Colombia* (Fondo Editorial Universidad EAFIT, 2003); Beatriz Urías Horcasitas, *Historias secretas del racismo en México*

(1920–1950) (Tusquets Editores México, 2007); Beatriz Urías Horcasitas, "Degeneracionismo e higiene mental en el México posrevolucionario (1920–1940)," *Frenia* 4, no. 2 (2004): 37–67; Laura Suárez, *Eugenesia y racismo en México* (Universidad Nacional Autónoma, 2005).

52. Stephanie Hunt-Kennedy and Melanie Newton, "The Hauntings of Slavery: Colonialism and the Disabled Body in the Caribbean," in *Disability in the Global South: The Critical Handbook*, ed. Shaun Grech and Karen Soldatic (Springer, 2016), 380.

53. Alexandra Minna Stern, "Buildings, Boundaries, and Blood: Medicalization and Nation-Building on the U.S.-Mexico Border, 1910–1930," *Hispanic American Historical Review* 79, no. 1 (February 1999): 64.

54. David Carey Jr., "Hygienic Determinism, Cultural Essentialism, and Public Health in Ecuador and Guatemala, 1900–1950," *Estudios Interdisciplinarios de América Latina* 34, no. 2 (2023): 14–43.

55. Gilberto Hochman et al., eds., *Patologías de la patria: enfermedades, enfermos y nación en América Latina* (Lugar Editorial, 2012); Stepan, *"Hour of Eugenics."*

56. MM, SA0746, Delegación sanidad de Tungurahua, Ambato, to Director de Sanidad, February 1, 1930.

57. The rise of devastating operations and other "somatic interventions" in mad people's bodies in Europe and the United States by the 1910s suggests that medical professionals increasingly situated madness in the body.

58. Suzanne Austin Alchon, *Native Society and Disease in Colonial Ecuador* (Cambridge University Press, 1991), 62n16. In sharp contrast, the association of goiter with mental disability was widely disavowed in El Salvador by this time. See Heather Vrana, "Endemic Goiter and El Salvador's Battle Against *Cretinismo,*" *American Historical Review*, 128, no. 4 (December 2023): 1587–617.

59. MM, SA0746, Delegación sanidad de Tungurahua, Ambato, to Director de Sanidad, February 1, 1930.

60. Plotkin, *Freud in the Pampas*, 15.

61. Natalia Molina, *Fit to Be Citizens? Public Health and Race in Los Angeles, 1879–1939* (University of California Press, 2006), 147.

62. Rivera-Garza, "'She Neither Respected nor Obeyed Anyone,'" 668.

63. MM, SA0699, Director General de Sanidad, Servicio Sanitario Nacional, Quito, December 23, 1939.

64. Molina, *Fit to Be Citizens?*, 147.

65. Baynton, "Slaves, Immigrants, and Suffragists," 562, 565 (quote); John McKiernan, *Fevered Measures: Public Health and Race at the Texas-Mexico Border, 1848–1942* (Duke University Press, 2012).

66. Elizabeth Mellyn, "Healers and Healing in the Early Modern Care Market," in *The Routledge History of Madness and Mental Health*, ed. Greg Eghigian (Routledge, 2017), 83–100; Yumi Kim, "Seeing Cages: Home Confinement in Early Twentieth-Century Japan," *The Journal of Asian Studies* 77, no. 3 (August 2018): 635–658; Ramos, *Bedlam in the New World*; Meyer, "Madness and Psychiatry."

67. MM, SA0767, Dirección General de Sanidad, Sangolquí, August 29, 1918 (quote); Burch, *Committed*, 3–4.

68. Estefanía Bautista-Valarezo et al., "Towards an Indigenous Definition of Health: An Explorative Study to Understand the Indigenous Ecuadorian People's Health and Illness Concepts," *International Journal for Equity in Health* 19, no. 101 (2020): 1–8; Irene Silverblatt, *Sun, Moon, and Witches: Gender Ideologies and Class in Inca and Colonial Peru* (Princeton University Press, 1987), 173; Natalie L. Kimball, *An Open Secret: The History of Unwanted Pregnancy and Abortion in Modern Bolivia* (Rutgers University Press, 2020); Marcos Cueto and Steven Palmer, *Medicine and Public Health in Latin America: A History* (Cambridge University Press, 2015), 14.

69. MM, AP1120, Informe cerca del predio La Concepción de Pifo, February 16, 1910. Similarly, early-twentieth-century "mental hospitals" in Lahore (present-day Pakistan) suffered poor conditions, which British officials considered "worse than jails." See Waltraud Ernst, *Colonialism and Transnational Psychiatry: The Development of an Indian Mental Hospital in British India, c. 1925–1940* (Anthem Press, 2013).

70. Rivera-Garza, "'She Neither Respected nor Obeyed Anyone'" 657.

71. Carey, *Health in the Highlands*.

72. Sylvia Sellers-García, *The Woman on the Windowsill: A Tale of Mystery in Several Parts* (Yale University Press, 2020), 39. In colonial Mexico, Ramos has observed, "nebulous terrain" demarcated "madness from inebriation." See Ramos, *Bedlam in the New World*, 124 (quote), 158.

73. Federico González Suárez, *Historia general de la República de Ecuador* (1890; reprint, Casa de la Cultura Ecuatoriana, 1969), 226.

74. Erin O'Connor, "Helpless Children or Undeserving Patriarchs? Gender Ideologies, the State, and Indian Men in Late Nineteenth-Century Ecuador," in *Highland Indians and the State in Modern Ecuador*, 56–71; Derek Williams, "The Making of Ecuador's *Pueblo Católico*, 1861–1875," in *Political Cultures in the Andes*, ed. Nils Jacobson and Cristóbal Alvojín de Losada (Duke University Press, 2005), 218, 222–23.

75. Natalie Lira, *Laboratory of Deficiency: Sterilization and Confinement in California, 1900–1950s* (University of California Press, 2021).

76. MM, SA0850, Ministerio de Prevision social y sanidad, Quito, May 15, 1940, Ambato, April 29, 1940. Unfortunately, the minister did not sign or otherwise indicate his name.

77. MM, SA0850, Delegado Sanidad a Ministerio de Sanidad y Hygiene, Ambato, April 29, 1940.

78. Molina, *Fit to Be Citizens?*, 147.

79. MM, SA0850, Delegado Sanidad a Ministerio de Sanidad y Hygiene, Ambato, April 29, 1940.

80. Adria L. Imada, "Family History as Disability History: Native Hawaiians Surviving Medical Incarceration," *Disability Studies Quarterly* 41, no. 4 (Fall 2021); Elizabeth O'Brien, *Surgery and Salvation: The Roots of Reproductive Injustice in Mexico, 1770–1940* (University of North Carolina Press, 2023); Lambe, *Madhouse*; Carlos S. Dimas, *Poisoned Eden: Cholera Epidemics, State-Building, and the Problem of Public Health in Argentina, 1865–1908* (University of Nebraska Press, 2022); Meyer, "Madness and Psychiatry"; Marcos Cueto, ed., *Saberes Andinos: ciencia y tecnología en Bolivia, Ecuador, y Perú* (Instituto de Estudios Peruanos, 1995); Marcos Cueto, ed., *Missionaries of Science: The Rockefeller Foun-*

dation and Latin America (University of Indiana Press, 1994); Cueto and Palmer, *Medicine and Public Health in Latin America*; Steven Palmer, *Launching Global Health: The Caribbean Odyssey of the Rockefeller Foundation* (University of Michigan Press, 2010); Steven Palmer, *From Popular Medicine to Medical Populism: Doctors, Healers, and Public Power in Costa Rica, 1800–1940* (Duke University Press, 2003); Diego Armus, ed., *Disease in the History of Modern Latin America* (Duke University Press, 2003).

81. Meyer, "Madness and Psychiatry," 195. In the Ottoman Arab world, violently mad people were similarly confined to hospitals. See Sara Scalenghe, *Disability in the Ottoman Arab World, 1500–1800* (Cambridge University Press, 2014), 98.

82. Ronn Pineo, "Misery and Death in the Pearl of the Pacific: Health Care in Guayaquil, Ecuador, 1870–1925," *Hispanic American Historical Review* 70, no. 4 (1990): 629–31; Lambe, *Madhouse*, 26; Meyer, "Madness and Psychiatry," 198; Ramos, *Bedlam in the New World*.

83. Plotkin, *Freud in the Pampas*, 16; Rodriguez, "Argentine Hysteric," 31.

84. Octavio Díaz, *Informe que a la Nación presenta el Ministro de lo Interior, Policía, Beneficencia, Obras Públicas, etc. en el año 1910* (Imprenta y Encuadernación Nacionales, 1910), xxii–xxiv.

85. MM, SA0891, Latacunga, October 27, 1931.

86. MM, AP 1120, Traversari to Sr don Juan Salvador, Jefe Político, January 22, 1910.

87. Foucault, *Madness and Civilization*.

88. Rivera-Garza, "'She Neither Respected nor Obeyed Anyone'" 661, 663.

89. Catherine Cox and Hillary Marland, "'He Must Die or Go Mad in This Place': Prisoners, Insanity, and the Pentonville Model Prison Experiment, 1842–52," *Bulletin of History of Medicine* 92, no. 1 (spring 2018): 78–109; Ramos, *Bedlam in the New World*, 114, 134–36, 167.

90. MM, AP 1120, Traversari to Sr don Juan Salvador, Jefe Polítoco, January 22, 1910.

91. MM, AP 1120, Traversari to Sr don Juan Salvador, Jefe Polítoco, January 22, 1910.

92. MM, AP 1120, Informe cerca del predio La Concepción de Pifo de Pedro Traversari y Manuel Jejon, February 16, 1910. Overcrowding marked asylums throughout Latin America. See Meyer, "Madness and Psychiatry," 204.

93. MM, AP 1120, Informe cerca del predio La Concepción de Pifo de Pedro Traversari y Manuel Jejon, February 16, 1910.

94. MM, AP 1120, Informe cerca del predio La Concepción de Pifo de Pedro Traversari y Manuel Jejon, February 16, 1910.

95. MM, AP 1120, Informe cerca del predio La Concepción de Pifo de Pedro Traversari y Manuel Jejon, February 16, 1910.

96. MM, AP 1120, Informe cerca del predio La Concepción de Pifo de Pedro Traversari y Manuel Jejon, February 16, 1910.

97. Carey, *Health in the Highlands*.

98. Lambe, *Madhouse*; Cueto and Palmer, *Medicine and Public Health in Latin America*, 189; Burch, *Committed*, 5; Pamela Block and Fátima Gonçalves Cavalcante, "Historical Perceptions of Autism in Brazil: Professional Treatment, Family Advocacy, and Autistic Pride, 1943–2010," in *Disability Histories*, 80.

99. Block and Gonçalves Cavalcante, "Historical Perceptions of Autism in Brazil," 79.

100. Rivera-Garza, "'She Neither Respected nor Obeyed Anyone,'" 671–72.

101. Burch, *Committed*, 8–9.

102. MM, AP 1120, Dr. Villavicencio informe sobre Lazareto Pifo, March 2, 1911.

103. MM, AP 1120, Dr. Villavicencio informe sobre Lazareto Pifo, March 2, 1911.

104. MM, AP0251, cartas: Eloisa C. de Betancourt; Dirección de la Junta Central de Beneficencia, Quito, June 4, 1943; Director de Junta Beneficencia de Milar, June 4, 1943.

105. MM, AP 1120, November 10, 1911.

106. MM, AP 1120, November 10, 1911.

107. Hunt-Kennedy, *Between Fitness and Death*, 2, 5, 13.

108. Carey, *Health in the Highlands*.

7

Disability, Colonialism, and Gendered Illness in the Aftermath of the 1773 Guatemala Earthquake

Martha Few

When a devastating earthquake struck Santiago de Guatemala at the end of July 1773, residents in this multiethnic colonial capital and the surrounding Maya towns in the Panchoy Valley would not have been caught wholly by surprise.[1] Repeated tremors in the days leading up to the major earthquake on July 29 provided early warning signs in this earthquake-prone region. It had already been a challenging summer, as the rainy season that year included strong storms in the weeks before the earthquake that caused the Pensativo River to breach its banks and flood the *barrios* (neighborhoods) on the eastern side of the city, as well as the city center, where the important markers of colonial authority and power were located: the central plaza, the palace of the president of the Audiencia of Guatemala, and the Cathedral. That Thursday afternoon in July when the earthquake hit, it knocked residents to the ground in the Santo Domingo and Candelaria barrios. People fled the city's buildings and homes and moved as quickly as possible into city streets and plazas for safety. The Audiencia president, don Martín de Mayorga, ordered that the doors to the city's jails be opened and the prisoners released, including the doors to the Casa Nueva women's prison.[2] Archival sources provide no information as to how patients residing in the city's four hospitals faired, though eyewitness accounts noted that the city's main hospital, the Hospital Real de San Juan de Dios, had extensive damage, and its roof caved in.[3]

Strong rains in the days following the quake hindered efforts to rescue trapped survivors and extract the dead from damaged homes and buildings. Significant aftershocks continued through the summer and into the fall, followed by a second major earthquake in December of the same year, again with more significant aftershocks. Numerous public health emergencies that began in the wake of the first quake in July intensified after the second major quake and continued to plague the area into the winter and spring of 1774. Challenges included lack of clean water, due to damage to the city's system of aqueducts and public fountains, and inadequate temporary housing, especially for the city's poor residents. Food shortages threatened the region as tributary Maya residents who lived in valley towns that provisioned the capital abandoned their homes and *milpas* (Maya-style cultivated fields), moving their families away from the dangerous built environments into the surrounding highland Maya communities or into the *monte*, the forested mountains and woodlands of Guatemala's western highlands.[4]

Earthquakes and other natural disasters created conditions for disease outbreaks such as those that emerged in the wake of these two major earthquakes during the latter six months of 1773 and spread through the region's multiethnic populations during 1774 and into 1775. Colonial officials attempted to reestablish the colonial order in the city as residents coped with rebuilding their lives and livelihoods. Elite residents, politicians, clergy, and others debated whether or not to rebuild or to abandon the capital and move to a new site.[5]

In the midst of these chaotic events and the ensuing social instability, two diseases emerged among the survivors that caused particular concern. *Tabardillo*, usually translated as "typhus," became a public health problem after the earthquake quickly spreading through local populations.[6] This illness caused symptoms of "pestilential fevers" and high death rates and tended to afflict and kill entire families and residents of the same household, especially those labeled by colonial officials as "the poor," the Maya, free and enslaved people of African descent, and people of multiethnic origin labeled "mestizos" and "*castas*" in the colonial record.[7] This particular tabardillo outbreak, however, reached members of Guatemala's elites, including the family members of *Regidor* (city council member) don Miguel de Coronado, whose son died from the illness, and multiple family members of both doña Rose de Herrarte and doña María Manuela Jérez.[8] One of the city's prominent medical doctors, Francisco de Azetuno, contracted tabardillo from treating the sick and died from the illness.[9] These instances when tabardillo uncharacteristically broke into the city's wealthier populations shows how the public health challenges in this postearthquake context affected all of the city's residents, not just the poor.

Medical doctors in the capital also noted the spread of a troubling new disease that they called *epidémica de la constitución* (epidemic of bodily constitution), which disabled people with "hysterical effects that cause great headache pains, delirium, and anxiety."[10] The name of this new disease reflected Galenic-humoral understandings of bodily constitution or makeup that underpinned medical theories at that time, with *constitución* referring to an individual's disposition (*temple*) and nature (*temperamento*).[11] Key members of the Audiencia's medical community characterized epidémica de la constitución as one that afflicted women, primarily ladina and Indigenous women who showed observable symptoms of mental or emotional distress caused by the trauma of the earthquakes.[12] Epidémica de la constitución could afflict women on its own or in addition to any new or lingering physical impairments or disabilities that shaped afflicted women's lives. Colonial officials in eighteenth-century sources used the term "ladina" to distinguish among the Maya by perceived levels of acculturation, the term signifying a racial-ethnic category of Indigenous and mixed-race people whom they deemed more Hispanicized in terms of language and culture, a way to separate them from monolingual Maya speakers and those identified by the colonial legal category *indio/a* ("Indian").[13]

A challenge for scholars working on disability and colonialism in the early modern period is developing a methodological strategy that draws on the rich insights of research in disability history, which has tended to focus on modern as well as US and European contexts and source bases, while at the same time take into account conceptions of health, disability, and disease operating in a colonial setting with distinct but overlapping European, Mayan, and African medical cultures and practices.[14] Colonial archives rarely provide insight or evidence from the perspective of the lived experiences and lives of individuals, so evidence for disability experiences must be gleaned from critical readings of sources produced in colonial contexts by colonial medical, political, and religious authorities for purposes of medicalization, surveillance, and the establishment and maintenance of racial-ethnic, gender, and social hierarchies of colonialism.[15] Some individual and community experiences of disability among this multiethnic colonial population may have been new in the case of those diagnosed with epidémica de la constitución. Others became visible only when the need to escape or flee the severe damage of the capital become necessary, or were exacerbated to the point of disability because of the difficulties faced in surviving and making a living in a partially destroyed city.

As colonial authorities, the clergy, and colonial elites struggled to address the effects of the earthquakes, support grew among city officials, the public health community, and professors in the medical school, the Universidad de San Carlos, for the establishment of epidémica de la constitución as a distinct illness category among female colonial subjects of Indigenous and mixed-Indigenous descent.[16] The illness category, though applied in this case just to women, responded to and acknowledged the stress and trauma that the events had on individuals, producing not just physical injuries but also debilitating mental and emotional responses encapsulated by the reported symptoms of "hysterical effects" (*efectos hystericos*). These effects encompassed a range of symptoms from generalized bodily pain and headaches to delirium (*delirios*) and anxiety (*inquietud*).[17] Certainly all sectors of colonial society, no matter the racial-ethnic group, economic status, or slave or free designations, experienced ongoing trauma from the earthquakes' devastation, trauma that caused temporary or permanent disability and debility. Yet the ad hoc Junta de Salubridad (Public Health Committee), established in the spring of 1774 by the Audiencia president and designed to address the public health crisis and create officially sanctioned medical instructions, singled out ladina and Indigenous women as being particularly susceptible to some of the most exceptional of these effects, pathologizing them in the process by grouping them under a kind of hysteria. Medical officials also linked the hysterical effects to the tabardillo (typhus) outbreak, suggesting the cases of Indigenous women's so-called hysteria were an additional, gendered effect of the disease.[18]

Descriptions during and after the 1773 earthquakes can provide some evidence of the disabling effects of surviving this earthquake, and of the generalized experiences of emotional distress, injury, and disease outbreaks. A report on the earthquake events that Juan González Bustillo, former president of the Audiencia, authored and sent to the king of Spain provides evidence of how residents experienced the events and the severe damage to the city.[19] González Bustillo toured the city after the first earthquake struck in July. He described seeing one resident after another struggling to emerge from the ruins of their homes and the city's buildings, covered in *polvo* (dust): "[Everyone] expressed great terror, and fear, and awe, at finding themselves in the midst of such peril. Some could be seen kneeling [in prayer], others prostrate on the ground, others calling on Heaven, asking God for his mercy, many making confessions, and many receiving absolutions."[20] The weeks after the initial quake were no less distressing. Firsthand accounts like González Bustillo's show that those who survived had to come to terms with the fact that "it was not possible to extract from [the rubble] those persons who were dying, [and] to free them from their ruined homes that they had not been able to escape from, or [to] help remove the dead." Audiencia president Mayorga, who initially had shown mercy to prisoners by releasing them from the city jails, feared the instability that act seemed to have caused and the general unrest and looting in the days following, so much so that he stationed troops in the capital's central plaza to guard the presidential palace and other important colonial and royal buildings.[21]

Natural disasters like the earthquakes can reveal that individuals' disability experiences in daily life caused advanced age, injury, incurable illness, or chronic disease. For colonial Guatemala and early modern Latin America, however, few female-authored sources such as diaries, letters, or other written materials survive in the archives.[22] An exception is a letter written by a woman who lived through the earthquake, Sister María Gertrudis de Yribe y Folgar, the abbess of the Capuchin convent in Santiago de Guatemala, who penned a private, personal letter to the abbess of the Capuchin convent in Oaxaca, Mexico, while the events remained clear in her mind.[23] The abbess referred to her friend only as "Marquita"; the two may have become friends earlier in their religious careers, likely as nuns together in a convent in Guatemala, given that the Oaxaca Capuchin convent was founded by nuns from the Guatemala branch of the Capuchin female order.[24] Colonial religious and political officials had named the July earthquake Santa Marta because it occurred on her saint's day, July 29, as "the most woeful tragedy that this world has ever seen."[25] As Sister María Gertrudis recounted to her friend, the main quake began around 3:15 in the afternoon and continued for three hours straight, "without taking more pause then the time it took to take a breath, and after this pause it continued with even more force."[26]

Sister María Gertrudis's account is exceptional because it provides one of a handful of extant informal, firsthand accounts of the 1773 earthquake written to friends and family. Moreover, her account provides a woman's perspective, that of a cloistered nun, whose connections to the outside world were mediated since she professed only through the *sala de torno* (a room that contained a revolving hatch, connected to a public entrance to the convent, that enabled cloistered nuns to pass objects in and out).[27] Where other residents of Santiago de Guatemala would have immediately fled their homes and buildings as the earthquake began, if they were able, the nuns would not have immediately fled because of this Capuchin convent's strict enclosure rules. Thus, the abbess described how she and the other nuns checked on one another and searched together for safe spaces inside the convent grounds, even as the buildings and walls crumbled into rubble around them:

> I was in the *sala de torno* when we saw the main entrance to the convent fall, and as best I could I fled from the *torno* with the others. We went to the door of the *confesionario* [the room where confessions were heard], and there we saw Madre Theresa sitting calmly on the steps of the fountain.[28] Everyone cried out to her to get out of there. And at that moment she took five steps to get a drink of water [from the fountain] because she was choking from the dust [*se ahogaba con el polvo*]. At that same moment a large section of the fountain broke off, and then the entire fountain itself rose up one *vara* into the air, and then slammed down, [falling] on the exact same place where the nun had stopped, just at her feet. We were thunderstruck-dazed (*atónitas*) to see that suddenly happen, and how our Lord saved her life.[29]

At this point in the night's events, the abbess and her fellow nuns expected to perish from the quake inside their convent. But then a loud sound caught their attention:

> All of us waited for something else to cause the earth to open and swallow us up. At this moment the bell rang with great violence. We went to look and saw that it was *su Ilustrísimo* [the archbishop], ordering us to flee [the convent]. Some of us resisted because it seemed to us that if we were going to die, it would be better for us to be enclosed in our convent, and not outside of it, but we were persuaded by our holy obedience, and so we opened the door [to the street].[30]

It must have taken much inner strength and faith for Sister María Gertrudis and her fellow nuns to leave the enclosure and join the throngs of people from all racial and ethnic groups and economic statuses, some injured, all very emotional as they tried to flee to safety through air filled with ash and debris from the city's destruction. Felipe Cadena, a Dominican friar and theologian who survived the quakes, recounted his surprise at seeing certain groups of people not usually seen on the streets, whose escape thereto "made visible to the public the highest status women in their domestic clothing, as well as the most secluded religious clergy." He also remarked on the exceptional appearance of "all of the communities and religious orders of nuns and *beatas* [lay sisters]" who sought refuge in the countryside to escape their destroyed convents and buildings.[31]

Sister María Gertrudis's account furthermore provides the experiences that an older woman with limited mobility faced during the earthquakes. Her letter reveals that she herself was either temporarily or permanently physically disabled with limited mobility even before the earthquake. I infer this from the letter where Sister María Gertrudis describes herself as unable to walk while the Capuchin nuns, all 28 of them, escaped together into the streets as their convent's walls fell around them during the subsequent aftershocks.[32] One of the men, Brother Francisco, "saw that I could not stand up or walk on my own, so he carried me from the building out into the street, and put me amid the rest of the nuns and *velos* (veiled ones) so that we could leave together.[33] A group of priests and lay religious men, along with extended family members of the nuns, showed up together at the convent to coordinate the nuns' escape from the building.

Priests and other male residents of the capital accompanied the Capuchin nuns as they made their way that night through the city's destruction to the designated meeting point for their religious order. A man named don Francisco Pacheco, the nephew of one of the Capuchin nuns, also noticed that the abbess could not walk well and that she repeatedly fell to the ground as she struggled through the rubble: "From Anca Street he consoled me by helping me up every time that I fell, seeing the awful state I was in."[34] Eventually Pacheco and another man, identified only as the *sacristán* (a male religious official), managed to commandeer a horse-drawn cabriolet and place the abbess inside to safely carry her to temporary housing at a cattle ranch outside the city. That night the nuns slept together on the floor of one of the ranch buildings.[35]

Personal letters written in the aftermath of other earthquakes around the same time, when they can be located, can serve to further flesh out individual experiences of disability and disaster.[36] In October 1815 in the town of San Miguel in what is now El Salvador, Joaquín María Palacios wrote a letter to don Lorenzo Moreno, a close friend and possibly the godfather to one of his children, about a "terrible earthquake" that had occurred a few months earlier, so strong that it knocked down the bell towers of the local church.[37] Palacios described the trajectory of the debilitating physical and emotional symptoms that he experienced in the wake of the event:

> Because of the many anxieties [*afanes*] and devastations [*asoliadas*] [caused by the earthquake] on 12 September, a strong *flución* [flux] attacked me. First came *un furioso frío* [a furious chill] that lasted six hours, so intense that I had to quickly write my last will and testament, and they anointed me [administered extreme unction].[38]

Like the abbess, Palacios saw the work of God as mediating his experiences and saving his life. Yet his subsequent illness, while not fatal, left him disabled, completely immobile and bed-ridden:

> Ultimately I lost all hope of surviving. But blessed be God, who turned away the illness in favor of health. Then one of my knees swelled up. They applied various poultices to it, and neither did these or any other treatments stop the flución. And because of this I have remained unable to leave my bed. I cannot move at all except to lay on my back face up, [and] because I have a knee that is so diseased, I cannot move myself except with assistance.[39]

From the context it is unclear exactly what this flución entailed except that the illness caused much swelling in his knee and other parts of his body. Moreover, the affliction did not respond to medical treatments and left him unable to move or even turn over in bed. So he asked his good friend and compadre to consult doctors that he knew in hopes of a cure:

> I beg of you, for God's sake, consult the best *facultativo* in the capital providing him this narration of my case, so that based on his judgement, [and] for my sanity [*sanidad*], you can send to me by return mail suitable medicines for treating [the illness].[40]

Both accounts provide compelling firsthand descriptions of disability caused or exacerbated by earthquakes around the turn of the nineteenth century, produced by literate members of the elite, materials more likely to be saved and later archived because of the writers' social statuses. The abbess in Guatemala and Palacios in El Salvador were enmeshed in social networks that they could depend on for their care, Sister María Gertrudis as a member of a religious community of nuns, and Palacios as a man with a compadre on whom he could rely for additional help and with the means to pay to have medicines sent to him. The sources also suggest the obvious:

that not only women but also men had physical and emotional responses to earthquakes in ways that are not usually transparent in archival documents, in contrast to epidémica de la constitución, conceptualized as a disease category that medicalized the debilitating trauma that primarily women experienced. This example indicates that men's trauma in the aftermath of natural disasters like earthquakes was not medicalized or even pathologized in the same way that women's experiences were.[41]

In Guatemala in 1773, the Audiencia and town council made containing the tabardillo outbreak the highest priority among a wide range of public health, housing, and provisioning challenges that lingered in the weeks and months after the two major earthquakes. Mayorga, as Audiencia president, created the ad hoc Junta de Salubridad in the spring of 1774 to address epidémica de la constitución and put the medical doctor Manuel Ávalos y Porras in charge. Ávalos y Porras quickly wrote and published a guide for city elites describing the disease's presentation and treatment.[42] Titled *Breve methodo de curar la enfermedad epidemica de la constitucion de este año de 1774, que el vulgo llama tabardillo* (Brief method for treating the disease epidémica de la constitución in this year of 1774, which the common people call tabardillo), the instructions were written for a reading audience of political and religious officials, Audiencia-licensed health care professionals, and *boticarios* (colonial government–sanctioned apothecaries). They spread the word of what was touted as the most medically up-to-date treatment for this new disease, which struck an alarming number of residents in the capital. To date, however, no firsthand accounts of epidémica de la constitución have emerged in the archive that allow an analysis of individual experiences of this disabling illness.

Even so, scholars can use sources produced by colonial medical, political, and religious authorities, such as this Audiencia-sanctioned treatment guide, to get a sense of the disabling aspects of the illness as it was experienced by Indigenous and ladina women. Care must be taken, however, to take into account that their disability and illness experiences were framed through the medicalizing lens of Guatemala's Enlightenment-era medical community as public health officials dealt with what seemed to them a new and pervasive illness with a range of symptoms.[43] The official treatment guidelines are here analyzed in conjunction with medical recipes and botanical writings that described various illnesses and treatments for tabardillo. Although the guides reflect eighteenth-century understandings of "hysterical effects," disorders of nerves (*nervios*), and other illness not named epidémica de la constitución, they describe similar symptoms in the context of other epidemic disease outbreaks and of miscarriages caused by violence and trauma and other extreme events experienced by women, particularly women of color, in colonial society.

In colonial Central America, licensed, university-educated medical doctors led efforts to construct and solidify disease categories that defined public health policy in the late eighteenth century. Starting in earnest in the 1760s and continuing until the Independence period of the 1820s, the colonial state commissioned medical treatment guidelines for the most pressing epidemic and infectious diseases. The authors, who generally were either officials in the Protomedicato (the bureaucracy in charge of regulating medicine in the Audiencia) or medical faculty at Guatemala's Universidad de San Carlos, designed and carried out public health campaigns that systematically addressed a broad array of epidemic and infectious diseases including smallpox, measles, typhus, whooping cough, and yellow fever. First, medical officials drafted the manuscript instructions; then they were copied and circulated among colonial officials, religious personnel, and local elites in areas experiencing disease outbreaks. If the treatments proved successful, the instructions were revised and then published by one of the capital's multiple printing houses in the form of small portable pamphlets. Each focused on a particular disease, which could then be easily sent or carried across Central America as needed.[44] The treatment guidelines would then be revised, updated, and quickly reprinted as needed in the aftermath of disease outbreaks, allowing a focus on afflicted populations including not only urban European-descended elites but also women, Indigenous people, and the urban and rural poor—wherever the disease struck. Moreover, doctors adapted medical recipe ingredients to particular local ecologies, or after an antiepidemic campaign gathered additional details regarding local diets or medical botany from local healers (*curandero/as*) and *parteras* (female midwives).[45]

When the Protomedicato's doctors designed the first smallpox inoculation programs tailored to the culturally diverse, predominantly Maya communities, for example, they had to take into account Maya medical cultures, the issue of language and cultural translation, and the local environments of Guatemala's western highlands. This adaptability can also be read in the title of one of the most important of these guides, published as a pamphlet by one of Nueva Guatemala's presses in 1794: José Flores's *Instruccion sobre el modo de practicar la inoculacion de las viruelas, y el metodo para curar esta enfermedad, acomodado a la naturaleza y modo de vivir de los indios del Reyno de Guatemala* (Instruction for the method of practicing smallpox inoculation, and how to cure this illness, tailored to the nature and way of life of the indigenous of the Kingdom of Guatemala).[46] Illness categories and treatments at this time were flexible, as particular outbreaks tested the boundaries of current understandings of disease categories and, at other times, broke through them entirely, necessitating significantly revised treatment guidelines and instructions. Furthermore, humoral medicine as practiced in the eighteenth century was structured by prescribing different treatments and methods according to age, gender, and other aspects of an individual's particular "nature" or "constitution" as healers sought to cure the sick by bringing the body back into balance.

Tabardillo expressed itself differently among the afflicted survivors of the 1773 earthquake than it had during earlier outbreaks that medical doctors were familiar with. This particular epidemic also included an observable cluster of digestive distress, spasms, delirium, and other symptoms that doctors believed particularly afflicted Indigenous and mixed-race women, and so they needed to rethink their treatment protocols and dietary guidelines.

Manuel Ávalos y Porras was the senior medical doctor in the capital at the time and a member of the medical faculty at the University of San Carlos, holding the chair in medicine, which came with the title Cathedrático de Prima Medicina.[47] Junta members, the Audiencia, and the city council looked to him to provide the medical leadership needed to address the outbreak and make treatment recommendations. Born in Guatemala, Ávalos y Porras attended medical school at the University of San Carlos in Santiago de Guatemala, where he was trained by José de Medina, then the chair in medicine and himself a University of San Carlos graduate.[48] In his seventies at this point, Ávalos y Porras was an experienced hand in antiepidemic efforts in Guatemala. As far back as the 1760s, he had coauthored colonial Guatemala's first official, government-sanctioned guidelines, titled "Observations on the Treatment Methods for Measles and Smallpox," in response to an epidemic of both diseases affecting the capital and surrounding communities.[49]

Interestingly, Ávalos y Porras constructed the title for the new medical instructions as an argument: "Brief Method for Treating the Disease Epidémica de la Constitución in This Year of 1774, Which the Common People

Call Tabardillo." He argued that common people (*el vulgo*) called the disease tabardillo, whereas, in his medical opinion, the illness included a significant variation labeled epidémica de la constitución. Ávalos y Porras did not elaborate further, however, in the body of the treatment instruction, nor did he ever concretely discuss whether these were two separate but overlapping illnesses. Today we know that epidemic typhus is transmitted by body lice that live and lay eggs in clothing, especially in the seams. After hatching, louse nymphs feed on human blood, molting three times over the course of two weeks to reach adulthood. The lice excrete typhus-infected materials that carry the disease to the skin; the disease in turn enters the human body when the afflicted scratches the insect's itchy feeding sites. It typically emerges within five to fifteen days after infection, causing headache, fever, and chills, followed by a distinctive rash.[50] Typhus epidemics were more or less regular occurrences in the lives of the peoples of colonial Central America and elsewhere in Spanish America during the colonial period, but nevertheless many remained awestruck by their rapid devastation and high death rates, including the disease's ability to kill an entire household in a matter of days.[51]

In Guatemala, typhus was a disease of the cold climates found in Guatemala's western highlands. It tended to break out in the winter and then fade in the spring and summer as temperatures warmed. It was also a disease of towns and urban areas, where residents lived in crowded conditions. Members of medical campaigns that addressed tabardillo outbreaks in the late eighteenth century described the sick as suffering from various fevers, including "furious fever," "epidemic fevers," "malignant fevers," "synochus," "fevers mixed with inflammation," "contagious fevers," "pestilential fevers," and "*fiebres petequales*."[52] All fell under the colonial-era disease category tabardillo (the term *tifus*, the modern Spanish word for typhus, was not used in colonial sources), yet, according to medical authorities, each of the variations to some extent required a different treatment.[53] Colonial families, including the highland Maya, cared for typhus patients in their homes. Because of this long-term experience with the disease over generations and its primary treatment in the home, there were plenty of opportunities for cross-cultural knowledge exchanges about the causes of typhus, how the disease spread, and how best to treat the afflicted and provide them the best chance for survival. It was not until an almost decade-long intermittent typhus outbreak from 1794 to 1804 in the predominantly Maya-populated regions of Guatemala's western highlands that formal colonial medical campaigns began to actively treat the disease in that part of the Audiencia.[54]

The 1774 epidémica de la constitución treatment guidelines did not begin with a description of the symptoms that the sick suffered from or any individual patient accounts; in fact, the medical instructions contained only recommended treatments, organized by gender and perceived levels of poverty. Perhaps Ávalos y Porras did not have time to produce more detailed instructions in this tense, time-sensitive public health situation. He may have assumed also that the target reading audience—mostly doctors, priests who manned temporary epidemic hospitals in the region, and government-licensed pharmacists—already had some familiarity treating the sick and their various symptoms. Interestingly, too, Ávalos y Porras prescribed therapies that focused not on counteracting the fevers that usually characterized tabardillo but on treating digestive difficulties, especially medical massages on the reproductive and digestive areas of the body, coupled with special diets, purging, and enemas.

Treatment recommendations for dietary and medicinal plant ingredients that best reduced symptoms in the sick varied in how expensive they were for caregivers and families to obtain. The instructions recommended that those caring for the sick first massage the body with animal fat (*cebo*) mixed with almond oil at key bodily locations and joints "repeatedly, with force, to warm up those parts": first the neck and feet, then the muscles around the knees, the entire length of the spine, and most important, the stomach. The group that the instructions labeled "the poor" could substitute a massage with ground tobacco and mustard on those same places, or they could use simple cooking oil mixed with toasted ground salt. If these materials were unobtainable or too expensive, those administering care could use any kind of animal fat mixed with salt and ground-up corn cobs.[55] The "very poor" might rely solely on animal fat together with a bit of ground rosemary.

Guidelines mandated certain dietary requirements, in this case the preparation of a healing beverage ideally composed of cacao seeds and water cooked with rue and cumin, served warm. This must be given to the sick without fail at 11 a.m., 5 p.m., and 11 p.m. so that they could regain their strength. The "very poor" could be treated with the same hot beverage but without the cacao seeds if too expensive for them to obtain. Finally, all typhus patients, including "the poor" and "very poor," required an enema performed 30 minutes after eating breakfast in order to help rebalance the body's humors.[56]

This treatment regimen reflects long-standing Galenic medical ideas whereby a healer could strategically adjust bodily humors using diet, healing potions, enemas, purges, massage, and therapeutic bloodletting in order to bring the body back into a healthful balance.[57] Other tabardillo treatment guidelines from the late colonial period, however, specified that typhus fevers should not be treated with heat, as these instructions indicated, but instead by something Galenically defined as "cold" to counteract the body's fevers.[58]

In the second section of the treatment guidelines, Ávalos y Porras warned that this outbreak of epidémica de la constitución in the aftermath of the earthquakes brought on "hysterical effects," headache pains, delirium, and anxiety. To treat these symptoms, the healer should first tie a strip of cloth tightly around the woman's ribs, then massage the stomach "and that which they call *arcas* (intestines), moving all the flatulent materials to the lower region." Next the healer massaged the uterus to relax the muscles in that part of the body. Once the intestines, uterus, and stomach area relaxed, the guidelines recommended, the healer should tie a band or sash tightly across the region and leave it there to keep the body relaxed. This treatment also involved a specific diet consisting of roasted chicken broth or a nourishing Maya drink called *atole*, made with ground corn mixed with beef broth or well-cooked beans with their broth (frijoles). Ávalos y Porras noted that "this works especially well for "Indians" (*indios*) and the very poor."[59] Here again the treatment focused on digestion difficulties and that area of the body. The massage may also have focused on the uterus, though this part of the instructions is ambiguous. The term *vientre* used there could mean either "belly" or "uterus," depending on the context, and here it is not clear. The strip of cloth tied around the ribs to calm the sick woman, however, is new and different in the context of tabardillo treatment.

Botanical details provide further clues as to how and why people might have lumped tabardillo and epidémica de la constitución together in Guatemala at the end of the eighteenth century. Knowledge of how to treat typhus with readily available plants and herbs in the Guatemalan highlands circulated in local medical cultures. In the highlands, most tabardillo patients were treated in the home by female family members who either gathered the necessary herbs themselves, grew them in their gardens, or knew which ones to trade for or purchase at local markets.[60] Interestingly, a number of plants thought to have curative or palliative properties for tabardillo patients were also believed to affect various aspects of female reproduction, a fact that underscores the gendered nature of the illness not only within colonial understandings of this disease but also in its prescribed treatments. Historian and naturalist Francisco Ximénez identified *cocolmeca* bark as a cure for tabardillo and its accompanying fevers *tercianarios* and *cuaternarios*.[61] Ximénez claimed to have himself experimented with this tree bark and so could confirm its beneficial use. He noted as well the bark's effects on female reproduction, that cocolmeca "makes barren women fecund" and restored healthy menstrual flows (and presumably could, depending on use, also cause intentional abortions).[62]

Among the medicinal plant samples that Francisco Geraldino, *alcalde mayor* (governor) of the province of Totonicapán, sent to be forwarded to doctors and scientists in Spain in the 1780s were leaves, sap, and bark from the Savino tree (*madera de Savino*), which grew along the area's riverbanks. When used as an ingredient in a healing poultice, medicinal bath, or curative drink made from the tree's bark, this plant cut short tabardillo and other "pestilential and malignant fevers by provoking sweat in the patient and restoring their body's humoral balance."[63] Geraldino warned, however, that medicines made from the tree's sap "should not be used on pregnant women because it is a very strong abortifacient [*aborto*]."[64] In-home treatments in this region likely used this plant not only to treat typhus but also to control menstruation and pregnancy.

Regrettably, Ávalos y Porras did not enumerate the "hysterical effects" in his instructions; he discussed in detail only the treatment. No further information is given about hysteria either as an illness category on its own or as part of the epidémica de la constitución, nor are any specific symptoms described in individuals. Repeated references to hysteria and "nervios" emerge in other genres of archival documents from colonial Central America, especially with regard to herbal and botanical treatments for the disease, but not in this case. Perhaps the reason is that the intended readership already knew how to recognize hysteria-related illnesses, which I have found reference to for the entire colonial period, though the sources do not always agree on a stable set of symptoms.

Evidence does exist in other contexts of persons suffering from illnesses labeled broadly as hysteria as a result of their having gone through some traumatic event, including an epidemic disease outbreak, an unexpected miscarriage, or interpersonal or colonial violence or punishment such as a public whipping. Eighteenth-century treatment guidelines for the first public health campaigns against measles, smallpox, typhus, and other diseases all included variants that produced concurrent hysterical symptoms. The 1769 treatment handbook for measles and smallpox (interestingly coauthored by Ávalos y Porras), for example, included a section on how to treat measles accompanied by hysteria: "If the patient suffered from measles and hysteria [*histeria*] simultaneously, the caretaker should incense the room with [the smoke from] burned shoes, feathers, or wool, whose smell would calm the patient; [in addition] place the herb crushed rue on the navel."[65] This source does not mention that measles with hysteria afflicted only women, and the guide provides no further detail on this matter. These sick persons, colonial doctors counseled, needed to be calmed, and this could be accomplished by producing smoke for the sick person to inhale by burning specific materials originally from animals: shoe leather from cattle, wool from sheep, and bird feathers.

Diagnoses of hysteria in legal cases described pregnant women who miscarried as a result of physical violence or public punishment enacted by colonial authorities. In a case from Guatemala's criminal court in the 1790s, three perpetrators were charged with beating a pregnant woman named Rosa Meyda while trying to collect a debt that she owed them. After the beating caused Meyda to miscarry, the two women and one man were charged with "homicide" (*homicidio*) of the fetus.[66] The two medical specialists who testified as part of the proceedings both noted Meyda's "hysteria" symptoms. Surgeon Nicolás Montúfar judged that Meyda's pregnancy had been in the later stages when she miscarried. He argued, however, that her miscarriage (*aborto*) occurred not because of the physical violence but because Meyda was "rather hysterical; because of the hysterical tendencies that she was inclined to suffer from."[67] The bodily symptoms included "strong hysterical shakes and jolts" that caused her to "regularly dislocate her jaw," something that Montúfar said he had seen in other pregnant women who miscarried.[68]

In contrast, surgeon Severino Luna diagnosed Meyda with a slightly different category of hysteria.[69] Luna had come to Meyda's home in the aftermath of the beating at the request of her husband. When he arrived, he found the woman in the midst of what he called a "hysterical privation" that included "violent spasms." He treated her with *ligaduras*, ropes or other binding material tied tightly around the muscles of a person who has "lost their senses," so that the bindings would calm her and cause her to "return to herself."[70] Tying a rope or sash around the spasming areas to relax a hysterical individual's body is similar to the therapy described in Ávalos y Porras's medical instructions for treating hysteria symptoms in cases of epidémica de la constitución. What tenuously ties these examples of hysteria together are traumatic events experienced by individuals and by local communities in the context of epidemic disease, natural disaster, and physical violence.

Ultimately, epidémica de la constitución did not solidify within Guatemala's professional medical practitioners as a medical category, and after these events, it disappeared from the historical record. Nevertheless, the trauma of exceptional events such as natural disasters—in this case, two severe earthquakes and significant aftershocks over a seven-month period—can provide important evidence of disability and impairment in the lived experiences of individuals and of specific social groups in colonial society. This insight is both frustrating and interesting: frustrating because failure to construct a new disease category leaves a dead end in the historical record, but interesting as well because it shows how colonial medical communities reacted to a new disabling illness that manifested in subject populations with observable clusters of symptoms after a natural disaster.

As a result, this rather unique historical example leaves many questions unanswered about researching and writing histories of disabilities in multiethnic colonial societies. It raises others, such as how, for example, Indigenous ideas shaped and were shaped by individual experiences of disability, and how this influence changed over time. Further research can bring other sources to bear, such as bilingual Maya-Spanish-language dictionaries produced by missionary priests in the colonial period. An anonymous Spanish-Kaqchikel–K'iche Maya manuscript dictionary, thought to have been penned in Guatemala sometime during the seventeenth or eighteenth centuries, includes the phrase *taue baꝁ mabe ru4ux labal ruma4[u]xto4* paired with the Spanish gloss "quando algun niño, o muger se espanta de algun temblor de tierra, o de otra cossa" (when a child, or woman, becomes scared from an earthquake or tremor, or from something else).[71] The Kaqchikel focuses on how earthquakes affect the heart (ru4ux, lit. "his or her heart"), the important metaphysical center and the site of one of three souls for the Kaqchikel that can be lost from experiences that cause extreme fright or fear, and must be cured by a Maya ritual specialist.[72] Scholar Servando Z. Hinojosa notes that among modern Kaqchikel, chronic *xib'iril*, that he translates as "soul fright" and "fright sickness," can occur as a result of the violence caused to individuals by natural disasters such as the 1976 Guatemalan earthquake.[73] Attention to these kinds of different culture experiences of disability in colonial Latin America can help inform broader histories and methodologies of disability history and the ways that colonial, Indigenous, African, and mixed-race peoples and cultures shape and are shaped by both individual and collective experiences.

NOTES

1. The basic outline of the 1773 earthquakes in Santiago de Guatemala come from Cristina Zilbermann de Luján, "Destrucción y traslado de la capital: La Nueva Guatemala de la Asunción," in *Historia General de Guatemala*, Tomo 3: *Siglo XVIII hasta la Independencia*, ed. Jorge Luján Muñoz (Asociación de Amigos del País / Fundación para la Cultura y el Desarrollo, 1995), 199; "Terremoto de Santa Marta," in *Diccionario Histórico Biográfico de Guatemala*, Flavio Rojas Lima (Fundación para la Cultura y el Desarrollo, Asociación de Amigos del País, 2004), 873; Laura E. Matthew, *Memories of Conquest: Becoming Mexicano in Colonial Guatemala* (University of North Carolina Press, 2012), 258–59; Mauricio Pajon, "Building Opportunity: Disaster Response and Recovery After the 1773 Earthquake in Antigua Guatemala" (PhD diss., University of Texas Austin, 2013); and Megan McDonie, "In the Shadow of the Volcano: Volcanic Landscapes, Indigenous Knowledge, and Cultural Exchange in Early Modern Mesoamerica" (PhD diss., Pennsylvania State University, 2020).

2. Juan González Bustillo, *Extracto ô relacion metodica, y puntual de los autos de reconocimiento, practicado en virtud de comisión del señor presidente de la Real Audiencia de este Reino de Guatemala* (Mixco, Guatemala, 1774), 15; Felipe Cadena, *Breve descripción de la Noble Ciudad de Santiago de los Caballeros de Guatemala; y puntual noticia de su lamentable ruina ocasionada de un violento terremoto* (Mixco, Guatemala, 1774), 10.

3. Cadena, *Breve descripción*, 8. For more on the five colonial period hospitals in Santiago de Guatemala, see Ramiro Rivera Álvarez, "Medicina y Primeros Hospitales de la Colonia," in *Historia General de Guatemala*, Tomo 2, ed. Jorge Luján Muñoz (Asociación de Amigos del País / Fundación para la Cultura y el Desarrollo, 1995), 361–66.

4. The 1773 earthquakes in Santiago de Guatemala (now Antigua) have received much historiographical attention because of the extensive destruction of city buildings and homes, and because colonial authorities eventually decided to abandon the city as the capital to build a new one, Nueva Guatemala (today's Guatemala City). Fascinating new and innovative approaches to the earthquake explore other aspects. On Indigenous knowledge of earthquakes and volcanism, see McDonie, "In the Shadow of the Volcano"; on sound history and the history of colonial music, see Diane Oliva, "Sonic Decency: Music in the Aftermath of Guatemala's 1773 Santa Marta Earthquake," *Journal of the American Musicological Society* 76, no. 1 (2023): 169–221. For an introduction to the range of published and archival sources available on this topic, see Lawrence H. Feldman, *Mountains of Fire, Mountains That Shake: Earthquakes and Volcanic Eruptions in the Historic Past of Central America (1505–1899)* (Labyrinthos, 1993).

5. For important comparative studies of eighteenth-century earthquakes in other parts of the Iberian world, see Charles F. Walker, *Shaky Colonialism: The 1746 Earthquake-Tsunami in Lima, Peru, and Its Long Aftermath* (Duke University Press, 2008); and Timothy D. Walker, "Enlightened Absolutism and the Lisbon Earthquake: Asserting State Dominance over Religious Sites and the Church in Eighteenth-Century Portugal," *Eighteenth-Century Studies* 48, no. 3 (2015): 307–28.

6. Archivo General de Centro América, Guatemala City, Guatemala (hereafter AGCA), A1-271-5919, Manuel Ávalos y Porres, "Breve methodo de curar la enfermedad epidemica de la constitucion de este año de1774," f. 1v–2 (hereafter Ávalos y Porras, "Breve methodo de curar la enfermedad epidemica de la constitucion," AGCA).

7. For more on tabardillo in the colonial period, see Martha Few, *For All of Humanity: Mesoamerican and Colonial Medicine in Enlightenment Guatemala* (University of Arizona Press, 2015), esp. ch. 2, "Typhus and the Landscapes of Maya Medicine," 96–132.

8. Carlos Martínez Durán, *Las Epidemias de tifus en Guatemala* (Tipografía Sánchez y De Guise, 1940), 22.

9. Martínez Durán, *Las Epidemias de tifus*, 32.

10. "En las mugeres ladinas [——]len causar maiores dolores de cabeza, delirios, e inquie[tud] los efectos hystericos." Ávalos y Porres, "Breve methodo de curar la enfermedad epidemica de la constitucion," f. 1v-2, AGCA. AGCA contains multiple copies of these medical instructions by medical doctor Manuel Ávalos y Porres, which implies that a number of handwritten copies were made and circulated to colonial officials, parish priests, and local doctors in the area. See also, for example, the Santiago's *Libro de Cabildo* records, AGCA, A1-1802-11806.

11. Real Academia Española, *Diccionario de Autoridades (1726–1739)*, under "constitución," https://apps2.rae.es/DA.html. European humoral theory, which continued to operate in late-eighteenth-century medicine, proposed that there are four human bodily dispositions and qualities: black bile or melancholy, yellow or red bile, blood, and phlegm, associated respectively with heat, cold, dryness, and wetness. In this theory, illness reflected an imbalance of the humors. For an excellent overview of humoral medicine, see Mary Lindemann, *Medicine and Society in Early Modern Europe* (Cambridge University Press, 1999). In colonial Guatemala, European humoral theories intersected with Indigenous medical cultures in interesting and complicated ways. See Few, *For All of Humanity*.

12. While other scholars of the 1773 earthquakes in Guatemala and their aftermath mention a tabardillo outbreak in their wake, I have not been able to identify any studies to date that mentioned or analyzed the disease category "epidémica de la constitución" as part of that outbreak. Martínez Durán's *Las epidemias de tifus* is currently the only medical history devoted solely to the tabardillo epidemic in the aftermath of the 1773 quakes. He labeled the epidemic using the modern term *tifus* (typhus). He did not, however, explore the issue of epidémica de la constitución in this work, or in his pioneering history *Las ciencias médicas en Guatemala: Origen y evolución*, 3rd ed. (Editorial Universitaria, 1964). Scholars who have written about the epidemic in broader studies of the 1773 earthquakes and the construction of the new capital, Nueva Guatemala, have tended to rely on Martínez Durán's work or have simply labeled the outbreak as *tabardillo* (typhus), applying

the modern disease category to the colonial outbreak, overlooking epidémica de la constitución.

13. In the colonial period, colonial officials also used the category "indio ladino" to describe those men and women they considered more Hispanicized, such as Indigenous language translators who participated in court proceedings, or inoculators and vaccinators in Indigenous communities who assisted in state-directed antismallpox campaigns in the late eighteenth and early nineteenth centuries. See, for example, AGCA A1-4929-42045, Santa Catarina Pinula (1660); and AGCA A1-191-3904, carta de Francisco Chamorro al Superior Gobierno, Santa Eulalia, 6 septiembre 1795, f. 10v. I explore this issue in depth in Few, *For All of Humanity*, esp. chs. 4 and 5.

14. For a discussion of the strengths and weaknesses of disability history to date, and what research on disability histories based in colonial and postcolonial Latin America contexts contributes, see the introduction to this volume.

15. My research over the years has explored this methodological issue in multiple contexts, including the history of religion, medicine and public heath and environmental history, as have many others who work on the history and ethnohistory of colonial Latin America. For my new work here on disability history, and in an attempt to meet the challenges posed by the colonial archive, I am inspired by, and build on, two pioneering works on the histories of enslaved women and men of African descent in Caribbean slave societies: Marissa J. Fuentes, *Dispossessed Lives: Enslaved Women, Violence, and the Archive* (University of Pennsylvania Press, 2018); and Stefanie Hunt-Kennedy, *Between Fitness and Death: Disability and Slavery in the Caribbean* (University of Illinois Press, 2020).

16. For more on the university, see John Tate Lanning, *The University in the Kingdom of Guatemala* (Cornell University Press, 1955).

17. Here and elsewhere when quoting from the original primary sources in Spanish, I leave them in their original orthography, uncorrected for accents, modernized spelling, or the like.

18. The linking of typhus and hysteria by colonial public health officials in the aftermath of the earthquake is investigated in depth later in the chapter.

19. González Bustillo, *Extracto ô relacion methodica*. In this formal, published report Bustillo compiled evidence and details from multiple political, religious, economic, and military sources; he was not interested in individual experiences. The target reading audience consisted of the king of Spain and royal officials who were assessing the damage to the capital and weighing whether to rebuild in the same spot or build an entirely new capital city in a different location. González Bustillo (1725–1797) held multiple political posts in Spain and colonial Spanish America, including that interim president of the Audiencia of Guatemala from 1771 to 1773, until Martín de Mayorga (1721–1783) took office, arriving just before the first quake in July 1773.

20. González Bustillo, *Extracto ô relacion methodica*, 14.

21. González Bustillo, *Extracto ô relacion methodica*, 16–17; Real Academia de Historia, "Martín Díaz de Mayorga y Ferrer," https://historia-hispanica.rah.es/biografias/14352 -martin-diaz-de-mayorga-y-ferrer.

22. For a discussion of this issue for colonial Guatemala, see Few, *Women Who Live*

Evil Lives: Gender, Religion, and the Politics of Power in Colonial Guatemala (University of Texas Press, 2002).

23. Luis Luján Muñoz, "Nueva información sobre los terremotos de 1773," *Anales d e la Sociedad de Geografía e Historia* 50 (January–December 1977): 195–226. By "private, personal letter," I mean an account or letter written by a survivor that, unlike a government report or correspondence, is not meant for professional or official use. Bustillo's report, for example, is a formal report to the king of Spain, and it was published. It provides a good general picture, but readers need to take into account that it was written in the context of strong debates about whether Santiago de Guatemala should rebuilt or should be abandoned as the capital of the Audiencia in favor of a new site.

24. Luján Muñoz, "Nueva información," 200.

25. Luján Muñoz, 207. The second major earthquake that year was known commonly as Santa Lucía because it occurred on her saint's day, December 13, 1773.

26. Luján Muñoz, "Nueva información," 207.

27. The Capuchin nuns here were a cloistered order, so they could meet visitors and exchange goods with them in the *sala de torno* only if shielded from them by screens, so as to keep with their order's enclosure restrictions (*clausura*). For a transcription of the order's rules and policies that the convent members in Guatemala followed, see Luján Muñoz, "El Monasterio de Nuestra Señora del Pilar de Zaragoza en la Ciudad de Guatemala, 1720–1874," in *Tesis de Licenciatura en Historia* (Humanidades, Universidad de San Carlos de Guatemala, 1973).

28. This was the pila, the main source of water to the Capuchin community for drinking, cooking, bathing, and washing clothes. Because this was a cloistered convent, it would have been located in an interior patio.

29. Luján Muñoz, "Nueva información," 207. A vara is a unit of measurement used in the colonial period to signify about thirty-two inches.

30. Luján Muñoz, "Nueva información," 207.

31. Cadena, *Breve descripcion*, 8–9, 10.

32. Luján Muñoz, "Nueva información," 199.

33. Luján Muñoz, "Nueva información," 207–8. "*Velos*" here likely refers to female novitiates who had not yet become professed nuns.

34. Luján Muñoz, "Nueva información," 209.

35. Luján Muñoz, "Nueva información," 209–10.

36. Besides Sister María Gertrudis's letter, as yet I have been unable to find any other private, personal accounts of physical or emotional illness written in the aftermath of the 1773 earthquake in Guatemala.

37. Esparragosa Papers (hereafter EP), private archive, "Carta de Juaquin M.a Palacios, San Miguel, 23 octubre 1815," n.p. This town is located near the volcano San Miguel, which remains active today. I am happy to share a digital copy of this letter on request.

38. "Carta de Juaquin M.a Palacios." Extreme unction was one of the rituals performed as part of the rites of death and dying in the colonial Catholic Church.

39. "Carta de Juaquin M.a Palacios."

40. "Carta de Juaquin M.a Palacios." Where the recipient lived is not included in the letter, so "the capital" might refer to the capital of the province, San Salvador, or to Nueva

Guatemala. *Facultativo* describes physicians and surgeons in the colonial period who hold academic degrees.

41. Thank you to Alex Herrera for suggesting how to clarify my point here.

42. Ávalos y Porres, "Breve methodo de curar la enfermedad epidemica de la constitucion," f1-2v, AGCA.

43. For more on the history of public health in Enlightenment-era Guatemala, see Few, *For All of Humanity*.

44. Few, *For All of Humanity*.

45. I analyze the history of this process in detail in Few, *For All of Humanity*.

46. Wellcome Collection, London, UK (hereafter WC), José Flores, *Instruccion sobre el modo de practicar la inoculacion de las viruelas, y metodo para curar esta enfermedad, acomodado a la naturaleza, y modo de vivir de los indios, del Reyno de Guatemala* (Nueva Guatemala, 1784). The content of this and other official antiepidemic treatment manuals also contain similar examples of adjustment and adaptation to Guatemala's majority Indigenous populations. I have written about this issue for the Audiencia of Guatemala from the 1760s to the 1820s, and across multiple diseases and illness, in Few, *For All of Humanity*.

47. Ávalos y Porres, "Breve methodo de curar la enfermedad epidemica de la constitucion," f. 1, AGCA.

48. Joseph de Medina (1680–1744) graduated from the University of San Carlos in 1712. In 1718 he occupied the chair in medicine at the University of San Carlos. He trained five *bachilleres* of medicine during his career, including Manuel Ávalos y Porras. Ávalos y Porras (1701–1775) was born in Santiago de Guatemala and when on to obtain his doctorate in medicine in 1734 from the same university. Martínez Durán, *Las ciencias médicas en Guatemala*, 217; "Manuel Ávalos y Porras" and "Joseph de Medina," in Rojas Lima, ed., *Diccionario Histórico Biográfico de Guatemala*, 147, 605.

49. AGCA, A1.7-271-5909, "Breve método que se ha de observar en la curacion de sarampion y viruelas" (Guatemala, 1769). The printed manual itself is unpaginated, but it can be found in this *legajo* of cabildo meeting records, just after folio 8v.

50. *Cambridge Historical Dictionary of Disease* (2003), under "Typhus, Epidemic."

51. Few, *For All of Humanity*, esp. ch. 2.

52. AGCA A1-194-4969, "Sobre tabardillos que se padesen en el pueblo de Santa Eulalia," ff. 1, 21; A1.24-6091-55306, "Apruebo las disposiciones que ha dado Vm y me comunica en oficio de 12 de Julio ultimo relativas a hacer extensiva en esa provincia la inoculacion de la vacuna," f. 44; A1-194-4969, "Metodo curativo observado con buen succeso en la curacion de la epidemia de fiebres petequales que ha padecido el Pueblo de Sta. Eulalia," ff. 5–6; 18; 18v. For the treatments found in "Metodo curativo observado con buen succeso en la curacion de la epidemia de fiebres petequales que ha padecido el Pueblo de Sta. Eulalia," f. 29, notice again that, even in the title of the prescribed treatment, the author tailored the guidelines to the illness experiences specifically for those in the Maya tributary town of Santa Eulalia in Jacaltenango parish, located at a high altitude in the Cuchumatán mountain range.

53. Few, *For All of Humanity*, 64.

54. For more details on the outbreak, see Few, *For All of Humanity*, 62–94.

55. Ávalos y Porres, "Breve methodo de curar la enfermedad epidemica de la constitucion," n.p., AGCA.

56. Ávalos y Porres, "Breve methodo de curar la enfermedad epidemica de la constitucion," f. 1v, AGCA.

57. For more on Galenic humoral medicine, see Few, *For All of Humanity*, esp. chs. 1 and 2.

58. In fact, Protomedicato-sanctioned treatments used in antityphus campaigns from the 1780s to the 1830s all cautioned against the consumption of "hot" foods like chile peppers and the use of Mesoamerican ritual steam baths, which they argued hastened death from the disease.

59. Ávalos y Porres, "Breve methodo de curar la enfermedad epidemica de la constitucion," f. 2, AGCA.

60. See Few, *For All of Humanity*.

61. Francisco Ximénez, *Historia natural del reino de Guatemala* (José Pineda Ibarra, 1967), 246. Ximénez also gave as alternative names for the plant *cocomecatl*, *palo de la vida*, and *palo de china*. Edward Polanco (personal communication with the author, October 26, 2012) suggests that this plant is *cocomecaxihuitl* in Nahuatl, where *xihuitl* refers to fire, year or plant, *yerba* (herb), grass, roughly translating as "afflicted-rope-herb" or "bitter-rope-herb."

62. Ximénez, *Historia natural*, 247–48. Olga Ruiz, an herbalist in Imuris, Sonora, judges this plant to be *Phaseolus metcalfei*, a root used locally for infertility, irregular menstruation, and inflammation of the reproductive organs. Olga Ruiz, personal communication with the author, October 2012. Thanks to Rebecca Masten Crocker for facilitating this communication.

63. AGCA A1-6088-55135, "En obedecimiento y cumplimiento de despacho y supremas ordenas y con arreglo a instruccion que ellas se cita y he hallado en este archivo, yo Dn. Francisco Geraldino," Gueguetenango, February 2, 1784, f. 35.

64. Geraldino, "En obedecimiento y cumplimiento," f. 36–36v.

65. *Método que se ha de observar en la curación de sarampión y viruelas*, 10v.

66. AGCA A2.2-166-3315, "Criminal contra Bonifacio Rogel, Bernadina Villalta, y Gervasia Pacheco por golpes que dieron a Marzelino Golpeado, y a su mujer Rosa [Meyda] de que resultó haver malparida esta," f. 9v. The fetus was called a *criatura* in the sources. I discuss extensively the language used to describe the fetus in cases of postmortem cesareans, miscarriages caused by violence, and other related materials in Few, *For All of Humanity*. See also Martha Few, Zeb Tortorici, and Adam Warren, *Baptism Through Incision: The Postmortem Cesarean Operation in the Spanish Empire* (University of Pennsylvania Press, 2020); Elizabeth O'Brien, "The Many Meanings of Aborto: Pregnancy Termination and the Instability of a Medical Category over Time," *Women's History Review* 30, no. 6 (2021): 952–70; and Nor E. Jaffary, *Reproduction and Its Discontents in Mexico: Childbirth and Contraception from 1750–1905* (University of North Carolina Press, 2016).

67. AGCA A2.2-166-3315, f. 1v: ". . . bastante [h]istérica según pareze, por ser propenza a padecer esas pribaciones estéricas (sic—should be [h]istéricas)." Although it can also mean "abortion," I interpret *aborto* in this instance as "miscarriage," given the context in the source.

68. Montúfar also testified that the beating caused "irritación de la cólera." In humoral medicine this translates as wrath, anger, spleen, and bile.

69. AGCA A2.2-166-3315, f. 10v.

70. AGCA A2.2-166-3315, f. 11.

71. John Carter Brown Library, Brown University, "Vocabulario copioso de las lenguas cakchikel, y [Q]iche," Manuscript, Anonymous, [Zapotitlan, Guatemala?: s.n. (*sin nomine*)], n.p. I've left the Kaqchikel in the original orthography.

72. David Carey Jr., *Health in the Highland: Indigenous Healing and Scientific Medicine in Guatemala and Ecuador* (University of California Press, 2023), esp. ch. 2; Servando Z. Hinojosa, *In This Body: Kaqchikel Maya and the Grounding of Spirit* (University of New Mexico Press, 2015), xvi–xviii, 8–10.

73. Hinojosa, *In This Body*, 9–10.

8

Disability Masquerade and Wounded Combatants in Civil War El Salvador

Heather Vrana

Arturo was head of the orthopedic hospital in Tequeque at the Chalatenango Front of the Salvadoran civil war in August 1984. It was his responsibility to make tough calls. When the order came to evacuate, who would walk, who would be carried, and who would be left behind? Which supplies were necessary, and which could be buried in a *tatu* and recovered later? When could those supplies be safely retrieved? Of course, his time as a combatant informed his decisions. But Arturo was also a *lisiado de guerra*, or wounded combatant (shortened to *lisiado* in popular usage). After a severe back wound injured his spinal column, Arturo had trained as a lay nurse (*sanitario*) and anesthetist. Medicine allowed him to continue to serve the revolution on the battlefront. A nurse who was also a lisiado, he knew how to clean wounds gently and patiently. His empathy made him a favorite among combatants. One day that August, just as the hospital received news of the army's invasion of the region, another lisiado, named Tomás, arrived from a hospital in El Tamarindo with a group of retreating nurses and hammock patients. Within minutes, yet another platoon arrived, at the end of a two-week trudge, with more wounded combatants from an even more distant front. In a flash, Arturo had to coordinate all these lisiados, nurses, surgeons, and other health volunteers and prepare an evacuation from the region as the army was invading.[1]

Arturo was one of many *compas*—the term used by combatants of the

I thank David Carey and the other contributors who helped me refine the arguments of this chapter at our summer workshop. A special thank-you to the three anonymous manuscript reviewers whose suggestions improved this chapter's focus and direction.

guerilla group FMLN (Farabundo Martí National Liberation Front) to refer to one another—whose health work shaped the course of the war. What we know about him comes from the *testimonio* of a Mozambique-born Belgian named Francisco Metzi. In *Por los caminos de Chalatenango con la salud en la mochila*, Metzi sought to "show a collective struggle and the individuals engaged in it, . . . who we are and how we live in the midst of a people's war in El Salvador." This view contested what he perceived as the disillusionment or misinformation that shaped how the war was understood.[2] In lisiados like Arturo and Tomás, Metzi saw moral authority, special knowledge, and a certain heroism. Such representations were not unique to Metzi, however. They characterized much of how the FMLN and its allies portrayed war-wounded people.

This chapter is about how the FMLN and people sympathetic to the organization represented lisiados in testimonio literature and propaganda films. It explains how these representations politicized disabled combatants (and to a lesser extent disabled civilians) to undergird the group's revolutionary project. It argues that this politicization worked through three key themes: exceptionalism and special knowledge, compulsory heroism, and embodied evidence of Salvadoran military cruelty. Together these themes formed the "disability masquerade" of the FMLN's wounded combatants. "Disability masquerade" is the term that disability studies scholars use for a political strategy for managing the "stigma of social difference" that "claims disability as a version of itself rather than simply concealing it from view."[3] Centering disability masquerade in wartime El Salvador allows lisiados' importance to the war effort to come into focus and permits us to understand how the masquerade itself shaped how lisiados experienced the war and postwar period.

Disability and Civil War

The Salvadoran civil war (1980–92) pitted the leftist FMLN against the government and military of El Salvador in a struggle over the deep social stratification that had characterized the nation's history. Across the 1970s, civic unrest and violent recrimination plus plainly fraudulent elections fed a growing opposition movement. In late 1980, five of the militant factions that had been part of this resistance joined to form a single force, the FMLN.[4] A month later, in January 1981, it launched what it called the Final Offensive, seeking to incite a civilian uprising against the government through guerrilla warfare. After this effort failed, a prolonged rural insurgency developed, punctuated by occasional fighting in the capital and other major cities. The war stretched over more than a decade and was marked by spectacular violence and deepening poverty, a leftist alliance fractured by distrust and tactical disagreements, fluctuations in US aid, failed peace talks, and the rising influence of the right-wing ARENA (Nationalist Republican Alliance) party. It ended only after the FMLN and the military recognized that total victory was impossible and, in late 1989, turned to the United Nations secretary general to negotiate a political end to the war. The peace process took several more years as the opposing sides clashed over the terms of the cease-fire, military and police reforms, social programs, and the reincorporation of former combatants, among other issues. The war's toll is usually measured in deaths and displacement. Overviews by historians, political scientists, and rights organizations routinely mention between 20,000 and 100,000 casualties, around 8,000 people disappeared, and 1 million people displaced. But these counts ignore the larger number of combatants and civilians who were disabled by the war. They also neglect the relevance of representations of war-related disablement and debilitation and how these representations served the war and later peace efforts.[5]

The disability studies concept of disability masquerade helps to explain the power of these representations. Coined by Tobin Siebers, "disability masquerade" refers to how disabled people exude, bring forth, flaunt, emphasize, and even exploit disabilities in ways that challenge compulsory able-bodiedness.[6] The masquerade allows people to manage disability stigma by claiming a version of disability rather than "passing" or "simply concealing it from view."[7] Often this version is linked to broader tropes and ideals, like "blind justice" or, as I discuss in this case, "revolutionary sacrifice." If, as Siebers writes, "the reasons for disability masquerading are political," then historians of disability ought to attend to those politics, drawing connections and distinctions across place and time and assessing how those politics have impacted disabled peoples' lives.[8] That is what this chapter intends to do. In doing so, it expands the concept of disability masquerade by emphasizing its political range. Notwithstanding its liberatory aims, the leftist FMLN articulated themes like special knowledge, exceptionalism, and compulsory heroism, themes that have bolstered a range of political projects and states, including colonialism, fascism, and liberalism.

This chapter falls between two well-studied areas—the Salvadoran civil war and histories of veterans—but addresses a topic that is itself largely ignored. The civil war dominates El Salvador's historiography. Most studies focus on political and social histories of the government or the left, refugees and immigration to the US, and the role of the US in funding the war. Nevertheless, this work does often point to the presence of disability in the past.[9] Mines and mortar explosions, gunshot wounds, painful dehydration, diarrhea, and deprivation appear, then give way to discussions of ideology, diplomacy, and attacks and counterattacks.[10] Similarly, disabled combatants are both everywhere and nowhere in testimonio literature and oral histories of the war. Nationalist and revolutionary histories and myths often invoke the body—individual and social, futural, fecund, and sacrificial—but do not acknowledge how these invocations shaped the past. Only the late Ralph Sprenkels paid attention to veterans' organizations in postwar electoral politics.[11] This chapter complements his work by outlining wartime representations of lisiados that shaped the social and political context of postwar veterans' organizing.

In some ways, the Salvadoran case resonates with the veterans' histories of the US and Europe that have proliferated in recent decades.[12] This research has primarily focused on representations of veterans in literature and popular culture, state programs for veterans, public healthcare systems (especially the formation of the UK's National Health Service), new medical technologies, the everyday challenges of rehabilitation and civilian life, and disability diagnoses associated with certain wars or weapons.[13] Themes of sacrifice, compulsory heroism, and overcoming as symbolic meanings of disability were as common in El Salvador as in Europe during and after the world wars and the US's many nineteenth- and twentieth-century wars. Yet the Salvadoran case is unique. First, lisiados' heroism was not easily marshaled to patriotic ends. Representations of disability bolstered the political claims of the FMLN, an insurgent organization at war with the government. In a stretch of the masculinist tropes of heroism, women and children could be lisiados de guerra. Whereas so much disabled veterans' history emphasizes the alienation experienced when "going home," all Salvadorans experienced the war and distinctions between civilians and combatants were not so easily drawn. No one sought to control or conceal disabled veterans' politics or their bodies, as was the case elsewhere.[14] News reports, whether from the military's press outlet or the FMLN's Radio Venceremos and Radio Farabundo Martí, kept casualties (including injuries and deaths) in the public's view. Disability histories of war outside the US and Europe offer more resonant case studies. For instance, the anticolonial politicization of certain disabilities, such as amputations in Turkey in the early 2000s, broken hands and arms after Yitzhak Rabin's orders to "break the bones" of stone throwers in the first intifada, and lower limb injuries after the Israeli Army's "shooting to cripple" tactic of maiming Palestinians in the 2014 war, suggests a similar association may have been made about El Salvador's lisiados.[15]

This case study joins recent disability studies research that points to the uneven growth of disability history and disability studies.[16] Specifically, it offers nuance to the earlier, "models" approach to understanding both disability's past and scholarship about it.[17] To begin with, many lisiados, like Arturo and Tomás, joined the FMLN's health brigades and so were both disabled people and medical authorities. Medicine offered some lisiados an opportunity that was socially and politically beneficial. This does not mean that medical cadres—disabled or not—were immune from ableism. But to assume the relationship between lisiados and medicine was antagonistic is ahistorical at best and unethical at worst. At the same time, it is untenable to view either war wounds or medicine as value neutral. In the context of war and often desperate illness and hunger, access to healthcare was critical and something people desperately wanted. For this reason, the FMLN made primary healthcare and war medicine central to its political work. More relevant to our understanding of the actual lived experiences of Salvadoran lisiados is how health was politicized and, at the same time, how representations of lisiados bolstered certain political projects, including the FMLN's insurgent struggle and the peace accords.

In addition to Metzi's testimonio, this chapter refers to those by Salvadoran doctor Eduardo Espinoza, who joined the FMLN early in the war and trained many of its health workers, and US doctor Charles Clements, who worked with civilians in the FMLN-held area of Guazapa from around March 1982 to 1983. Clements's testimonio was published in 1986 in an effort, like Metzi, to shape people's understanding of the ongoing war. Espinoza, on the other hand, published his memoir in 2007, fifteen years after the war ended. This chapter also draws on FMLN films and print publications, especially two propaganda films that highlight lisiados and the popular healthcare system. The first, *Todo el amor*, features lisiados who were evacuated to an encampment near Havana, Cuba, for rehabilitation. The second, *La salud al frente*, discusses the healthcare system in Morazán, emphasizing both combat medicine and community preventive medicine efforts. Most film analyses of disabled veterans address fiction films. But documentary films, especially these propaganda films, make different truth claims. The FMLN called Salvadorans to arms by framing war-related disability as continuous with the debilitation of poverty and inequality. When it then linked war-related disablement to Yankee intervention and foreign interests, the group effectively framed anticolonial and revolutionary struggles as wars over debility and disability.[18]

The capacity of each side to treat casualties, including the war-wounded, was especially salient. However, the ways disability figured into revolutionary medicine are not well understood even as war wounds and disablement were an important part of Cold War science, technology, and medicine, a historical subfield presently enjoying a burst of exciting scholarship.[19] To Cold War historians, this chapter suggests that disability can be a useful lens for examining some of the key questions of popular mobilization, counterrevolutionary violence, foreign intervention, international solidarity, and historical memory. Better understanding lisiados and disability contributes not only to ongoing discussions in disability studies and history about care, cure, and public health, but also to debates in social movement history about the civil war's conclusion.

This chapter's film and text archive yields insights that may not have been apparent in oral histories. For one, as contemporary sources (except for Espinoza's testimonio), the films and texts indicate the political importance of disability for the FMLN during the war. Too, they lend an appreciation of the range of combatants who were injured in combat or disabled by combat conditions, which is especially significant absent a comprehensive national census of disabled combatants.[20] These sources also convey the agency of lisiados. Wartime medicine and its representations in disability masquerade provided avenues for disabled combatants like Arturo and Tomás to shape not just the popular health system but also the FMLN's narrative of the war itself. If the civil war was, in anthropologist Sandy Smith-Nonini's terms, "a war against health," then the FMLN would fight *for* and *with* health.[21]

"Unconscious of the Limits of Suffering"

Disparities in health and access to healthcare were fundamental to Salvadoran militants' rationale for taking up arms.[22] Some used disability masquerade to underscore the justness of their struggle. In 1981, FMLNaffiliated university students in the General Association of Salvadoran University Students (Asociación General de Estudiantes Universitarios Salvadoreños, or AGEUS) published a pamphlet entitled *Healthcare in El Salvador, Another Reason for the Popular Struggle*. In it they declared: "The health conditions in which the people of El Salvador have lived during the fifty years of military tyranny and fierce oligarchic domination and exploitation have created a terrible scene of suffering, pain, death, and sickness for the Salvadoran people."[23]

The authors posited that disabled and debilitated Salvadorans were proof of the Salvadoran government's cruelty. Like representations of disability in socialist fiction film and literature in which "bodily sufferings of numerous proletariat subjects, such as illnesses, injuries, scars, and deaths, are always ascribed to imperialist abuse or the torture of the ruling class in the oppressive old society," the AGEUS text explained how decades of inequality had debilitated Salvadorans.[24] The "suffering, pain, death, and sickness" of poor and working Salvadorans became evidence of the government's abuse and the FMLN's righteousness.

The AGEUS pamphlet continued, "We find ourselves before the heroism of a people who, unconscious of the limits of suffering, insist on directing their own destiny and responding to their health problems with an unbreakable determination to win the final victory and to set up a truly popular and revolutionary government."[25] In other words, the revolution would be a triumph brought about by those who suffered, who were in pain, who were sick, even those who died. This was akin to the "supercrip" types discussed at length by disability studies scholars.[26] Only, in this case, compas would overcome suffering to fight a revolution, and structural barriers to health were foregrounded. The war would be fought *for* and *with* health and healthcare.

At the start of the war, El Salvador's doctor-to-patient ratio was the lowest in Latin America. Eighty percent of rural peasants had no potable water and 60 percent had no access to health services. Making matters worse, just before the war, the nation's health budget was cut by 50 percent. Then, as the war deepened, the government withdrew resources from the health ministry to better fund the military. Three out of four children experienced malnutrition.[27] The Salvadoran state had actively constructed a population of citizens who were unable to help themselves and faced structural barriers to their ability to be healthy yet were dependent on state intervention.[28]

The FMLN quickly developed the infrastructure and expertise necessary to improve medical care for combatants and rural and poor Salvadorans who experienced exclusion, neglect, and malpractice. This health system did not have a formal name. Its structure was largely left to each of the five organizations that composed the FMLN and that responded to the needs and resources of each combat region. Practitioners came from a wide range of backgrounds and expertise, from formal institutional medicine to community medicine, and counted Salvadoran physicians and nurses, foreign physicians and paramedics (including Mexicans, Venezuelans, Belgians, Germans, and Americans), and community health promotors among its ranks. This popular health system became vital to combatants and civilians, especially as the war progressed and the Ministry of Health pulled most of its staff from regional hospitals, leaving Salvadorans without access to basic healthcare infrastructure. The war aggravated debilitating chronic conditions and further limited access to an already insufficient healthcare system. It also created thousands of new *lisiados* wounded in combat. With healthcare in serious demand, the FMLN could use its popular health system to demonstrate to civilians that the guerrilla was willing and able to improve their lives.[29] The FMLN also linked the popular healthcare system to the broader social transformations it sought to make, whether at home, on the battlefield, or in rehabilitation.[30]

All of this history is apparent in the undated FMLN film *La salud al frente*, which documented the popular healthcare system in Morazán. *La salud al frente* reflected elements of direct cinema (long shots and synchronous sound) and dramatic documentary (montage, heavy editing, voiceover, asynchronous sound) alongside some elements of Latin American "Third Cinema."[31] Long shots of wounded combatants carried in hammocks, health brigade trainees receiving instruction, individual consultations with civilians, and the maintenance and collection of medical supplies all reinforced the disability masquerade that represented debilitated and disabled bodies as evidence of the Salvadoran military's and government's cruelty.

In an interview early in the film, a *brigadista* says, "We can say that we have a structure for health that improves the conditions of health of our *pueblo*. That offers medical attention not only to our guerrilla organization but also to our entire organized population [*población organizada*] and even to some who are not organized because we offer health services to the entire population who asks for it."[32] To illustrate his point, the film cuts to a noncombatant woman and her daughter who are meeting with an FMLN *médico* for a consultation. The recorded audio is difficult to hear, but they begin talking about the daughter's feet, then they talk about her stomach. She is embarrassed to discuss symptoms, but the doctor is unflappable and hands over a bottle to her *mamá*. She has worms (*lombrices*), and, he says plainly, the health post is out of the medicine that can kill the worms. The medicine he can give them, seemingly bismuth subsalicylate, is *"para calmar la diarrea, no para curarla"* (to relieve her diarrhea, not to cure it). The girl smiles shyly behind her hands and listens while the doctor tells her mother to return in 15 days with something to drink in case they have better medicine. The médico has clearly explained this lack of medicines many times. "We have challenges [*Nosotros tenemos dificultades*]," he says. Diarrhea from a lack of potable water was easier to relieve than to cure, given the conditions of rural life and war. The film plainly demonstrates the government's neglect and its effect on poor Salvadorans as it showcases the FMLN's attempts to heal them. Indeed, FMLN medics spent a good deal of time addressing the stomachaches, diarrhea, foot pain, infections, sexual health problems, and malnutrition that assailed poor rural communities.

During another consultation scene, a voiceover explains that people in these rural zones had never had access to a permanent doctor. Instead, they were required to walk long distances to arrive at the nearest *puesto de salud* (health post). The voice proudly states, "Today it is the revolution which in the middle of war has endowed this zone with a true health system: three hospitals, four mobile clinics, and dozens of doctor's offices" in Morazán for combatants and civilians, "without distinction."[33] The film returns to this point in a later voiceover during a training scene at the field Medical School: "There is no division between the military health service [*servicio de sanidad militar*] and public health [*salud pública*]."[34] Civilians would receive the same quality of care as combatants, in sharp contrast to the unequal health system outlined by the AGEUS students' booklet. The very brigadistas who rescued compas injured in combat organized courses on hygiene and nutrition in the civilian communities.

Despite the rosy picture painted by much of the film, disability masquerade helps make sense of the unequal nature of these encounters. In one scene, the camera pans across a group of people who seem to be waiting for a consultation, then follows a naked toddler with a distended belly as they walk across a dirt floor. A voiceover states: "Because of the subhuman conditions of housing, nutrition, and hygiene, the population has suffered cer-

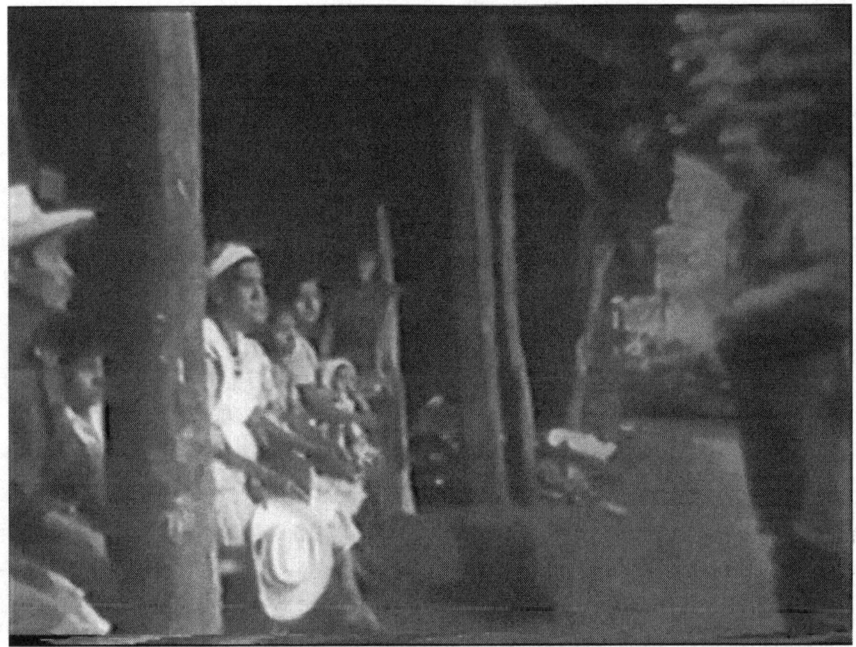

This film still shows an FMLN médico (*right*) with glasses and dark brown hair, wearing a long-sleeved button down shirt and long pants as he speaks to a small crowd of campesinos seated under the awning of a building constructed of dark wood with a dirt floor. The crowd is mostly children and two adults who wear hats and simple dresses. They face the médico as he speaks. Sistema Radio Venceremos, *La salud al frente*. Museo de la Palabra y la Imagen (MUPI).

tain endemic illnesses. The popular health system seeks to get to the root of these illnesses [by] building awareness in the population about the means of prevention." The film unsubtly displays scenes of debilitation, offering a version of campesinos' suffering as subjection, then posits popular healthcare's community work as a solution. Another shot pans across community members sitting in a row while listening to a lecture on hygiene and nutrition from the FMLN médico who treated the girl shown earlier with diarrhea. He tells them that the common illnesses they suffer from are "primarily due to many things; one of them is poor nutrition to which we have been subjected here . . . traditionally eating only a little bit of tortilla, a bit of corn, or beans."[35] This disability masquerade does not ask for campesinos' perspectives, nor does it consider that campesinos might resist the brigadistas' ideas. It presents their debilitation as the result of more than just neglect: it is evidence of the government's active subjection of campesinos.

The film closes with a powerful sequence of scenes. First, folkloric music plays while a voiceover states that stashes of medicine are as important as those of arms and ammunition. A pile of medical supplies lies on the ground, and the voiceover adds that the pueblo brings medicines to the front through "thousands of channels." It continues: "Thanks to it [the pueblo] and to the support of international solidarity, the system of popular health has been able to function. . . . So far . . . because the enemy has decided to unleash total war." The film cuts abruptly from the pastoral scene of a young woman sorting medical supplies in the forest to an urban aerial bombardment.

La salud al frente represents poor communities' debilitation and war-related disabilities as evidence of the cruelty of the government and its US allies and contrasts this destruction with the FMLN's popular healthcare system. By teaching medicine to campesinos and providing medical resources to communities that had never had a doctor, combatants squared off against national militaries, special forces, police, and paramilitary groups in a battle not only for hearts and minds but for guts and limbs as well. In fact, *La salud al frente* concludes by returning to a young brigadista who looks just off camera and invites democratic nations to help the FMLN by sending medicine and medical equipment, because "we do not have it." The film ends on his words: "They are invited to contribute, you know?" The film's disability masquerade finds proof of the government's cruelty in the bodies of poor Salvadorans and in the FMLN health cadres' dogged efforts to bring health to the people and bring them into the health system, the practice of the revolution's principles.

"We Will Offer Our Blood Proudly"

The FMLN's disability masquerade also responded to debilitating poverty and war injury through compulsory heroism. The widely circulated pamphlet *Los 15 principios de combatiente guerrillero* (The 15 principles of the guerrilla combatant), approved by the General Command in 1985, spelled out the government's cruelty in general terms. Some of the principles acknowledged "hardships," evoked "the memory of our heroes and martyrs," and proclaimed the willingness to "offer our blood proudly."[36] Such statements underlined that disability was a serious concern for many who lived through the war. Combatants were guided to expect to be treated with honor, respect, care, and attention when they were wounded. As lisiados, they would overcome individual war wounds through comradely spirit and, sometimes, international solidarity.

Approximately 500 Salvadoran lisiados went to Cuba for medical treatment and rehabilitation.[37] Some recuperated at the 26 July encampment just outside Havana, where they underwent surgeries and physical and occupational therapy, received medicines, and recovered in an atmosphere of revolutionary camaraderie.[38] The media unit of the People's Revolutionary Army (ERP) faction of the FMLN produced and distributed the film *Todo el amor*, about the encampment and its residents. The film teaches its audience about Cuba's medical solidarity and the experiences of young people disabled in the war. It may have also educated civilians at home about what kinds of bodies would return from the war.[39] It is unclear whether or to what extent disabled combatants were involved in its filming and production, but the film begins with a salute to "these ninety-eight national heroes who with the satisfaction of a duty fulfilled depart to fight new battles on other battlefields [*terrenos de lucha*]."[40] It represents rehabilitation unequivocally as a compulsory and heroic act but does not emphasize physical disability over emotional trauma or elevate combat wounds over those caused by torture. Long shots in montage establish themes like combat, rehabilitation, and daily life, but the film jumps from one place and time to the next, following lisiados from the battlefield, to field hospitals, to their transfer to San Salvador and eventual airlift to Cuba's José Martí airport, then through rehabilitation in Havana.

After the lisiados' arrival at the 26 July encampment, the film turns to interviews with young people who describe how they were disabled. Most were injured by mines that exploded and injured their feet and hands. The camera usually focuses on the interviewee's face, then tracks down their body to the injury or amputation. Some of the interviewees seem to be as young as 11 or 12, others in their early twenties. Some shots show *lisiados* with significant burns under wrapped arms, feet, hands, and heads. One young teenager, wrapped in gauze and perched in a wheelchair, holds a cigarette with a long ash. He looks wordlessly at, or maybe past, the camera. Another stares blankly at the camera from his wheelchair. The film then cuts abruptly to a combat scene. Gunfire whizzes past the camera. Two combatants, or maybe civilian porters, carry a young boy in a hammock stretched on a long tree branch, a technology termed "the people's ambulance." Then the film returns

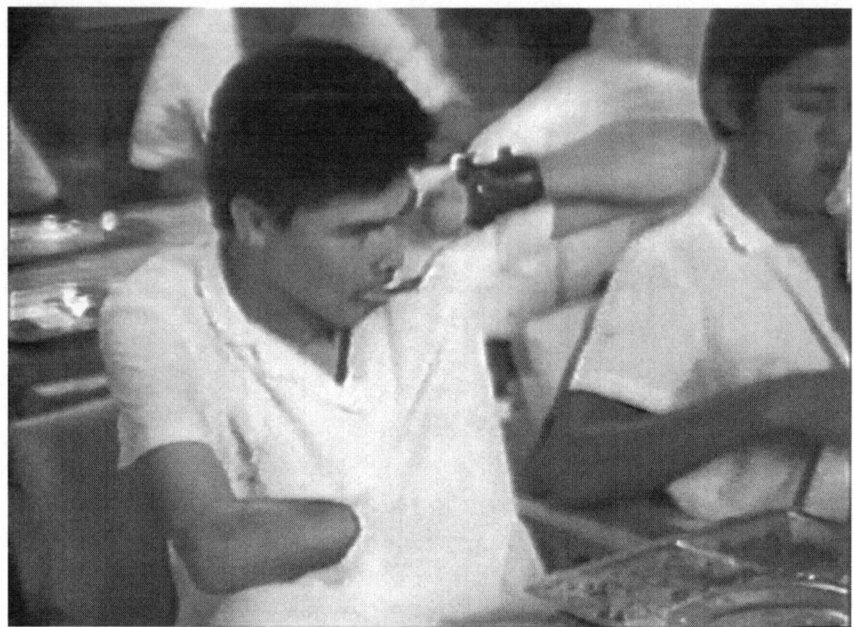

In this film still, two young men wearing white short-sleeved button-down shirts sit at a cafeteria table, eating lunch. The young man on the right wears his shirt unbuttoned to the chest, while the young man on the left is eating a bite of food from a metal tray. The young man who is eating has a right forearm amputation and a left hand amputation. To eat, he uses a spoon attached to his left wrist by a strap. Behind these two young men, several other people are also sitting at tables and eating from metal trays. Sistema Radio Venceremos, *Todo el amor*. MUPI.

to the blank-staring teen. This sequence tells a cyclical story: rehabilitation, injury, mortars, then live fire, then back to injury and rehabilitation.

Much of the film suggests how lisiados and their comrades negotiated the overlapping experiences of being wounded and being disabled.[41] A series of scenes of everyday life begins with a Salvadoran compa who explains to a group of lisiados the importance of recuperation. He affirms that they are playing a role by healing and that their main objective is to recover and then return to the struggle, albeit in the areas that now suit them. He says that in order to heal, one has to *want* to heal. His words make explicit the point of the subsequent scenes, which are long shots of the activities that filled each day for the lisiados: physical therapy like stretching, walking, doing pull-ups,

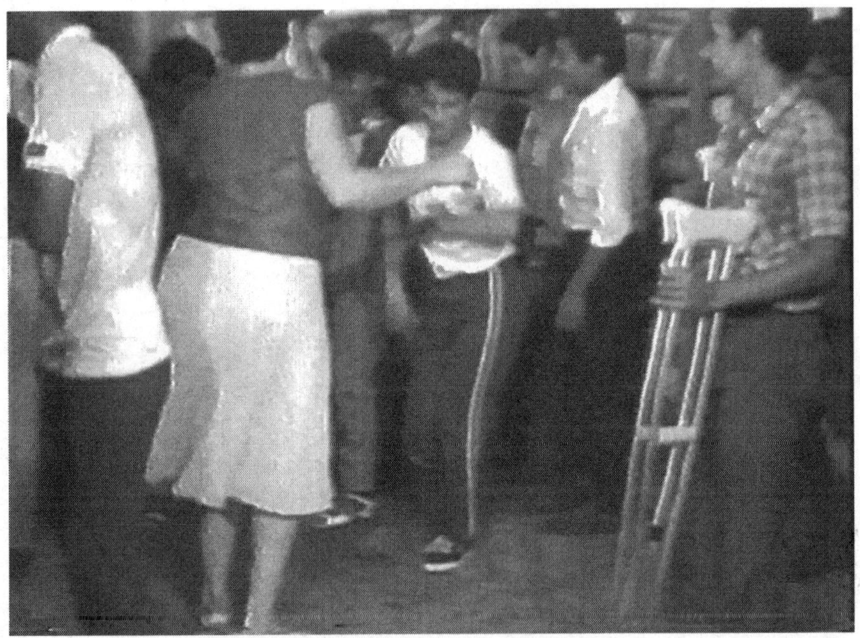

This film still shows a group of people, some standing and others dancing. In the center of the frame, a man wearing a white T-shirt, blue track pants with a white stripe, and a black sneaker, whose right leg has been amputated below the knee, dances to a *cumbia* with a woman in a red blouse and white skirt. In the right foreground, a man in a checkered shirt and gray pants holds the man's crutches while he dances. Sistema Radio Venceremos, *Todo el amor*. MUPI.

and practicing with new orthotics; occupational therapy like practicing writing; the care and community work of preparing concrete and laying bricks; and group meals in the cafeteria. Lisiados also made prosthetics for these activities. Many scenes show combatants leaning over trays heaped with food or resting against a wall with a piece of bread and a drink. Food was, apparently, plentiful at the 26 July encampment.[42]

So was fun. Young lisiados played a lot of soccer. They practiced guitar, learned to read and write, made wooden assault rifles, prepared and performed skits, and explored parks and tourist sites in Havana. They dressed up to go to dance parties. Often, the camera lingers on lisiados' extraordinary bodies as they do these recognizably ordinary things.[43] In activities akin to the everyday world-making that Zoë Wool describes as having taken place at Walter Reed hospital, lisiados and nurses at the encampment celebrated the figure of the heroic lisiado despite and by means of the painstaking and painful efforts to recover from injuries while enacting everyday ordinary life in a spectacular and exceptional space.[44]

The film's disability masquerade presents the lisiados as evidence of the military's cruelty and their rehabilitation as acts of compulsory heroism. In one interview, a boy explains that his sacrifices were worth it because the guerrilla is seeking to build a more just society where no one has more than anyone else and everyone has their health and the opportunity to study. He says that he has been disabled and his father killed, but their spirits would reside with the pueblo forever. Next, the camera focuses tightly on the face of a young man who solemnly says, "I am this way—well—blind and I am missing a hand, but I did it consciously. . . . I gave my drop of blood [*dí mi gota de sangre*] to attain liberation for a people. This is the pride that makes me stronger, that makes me feel satisfied with my head held high."[45] In fact, the film itself was dedicated to four lisiados (Luis, Manuel, Will, and Anibal) who were killed by the US-trained Ramón Belloso Battalion as they awaited medical transport through the auspices of the Catholic Church and the International Committee of the Red Cross (ICRC) in Chorro Blanco, Chalatenango. The film's dedication underlines the FMLN's call for all lisiados to continue to offer their drops of blood to the revolution. Its disability masquerade offered representations of combat medicine and rehabilitation that fused individual sacrifice with collective experiences and even shaped foreign diplomatic relations.[46]

Medic Eduardo Espinoza's testimonio, published decades after the war, also emphasizes compulsory heroism for lisiados. Espinoza joined the Farabundo Martí Popular Liberation Forces (FPL) in August 1975, compelled by witnessing the July 30 massacre of secondary school and university students. Espinoza and his friend were attacked by National Guard troops when they ran to offer first aid to the wounded as medical students. Espinoza remembered, "From then on, I steeled myself and increasingly devoted myself 'to the struggle.' I cared for the wounded, I taught combatants first aid, I designed advanced health courses, I trained for the physical rigors of war, I recruited colleagues and organized them into support collectives, and I read piles of books and broadsides."[47] After working within the clandestine urban guerrilla forces, Espinoza transferred to the San Vicente (also called Chinchontepec) volcano in December 1980. He became responsible for organizing the FPL's medical and hospital services.

Espinoza's testimonio, *Relatos de la Guerra* (published in English as *The Liberation Struggle in El Salvador*), discusses the emblematic sacrifices and heroism of several lisiados. Lisiados appear in Espinoza's testimonio often to demonstrate the impossible moral questions raised by war. For instance, Javiercito, a combatant at just 14 or 15 years of age, blacked out during an air raid and woke up in a guerrilla hospital with both of his legs amputated above the knee. Espinoza remembers how "Javier shrieked that he wanted a gun to kill himself."[48] But he decided to live and later directed a collective that repaired the FMLN's communication radios. After the war, he joined the Dimas Rodríguez Cooperative for disabled veterans and urged Espinoza to donate the proceeds from his testimonio to the cooperative's scholarship fund for children of lisiados. Espinoza writes, "I don't know how he got over it, but he did and very well."[49] Another lisiado, named Nacho, had entered the healthcare structure after a 120 mm mortar shell damaged his sciatic nerve and altered his gait and his walking speed. When an armed forces attack became eminent, Nacho was ordered to leave the field hospital with a column of the wounded. He preferred to stay but instead heroically and effectively led the evacuation of a group of thirty combatants with minor injuries and seven who were unable to walk and were carried on hammocks.[50]

Combatants in critical care or who were nonambulatory were particularly vulnerable. Later in the same hospital evacuation, Espinoza's and Nacho's columns reconnected only to confront another difficult choice. The medical staff numbered just 28 to 14 *lisiados*, and each wounded combatant required at least two carriers. To flee would have required the group to move without guards at the front or rear of the column—unacceptable—or to abandon one patient—terrible. Espinoza had to determine which of the non-ambulatory patients would be left behind. He chose Donaldo. At just 17 years old, Donaldo had been in a coma since an operation to repair his abdomen, which was filled with blood after a bullet split his liver, perforated his intestines, and destroyed most of his right kidney. He survived the six-hour surgery but went into shock and a coma, then developed sepsis, and then kidney failure. Espinoza ordered Donaldo to be carried a 100 yards into a coffee field with a slow-drip antibiotic in his IV in case he survived the attack.[51]

Even the hammock patients, who were supposed to be carried in that *guinda* (the Salvadoran word for a strategic retreat), wound up camouflaged and hidden after the civilians who were sometimes relied on to carry hammocks and equipment fled before the lisiados arrived at a rendezvous point.

They hid only about 30 feet from where enemy troops passed. One of them, a teenage combatant named Trinchera, had been shot in the femur and then developed chronic osteomyelitis, then refractured his femur, making him Espinoza's "most veteran patient," whose "chronic illness had made him part of the everyday landscape of the Hospital del Frente." As they waited, Espinoza, Trinchera, and another member of the hospital staff agreed they would save three bullets for themselves so they could not be taken prisoner.[52] As Uriel, a disabled combatant in Chalatenango and a key figure in Metzi's testimonio, recalled, "Whenever we thought things were getting really tough and that the chances of getting out were slim, we just joked about it."[53]

Disabled combatants and civilians were usually at greater risk than their counterparts during attacks and guindas: a difficult reality that the *testimonios* do not elide but instead present as heroic sacrifice. Dr. Charles Clements's testimonio tells of Miguel, who was disabled with arthritis and thus hesitant to leave his village of Copapayo on a guinda. Because he could not flee, he was wounded in an attack by the Ramón Belloso Battalion and bled to death, testimony to the armed forces' cruelty as they killed an old man. Clements recalled that a health worker named Jasmine instructed sanitarios who were following troops in an invasion of San Salvador from Salitre that the wounded "must not be deserted, . . . but sometimes it would be impossible to evacuate them." Clements continued, "Jasmine didn't say to kill the wounded or leave them alive. But she did point out that no injured prisoner was known to survive capture and that everyone realized what might be in store for them in such a case. The government troops are especially cruel to the wounded."[54] This certainty was echoed by Uriel: "We knew if they captured us alive, they would torture the living hell out of us. Those bastards would make mincemeat of us."[55] In the FMLN's disability masquerade, lisiados responded to the Salvadoran military's cruelty with sacrifice and heroism. Sometimes cruelty, sacrifice, and heroism endowed lisiados with special knowledge that made them good caregivers and allowed an exceptional connection to fellow lisiados.

"The Trauma of Feeling Your Whole Life Collapse Around You"

Clements's book *Witness to War* is one of the best-known testimonios about the war published in the US. Its purpose was to educate US citizens and persuade them to demand that their government end its reckless pursuit of proxy wars. Like the FMLN texts, it represents disabled or debilitated Salvadorans as evidence of the terrible conditions of war. Unlike the other texts discussed in this chapter, however, it does not invoke compulsory heroism. Instead, it emphasizes the exceptional moral authority or special knowledge of lisiados. Clements even frames his own arrival at the Salvadoran war front in terms of his disability: After he experienced a crisis of conscience following numerous missions in Vietnam, the US military ordered Clements to six months' psychiatric confinement, then recommended him for psychiatric discharge. He describes this period in his life in terms of "the trauma of feeling your whole life collapse around you." Ineligible for a pension because the Air Force Evaluation Board determined he had been only "ten percent disabled" in combat, not the 30 percent that would have qualified him, he decided to attend medical school.[56] As with Arturo and Tomás, then, Clements's career in medicine was launched by his own experience with war-related disability. Also like the lisiados whom he and others wrote about, Clements derived his moral authority from his own experiences in war. The final section of this chapter discusses this third form of the FMLN's disability masquerade and how it shaped lisiados' experiences of the war.

In his testimonio and in conversation, Clements reports coming to consciousness over the Salvadoran war after meeting disabled war refugees at a family medicine clinic in Salinas, California, where he was a resident.[57] In *Witness*, Clements calls them "hysterics, depressives, catatonics, paranoiacs—human being after human being whose mind had been tormented by terror." Like the first form of disability masquerade discussed in this chapter, these lisiados' very bodies and minds were evidence of the government's cruelty. Clements, along with colleagues Bill Monning, Dave Evans, and others, was determined to speak out against the war and, when those efforts fell flat, to offer healing and "bear witness."[58] To this end, he organized delegations of Vietnam veterans to tour El Salvador, Nicaragua, and Honduras. Evans, a former Marine, joined a 1985 delegation. By then in his mid-thirties, he had become a double amputee at age eighteen after an ambush that destroyed both of his legs.

In the many narratives of his life that he shared with journalists, politicians, ethnographers, and filmmakers, Evans recounted how prosthetics work gave him the opportunity to meet other disabled veterans.[59] A part-time job cleaning at the J. E. Hanger prosthetics clinic in Charleston, South Carolina, turned into an apprenticeship, then a career. Like Clements, Metzi, and Espinoza, Evans pointed to war disability as an entry point into medical practice. In Evans's disability masquerade, being war wounded made him an especially skilled practitioner. He often recalled how the reticence of depressed or discouraged victims of land mines (and the limitations of his poor Spanish) was surmounted by the dramatic reveal of his own prosthetics.[60] Evans would walk and run or, in some versions of the story, skip or dance down hospital wards, then take off one of his prosthetics and pass it around.[61] Injured veterans (Evans sometimes went to Salvadoran military barracks) and civilians wept tears of joy. Without words, Evans could show them that he knew what they were going through and that their lives could be different. On these occasions, Evans's disability masquerade was a jubilant version of his disability that built affinity among lisiados and spurred their interest in prosthetics. By his own estimate, Evans fit around 20,000 people with prosthetics over his career.[62]

Metzi wrote of several lisiados who organized technical teams, especially in orthopedics and explosives in the combat zone of Chalatenango. Tomás trained as a lay nurse after a wound that caused nerve damage in his leg and became head of a hospital in El Tamarindo. Arturo, whose story opens this chapter, became a nurse and anesthetist in the zone after a severe injury to his spinal column.[63] Uriel was transferred to Chalatenango for treatment after a bullet destroyed his hip and penetrated his small intestine seven times. Metzi remembered that nearly everyone preferred Arturo to the other lay nurses who had not been injured: "Some of the lay nurses thought you had to be really rough to cleanse a wound properly. We said, 'They don't know how much it hurts.' Arturo was really patient though. He'd been there. He had a softer touch, like almost all those who had been wounded themselves."[64]

A short interview with Uriel that appears in Metzi's testimonio seems to offer the reader more immediate access to the war experience. Its disability masquerade positions Uriel as an authority who is a lisiado but also gestures toward a broader group of lisiados who recognized in Arturo special skills. Eventually, Uriel left the front for rehabilitation in France as part of an ICRC-mediated exchange of lisiados for army officers.[65] Comparing the hospitals in Chalatenango (or Chalate for short) to those in France, he told Metzi, "About the only thing the medical teams in Chalate can rely on is their desire to do something. But for the wounds we get there, the *compas* need a hell of a lot of medical equipment that they just don't have. But the truth is, they do everything they possibly can for us."[66] No small part of this desire came from the experiences and special knowledge of lisiados who continued with the revolution as part of the health system.

Uriel went into technical work in explosives after his recuperation. When Metzi asked whether he ever considered health work, he replied that he had thought about it for a little bit, but "above all, I felt constantly disappointed to see that other injured people recuperated and returned to combat and I am just here." A man he called "one-legged Juan" was already involved in the explosives workshop, and they got along really well. Soon, other lisiados joined them. Of Juan, Uriel remembered, "He raised our morale, and didn't let us get down or brood over our handicaps. He was a real example, especially with his amputated leg and all. We felt if he could do it, why couldn't we? He was a great comrade, a really extraordinary person."[67] Uriel, Juan, and others seem to have formed a community of lisiados in the explosives shop, where they made the very kinds of devices that may have disabled them, perhaps even reinforcing the disability masquerades of special knowledge and compulsory heroism as they worked.

Other disabled combatants who remained near the front wove fishing nets, helped the sanitarios by washing bandages and preparing treatments, and made the hammocks used to transport wounded combatants. Edwin did all these critical tasks, tended the vegetable patch, and made crutches for himself and a friend during the more than eight months that he was in a cast after his tibia was shattered. Another combatant, Isaias, had the unusual experience of reentering combat after serious injury. His lungs, diaphragm, and intestines were seriously injured, and his recovery was complicated by septic shock and paralysis caused by a piece of shrapnel. He proudly remembered that no one thought he would survive. Once stabilized at the front, Isaias transferred to the FMLN's Military School (Escuela Militar), where he worked in instruction and propaganda, all the while doing a battery of rehabilitative exercises and massages. He reentered combat with a platoon of his trainees and later rejoined a commando unit.[68] The narrative of his exceptional case features several aspects of the FMLN's disability masquerade: special knowledge and moral authority, compulsory heroism, and embodied evidence of the military's cruelty.

However, the course and meaning of lisiados' lives after the war's end was less straightforward. An eponymous film discusses the work of Victoria, the nom-de-guerre of Christa Baatz, a West German orthopedist who joined the FPL's medical team in 1984.[69] In the film, one of Victoria's patients, interviewed in a hammock shop where he worked in Arcatao, says, "I have a good job, you know, appropriate for a lisiado where one can work, well, without much movement . . . because there are a lot of jobs . . . agricultural jobs that are not suitable for a lisiado."[70] Toward the end of the film, the interviewer speaks to a longtime combatant while Victoria wraps his left arm from bicep to hand in a thick white cast. The interviewer asks what the lisiado would do if a ceasefire were declared tomorrow. The man acknowledges that the FMLN is involved in serious talks. Still, he has a clear sense of why he was fighting. If the war were to end, though, he might like "to study and prepare himself better." If not, he shrugs, he would "find some kind of work."[71]

These words recall those of the young lisiados in *Todo el amor*. Toward the end of that film, one young woman wonders, "How will I continue giving my small part [*mi grano de arena*]? How will I continue supporting the revolution?" Maybe she can be a teacher, she reflects. A young man blinded by a military doctor says he is thinking how, "despite the difficulty that I have, I could take a course in poetry." Another young boy says that he wants to be an educator to teach kids how to read because "to share something that one knows or to teach is the most beautiful thing there is." As he imagines how beautiful a "liberated El Salvador" would be, the camera focuses at middle distance on two lisiados who use crutches to stroll down the beach.

Another young lisiado, Chiquillada (the nom de guerre of Israel Quintanilla), arrived in Cuba for rehabilitation after occupying the Metropolitan Cathedral for 45 days with a group demanding medical evacuation. He had joined the FMLN as a teenager just after his father died, motivated more by the opportunity to meet young women than by the political content of the meetings that his older brothers organized. In May 1988, a mine exploded, and his leg was injured and, later, amputated. He and his comrades remained in Cuba until the 1992 peace accords were signed, though returning to El Salvador "was their greatest hope." This hope was tempered by a huge concern: "The question was what we would do once we returned to the country. I had always depended on my parents, then the party [FMLN]; I did not know how to behave as a person."[72] Like many young people who joined the FMLN, Chiquillada had no adult experience outside combat. Not only did the material conditions that lisiados confronted present real problems, but wartime representations—including the three dominant forms of disability masquerade discussed at length in this chapter—fell short of securing a postwar future for them.

Conclusion

Representations of disabled combatants and civilians and of the meanings of health, injury, and rehabilitation were impactful during and after the Salvadoran civil war. In testimonio literature and FMLN films, disabled people's experiences took on certain political meanings: they became evidence of suffering at the hands of an unjust state, a social problem to be solved, a source of exceptional knowledge, and a call to compulsory heroism and solidarity. Centering the FMLN's disability masquerade readily demonstrates lisiados' significance to the FMLN's war effort, whether through rhetorics of sacrifice that invoked compulsory heroism or through their representation as living testament to the violence of the Salvadoran government and its military. *La salud al frente*, for instance, presented responses to disability within the popular health system, including preventive medicine and hygiene and nutrition courses, the training of local health providers, and the solidarity of international physicians and paramedics as a microcosm of the larger social and economic transformations that the revolution sought to affect.

In this first form of disability masquerade, the FMLN's healthcare work was set against the government's extermination. The FMLN's sanitation, hygiene, and nutrition education campaigns, its literacy and training programs for local practitioners, and its approach to disabled combatants were also a defense against the Salvadoran government. For disabled Salvadorans, these resources offered not only relief but also an opportunity to shape the revolutionary present and forge a new future. Representations of the health cadres and of their work for, with, and often by lisiados formed a vital part of the FMLN's disability masquerade. Still, combat conditions were terrible, and disabled combatants were more vulnerable to sickness, attack, and abandonment than their comrades. Heroic representations of lisiados, which were common, could highlight but not ameliorate these realities. Compulsory heroism is the second form of disability masquerade this chapter highlighted. Unlike other forms of disability heroism, including supercrip types, this masquerade did not elide but instead highlighted structural barriers and neocolonial extraction. Finally, the third masquerade highlighted by this chapter is that of lisiados' special moral status or exceptional knowledge, exemplified by the talented health brigade workers and Evans's dash around hospital corridors. Together, these types of disability masquerade bolstered the FMLN's war effort at home and abroad. They politicized disability.

This politicization, of course, shaped how veterans could organize after the war. The final peace accords signed at Chapultepec Castle in Mexico City in January 1992 acknowledged that the incorporation of former combatants into civil society was crucial for a lasting peace.[73] But peacetime El Salvador fell far short of the young lisiados' dreams. The peace accords ensured that human rights would become the dominant framework for disability politics, but their implementation was complicated. For one thing, incorporation into normal life, which was narrowly defined as one's capacity to work, became the standard by which disability and rehabilitation were measured. Also, the accords were vague about how lisiados would be supported. For instance, no special benefits were provided for young combatants, and no official program acknowledged the health training lisiados and other brigadistas received during the war. Their knowledge and experiences as lisiados were no longer specially valued. Compulsory heroism collapsed, and lofty ideological principles for which some had fought fell flat as party leadership began to reverse their positions and the five factions splintered. Some FMLN leaders gained wealth, while rank-and-file *lisiados* struggled, undermining the masquerade that presented lisiados' bodies as evidence of the government's ineptitude and the military's special cruelty.

Almost a year after the signing of the peace accords, a legislative decree established a fund (later named Fondo de Protección de Lisiados y Discapacitados a Consecuencia del Conflicto Armado [FOPROLYD]) for both armed forces and FMLN veterans with physical and mental disabilities who had been directly injured and disabled in the war and those who had been disabled or injured in logistical, administrative, training, or similar roles.[74] Minors and dependents who had lost parents in the war were covered until they reached 18 years of age. Parents who had lost children were also included. Benefits could include money, equipment (like orthopedic devices), pharmaceuticals, and a range of medical, mental health, and clinical laboratory resources. FOPROLYD's upper management and a technical commission were charged with determining who was eligible to receive these benefits. In practice, they were slow to come.

After years of waiting for the government to fulfill its obligations, disabled veterans formed new organizations to advocate for their needs.[75] The first among these was the Asociación Salvadoreña de Lisiados y Discapacitados de Guerra (ASALDIG), which was granted a seat on the FOPROLYD's board. However, divisions within the group along the old factional lines of the ERP and FPL undermined its ability to effectively pressure the government and FOPROLYD. Ultimately, group members from the FPL left and formed a new group, the Asociación de Lisiados de Guerra de El Salvador (ALGES), which was formally recognized in July 1997 and became the FMLN's official organization of lisiados. Into the late 1990s, the group expanded to include former military and civilian war-wounded.[76] Enemies in war, in peace, they faced many of the same challenges. Both sides felt "unrecognized, neglected, and forgotten by those who in times of war had praised their achievements and sent them into battle."[77] "Now," one former FMLN combatant declared, "we are equally screwed [*jodidos*]. Some of us remain lame [*patojos*], others in wheelchairs or blind, some deaf and others without arms."[78] In addition to expanding its membership, ALGES also expanded its projects to include creating municipal jobs for disabled veterans and their family members, promoting sustainable farming opportunities, and opposing the privatization of water. Meanwhile, ASALDIG continued to struggle and splintered into several other organizations.

In sum, disabled combatants were crucial to the war effort, at home and abroad. They were also valuable in testimonio literature and FMLN films, where their sacrifices—especially those of young people—demonstrated the transcendence of the struggle. In peacetime, these meanings and purposes changed. Under the terms of the peace accords, much of the transformative power of popular health and lisiados' place within it was lost.[79] Like other veterans, some Salvadoran lisiados struggled to find economic and social stability. Others cannily worked within the legal framework of the postwar period to advocate for themselves and other disabled veterans in organizations like ALGES and ASALDIG.[80] Some were able to maintain and even expand the bonds of solidarity that had guided them in the war years by looking back critically on the FMLN's disability masquerade. Others moved forward by providing lisiados with much-needed resources like income, equipment, and therapy following the rights-based language of the peace accords. In ALGES, lisiados built a postwar identity as disabled veterans. In a 2007 interview, Chiquillada, by then president of ALGES, declared, "The fact that a comrade has a disability does not mean that he cannot contribute as a person, in his family life, at work, and in society in general. We still have great challenges, and [if we are] organized in ALGES, we will meet them."[81]

So far, triumph has been illusory. El Salvador stands out among Central American nations for the long-standing prominence of disabled veterans of both sides of the conflict in culture and politics, in contrast to Guatemala, where military veterans command political power and guerrilla lisiados are ignored, and Nicaragua, where only pro-Ortega lisiados have a voice. Yet life remains difficult for lisiados. The persistence of poverty and inequality has meant that growing numbers of Salvadorans moved from the countryside to the city, to coastal areas like the Bajo Lempa where sugar production devours the land, or onward to the US, where their futures could be even more uncertain. "Tough on crime" policing that targets gangs and drug trafficking has shaped a deportation-immigration circuit in which gangs like MS-13 and Barrio 18 flourish. In recent years, a series of legislative reforms have weakened protections and provisions for veterans. In so many ways, the failures of peace have brought new wars, and these wars have created more lisiados de guerra.

NOTES

1. Francisco Metzi, *The People's Remedy: The Struggle for Health Care in El Salvador's War of Liberation* (Monthly Review Press, 1988), 128–44.

2. Metzi trained as a biologist, hospital orderly, and nursing aide before coming to El Salvador, where he served with the Farabundo Martí Popular Liberation Forces (FPL) between 1983 and 1985.

3. Tobin Siebers, "Disability as Masquerade," *Literature and Medicine* 23, no. 1 (Spring 2004): 5, 8.

4. These factions were the People's Revolutionary Army (ERP, based in Morazán), Farabundo Martí Popular Liberation Forces (FPL, based in Chalatenango and San Vicente), National Resistance (RN, centered on Suchitoto and the northern slope of the Guazapa volcano), Revolutionary Party of Central American Workers (PRTC, based mostly in Usulután), and the Armed Forces of Liberation (FAL, based on the southern slope of Guazapa). For an overview, see Erik Ching, *Stories of Civil War in El Salvador* (University of North Carolina Press, 2016), 37–40.

5. This chapter privileges combatants with physical disabilities, though the war caused psychosocial trauma that was and is disabling. Ignacio Martín-Baró offers a clear contemporary picture of the trauma experienced by civilians in four communities, in "Political Violence and War as Causes of Psychosocial Trauma in El Salvador," *International Journal of Mental Health* 18, no. 1 (Spring 1989): 3–20.

6. Siebers paraphrases Barbara Christian to write about how narrative is where theory takes place. Together they guide me to look beyond description of disabled people in the past in order to understand what these descriptions *did* or to what effect they were invoked and, in turn, how these representations shaped disabled combatants' lives.

7. Siebers, "Disability as Masquerade," 5, 8.

8. Siebers, "Disability as Masquerade," 7.

9. See Jeffrey L. Gould, *Solidarity Under Siege: The Salvadoran Labor Movement, 1970–1990* (Cambridge University Press, 2019); Aldo Lauria Santiago, *Landscapes of Struggle: Politics, Society, and Community in El Salvador* (University of Pittsburgh Press, 2004); Rafael Menjívar Ochoa, *Tiempos de locura, El Salvador, 1979–1981* (FLACSO El Salvador, 2005); Ching, *Stories of Civil War in El Salvador*; Ching and Héctor Lindo-Fuentes, *Modernizing Minds in El Salvador: Education Reform and the Cold War, 1960–1980* (University of New Mexico Press, 2012); Joaquín Chavez, *Poets and Prophets of the Resistance: Intellectuals and the Origins of El Salvador's Civil War*; Aldo Guevara, "Military Justice and Social Control: El Salvador, 1931–1960" (PhD diss., University of Texas, 2007); Susan Bibler Coutin, *The Culture of Protest: Religious Activism and the U.S. Sanctuary Movement* (Westview Press, 1993); Elisabeth Jean Wood, *Insurgent Collective Action and Civil War in El Salvador* (Cambridge University Press, 2003); Molly Todd, *Beyond Displacement: Campesinos, Refugees, and Collective Action in the Salvadoran Civil War* (University of Wisconsin Press, 2010); Leigh Binford, *From Popular to Insurgent Intellectuals* (Rutgers University Press, 2022).

10. See William Stanley, *The Protection Racket State: Elite Politics, Military Extortion, and Civil War in El Salvador* (Temple University Press, 1996); Gould and Lauria Santiago, *To Rise in Darkness*; Gould and Carlos Henríquez Consalvi, dirs., *La palabra en el bosque* (Films Media Group, 2012).

11. Ralph Sprenkels, *After Insurgency: Revolution and Electoral Politics in El Salvador* (University of Notre Dame Press, 2018).

12. Susan Burch and Ian Sutherland, "Who's Not Yet Here: American Disability History," *Radical History Review* 94 (2006): 127–47.

13. David A. Gerber, ed., *Disabled Veterans in History* (University of Michigan Press, 2012); David Serlin, "The Other Arms Race," in *The Disability Studies Reader*, ed. Lennard J. Davis (Routledge, 2006), 49–65; Zoë Wool, *After War: The Weight of Life at Walter Reed* (Duke University Press, 2015).

14. John M. Kinder, *Paying with Their Bodies: American War and the Problem of the Disabled Veteran* (University of Chicago Press, 2015).

15. Salih Can Açiksöz, *Sacrificial Limbs: Masculinity, Disability, and Political Violence in Turkey* (University of California Press, 2020); Jasbir K. Puar, *The Right to Maim: Debility, Capacity, Disability* (Duke University Press, 2017). As these far-reaching connections demonstrate, an overview of disability in anticolonial and revolutionary movements and states would be fruitful.

16. Nirmala Erevelles, *Disability and Difference in Global Contexts* (Palgrave Macmillan, 2011), 19–20; Mel Y. Chen, Alison Kafer, Eunjung Kim, and Julie Avril Minich, "Introduction: Crip Genealogies," in *Crip Genealogies*, ed. Mel Y. Chen, Alison Kafer, Eunjung Kim, and Julie Avril Minich (Duke University Press, 2023), 13.

17. For more on the "models" approach, see this book's introduction.

18. For a discussion of the distinction between these terms, see this book's introduction.

19. See, especially, Anne-Emanuelle Birn and Theodore M. Brown, eds., *Comrades in Health: U.S. Health Internationalists, Abroad and at Home* (Rutgers University Press, 2013); Birn and Raúl Necochea López, eds., *Peripheral Nerve: Health and Medicine in Cold War Latin America* (Duke University Press, 2020); Audra Wolfe, *Freedom's Laboratory: The Cold War Struggle for the Soul of Science* (Johns Hopkins University Press, 2020).

20. In January 1993, the United Nations Development Program, the National Commission for the Consolidation of Peace (Comisión Nacional para la Consolidación de la Paz), and the Program for the Productive Reinsertion of War-Wounded and -Disabled (Programa de Reinserción Productiva de Lisiados de Guerra) conducted a national census of civilians and military and guerrilla veterans to determine the degree of need for assistance programs. But the census seemed only to survey 30,854 people (of whom 12,114 were determined to be wounded by the war). Among these, 2,219 were civilians, 5,720 were ex–armed forces combatants, and 4,155 were ex-FMLN combatants. The census also counted 18,662 family members of fallen combatants. FOPROLYD (Fondo de Protección de Lisiados y Discapacitados a Consecuencia del Conflicto Armado), "Reseña Histórica, 1992–2018," 11, accessed June 1, 2022, https://www.fondolisiados.gob.sv/wp-content /uploads/2020/09/resenahistorica.pdf.

21. Sandy Smith-Nonini, *Healing the Body Politic: El Salvador's Popular Struggle for Health Rights from Civil War to Neoliberal Peace* (Rutgers University Press, 2010), 19, 73–74, 98–121.

22. Counterrevolutionary health plans also emerged in response to broad-based demands for healthcare but are outside the scope of this chapter. I address those plans in my forthcoming book.

23. Asociación General de Estudiantes Universitarios Salvadoreños (AGEUS), *Salud en El Salvador: Otra razón para el combate popular* (1981).

24. Zihan Wang, "Disability, Revolution, and Historiography: Grandma Mao Zhi in *Lenin's Kisses*," in *The Routledge Companion to Yan Lianke*, ed. Riccardo Moratto and Howard Yuen Fung Choy (Routledge, 2022), 239.

25. AGEUS, *Salud en El Salvador*.

26. For an overview and reevaluation of this type, see Sami Schalk, "Reevaluating the Supercrip," *Journal of Literary and Cultural Disability Studies* 10, no. 1 (2016): 71–86.

27. Alfred Gellhorn, "Medical Mission Report on El Salvador," *New England Journal of Medicine* 308, no. 17 (1983): 1043–44. See also Smith-Nonini, *Healing the Body Politic*; Luis A. Avilés, "Modernized Injustice: The Reform and Modernization of the Salvadoran Health Care System" (PhD diss., Johns Hopkins University, 1998).

28. See Heather Vrana, "Endemic Goiter and El Salvador's Battle Against *Cretinismo*," *American Historical Review* 128, no. 4 (Dec. 2023): 1587–1617.

29. Healthcare cadres of Algeria's National Liberation Front made similar claims. See Jennifer Johnson, *The Battle for Algeria: Sovereignty, Health Care, and Humanitarianism* (University of Pennsylvania Press, 2016).

30. Of the many elements that shaped popular health, three were most important: Christian Base Communities (Comunidades Eclesiales de Base [CEBs]), informed by libera-

tion theology; the University of El Salvador (Universidad de El Salvador [UES]) medical school and professional medicine; and internationalist physicians. Churchwomen brought medicines along with food to CEBs and taught sanitation and nutrition in literacy classes. The influence of university-trained practitioners expanded around 1980 when growing numbers of faculty and students joined lay catechists after the military invaded and occupied the UES medical and dental schools. See Smith-Nonini, *Healing the Body Politic*, 49–51, 54–58; see also Consejo de Mujeres Misioneras por la Paz, *La semilla de cayó en tierra fértil* (Consejo de Mujeres Misioneras por la Paz, 1996).

31. John Hess, "Collective Experience, Synthetic Forms: El Salvador's Radio Venceremos," and John Mraz, "Santiago Alvarez: From Dramatic Form to Direct Cinema," in *The Social Documentary in Latin America*, ed. Julianne Burton (University of Pittsburgh Press, 1990).

32. Sistema Radio Venceremos, *La salud al frente* (Museo de la Palabra y la Imagen [MUPI]), n.d.

33. Sistema Radio Venceremos, *La salud al frente*. See also Michael Terry and Laura Turiano, "Brigadistas and Revolutionaries: Health and Social Justice in El Salvador," in *Comrades in Health*, ed. Anne-Emanuelle Birn and Theodore M. Brown (Rutgers University Press, 2013), 226. On Chalatenango, see Smith-Nonini, *Healing the Body Politic*, 6.

34. Sistema Radio Venceremos, *La salud al frente*.

35. A USAID-funded health survey cited by Sandy Smith-Nonini reported that about half of all illnesses and a quarter of all deaths in children were caused by diarrhea and intestinal disorders. The same report found that "poor rural sewage facilities and lack of potable water were the leading contributors to child morbidity." Another 18 percent of childhood illnesses were caused by preventable respiratory infections. See Asociación Demográfica Salvadoreña and US Centers for Disease Control, *Encuesta Nacional de Salud Familiar* (FESAL-88), quoted in Smith-Nonini, *Healing the Body Politic*, 34.

36. Comandancia General del FMLN, *Los 15 principios del combatiente guerrillero* (El Salvador, 1985). See also John L. Hammond, "Popular Education in the Guerrilla Army," *Human Organization* 55, no. 4 (Winter 1996): 436–55.

37. This estimate does not include the numerous lisiados who entered Cuba without documentation or Red Cross intervention. On Cuban medical diplomacy, see Julie Feinsilver, "Cuba as a 'World Medical Power': The Politics of Symbolism," *Latin American Research Review* 24, no. 2 (1989): 1–34; John M. Kirk and H. Michael Erisman, *Cuban Medical Internationalism: Origins, Evolution, and Goals* (Palgrave Macmillan, 2009); Cheasty Anderson, "South-South Cooperation as a Cold War Tonic," in Birn and Necochea López, *Peripheral Nerve*. Salvadoran lisiados occasionally required surgery in Moscow, a subject that historians have not addressed; see "El Salvador: La deuda con los Lisiados de guerra," *El Proceso México* (Mexico City), February 1, 2003.

38. See Vrana, "All the Love: Transnational Youth and Disability in El Salvador's Civil War," *Social History* 48, no. 1 (2023): 162–83. The 26 July rehabilitation camp housed combatants from the ERP and the FPL. Bob Whitney, a Canadian solidarity activist who visited the encampment and a hospital in Havana for more serious cases, recalled that serious injuries and the need to heal quickly diminished partisan divisions. Bob Whitney, interview with the author, March 6, 2021.

39. Thanks to Gabriela Soto Laveaga for this insight.

40. Sistema Radio Venceremos, *Todo el amor* (MUPI, n.d.).

41. A single word, "lisiado," is used throughout the film and in combatants' and veterans' writings to describe both being wounded and being disabled.

42. Lisiados planted and tended gardens and raised farm animals in an effort to become self-sufficient and less reliant on Cuban hospitality. Bob Whitney, interview with author.

43. See Sharon L. Snyder and David T. Mitchell, *Cultural Locations of Disability* (University of Chicago Press, 2006), 173; Catalin Brylla and Helen Hughes, eds., *Documentary and Disability* (Palgrave Macmillan, 2017).

44. Wool, *After War*.

45. Sistema Radio Venceremos, *Todo el amor*.

46. Two famous revolutionary doctors—Salvador Allende and Ernesto "Che" Guevara—credited medical training and work among debilitated and disabled people as turning points in their developing radical consciousness. But medicine was often a conservative field. Some students and faculty at the UES became involved in the revolutionary left, while others supported the military.

47. Eduardo Espinoza, *Relatos de la guerra* (Secretaría de Arte y Cultura, 2007), 32–33.

48. Espinoza, *Relatos de la guerra*, 22.

49. Espinoza, *Relatos de la guerra*, 22.

50. Espinoza, *Relatos de la guerra*, 51.

51. Espinoza, *Relatos de la guerra*, 58–59.

52. Espinoza, 62–63. In fact, Espinoza had already been imprisoned twice.

53. Metzi, *The People's Remedy*, 152.

54. Charles Clements, *Witness to War: An American Doctor in El Salvador* (Bantam Books, 1984), 56.

55. Metzi, *The People's Remedy*, 152.

56. Clements, *Witness to War*, 118.

57. Dr. Charlie Clements, interview with the author, May 20, 2024. Clements published *Witness to War*, embarked on speaking tours, cofounded the Salvadoran Medical Relief Fund, and organized countless delegations of Vietnam veterans to El Salvador; meanwhile the US government sent Vietnam veterans to advise the Salvadoran army.

58. Clements, *Witness to War*, 7, 9–10.

59. He would go on to direct Medical Aid to El Salvador's Prosthetics Project. "The Rambo Antidote," *Mother Jones* (January 1989): 30.

60. *Central American Studies and Temporary Relief Act of 1987: Hearings on H.R. 618 and H.R. 1409 Before the House Subcommittee on Rules of the Committee on Rules*, 100th Cong. 98 (1987).

61. Douglas Imbrogno, interview with the author, March 30, 2024; Clements, interview with the author, May 20, 2024. See also "Land Mines Take Toll in El Salvador," *Washington Post*, September 16, 1985; Douglas Imbrogno, "Hero of the Open Heart: The Long, Strange Trip of Dave Evans' Notable Life," WestVirginiaville.com, August 4, 2021, https://westvirginiaville.com/2021/08/dave-evans/.

62. Imbrogno, "Hero of the Open Heart."

63. Metzi, *The People's Remedy*, 128–29.

64. Metzi, *The People's Remedy*, 151.

65. Metzi, *The People's Remedy*, 135–36. In Guazapa, Clements became a liaison for the ICRC. See Clements, *Witness to War*, 166–168, 173, 182. Countless clandestine avenues for lisiados' evacuation to Nicaragua and Cuba remain protected information among the compas.

66. Metzi, *The People's Remedy*, 153–54.

67. Metzi, *The People's Remedy*, 152.

68. Metzi, *The People's Remedy*, 156–57.

69. ALGES (Asociación de Lisiados de Guerra de El Salvador), "Homenaje," Facebook, posted April 28, 2015, https://www.facebook.com/alges89/posts/804301442980340/.

70. Leo Gabriel, *Victoria* (MUPI, 1991). On rehabilitation programs for laborers under revolutionary governments, see Jeff D. Grischow, "Kwame Nkrumah, Disability, and Rehabilitation in Ghana, 1957–66," *Journal of African History* 52 (2011): 179–99. On deaf culture in the USSR, see Susan Burch, "Transcending Revolutions: The Tsars, the Soviets, and Deaf Culture," *Journal of Social History* 34, no. 2 (Winter 2000): 393–401; and Claire L. Shaw, *Deaf in the USSR: Marginality, Community, and Soviet Identity, 1917–1991* (Cornell University Press, 2017).

71. Gabriel, *Victoria*.

72. ALGES, "Contando La Historia . . . Israel Quintanilla," October 9, 2007, http://www.alges.org.sv/contando-la-historia-israel-quintanilla.

73. Government of El Salvador and FMLN, "Peace Agreement," January 16, 1992.

74. Asamblea Legislativa de El Salvador, Artículo 29, "Ley de Beneficio para la Protección de los Lisiados y Discapacitados a Consecuencia del Conflicto Armado," December 13, 1992.

75. A similar process occurred in Nicaragua. See Stephen Meyers, "History and Divisions in Nicaragua's Disability Rights Movement," *Current History* 121, no. 832 (February 2022): 63–68.

76. Sprenkels, *After Insurgency*, 376n9.

77. ALGES, "Entre la guerra y la paz: Testimonio de una vida," April 3, 2008, http://www.alges.org.sv/entre-la-guerra-y-la-paz-testimonio-de-una-vida.

78. ALGES, "Entre la guerra y la paz."

79. See Smith-Nonini, *Healing the Body Politic*.

80. On veteran organizing, see Neil J. Diamant, "Veterans, Organization, and the Politics of Martial Citizenship in China," *Journal of East Asian Studies* 8, no. 1 (2008): 119–58.

81. ALGES, "Contando la historia."

With Us, Not About Us

Julie Avril Minich

Reading *Histories of Disability in Latin America*, I thought about the literary critic Kandice Chuh and her irritation with the scholarly compulsion to identify what objects of knowledge—texts, works of art, historical documents, fields of study—are *about* (in other words, the everyday, uncritical work of categorization we perform whenever we offer input on doctoral exam lists, create new course titles, or propose new faculty lines). Ordinary as it is, this impulse, which Chuh calls *aboutness*, "buttresses the institutional forms of knowledge and ignorance that bear the organizational architecture of bourgeois liberalism in ways that produce or intensify a kind of silo mentality that holds knowledge formations apart from each other."[1] Recalling Chuh's manifesto against aboutness, I realized that what I love most about *Histories of Disability in Latin America* is that it's not about disability. Instead, it's a book that participates in the creation of disability history without reifying the aboutness of disability studies. That is, this volume requires us to rethink disability history: whom we imagine as its main protagonists, where we expect to find its archives, which conceptual frameworks we understand as most suitable for its interpretation.

When I first encountered disability studies as a graduate student in the early 2000s, two things happened. The first is that—like many scholars exploring disability studies for the first time—I realized the truth of Douglas Baynton's famous assertion that "disability is everywhere . . . once you begin looking for it."[2] This was profoundly transformative for me as a literary critic: Texts whose interpretations I believed I had exhausted took on exciting nuances and unexpected aesthetic possibilities when examined through the lens of disability. Every aspect of my work suddenly opened to new ideas.

At the same time, however, something else seemed to close down these intellectual opportunities: a need to write about disability *in the right ways*—that is, in ways deemed conducive to the aims of a disability rights movement largely focused on securing recognition on the terms of Western capitalist nation-state formations.[3] I remember nervously telling a well-known disability scholar (someone I desperately wanted to impress) about my dissertation only to be confronted with the question: "But how many of the authors you write about are *actually* disabled?" My response—that many of the writers did not call themselves disabled but wrote about profoundly disabling experiences—did not seem to inspire further interest in my work.

What I did not know to say at the time was that many of the writers included in my dissertation—US-based Latinx writers—do not call themselves disabled because disability is not an identity available to all people in the same way. In their introduction to this volume, editors David Carey Jr. and Heather Vrana offer terms like *rusipanik Ajaw*, *ruloq'ob'al Ajaw*, *Huihuilaxpol*, *aoccan niyehuati*, and *cecepoac* that cannot be translated directly as "disability" and that predate the colonial constitution of what we now call "Latin America" but that nevertheless continue to inform the way social value is distributed among different bodyminds throughout the region. Similarly, Sami Schalk offers a list of reasons why cultural workers who have played a pivotal role in the development of US-based Black disability politics may not themselves identify as disabled: "These reasons may include lack of access to official disability diagnoses, services, and resources (in other words, not being legally or medically recognized as disabled); the traumatic or oppressive circumstances of their disablement; internalized ableism; identification with disability-specific rather than disability-general communities (i.e., Deaf, autistic, Mad, etc.); the potential for a disability label to further their marginalization; or identity development in communities of color and families of origin in which politicized or celebratory concepts of disability did not exist."[4]

As Julie Livingston has observed, use of the term "disability" often implies the adoption of an identity that is not necessarily embraced by all people who experience physical, cognitive, or emotional impairments; disability is "both biologically grounded and socially parsed, an umbrella term that denotes different things in different places and at different times."[5] Because disability designates an identification that does not travel easily into all cultural and historical contexts, Livingston famously adopted the term "debility" to address how "impairment and disfigurement arise out of particular junctures—the rise of mining and mining accidents, for example—and thus it gives us insight into a people's historical experience and changing assumptions about personhood and self."[6] Debility has, in turn, been widely adopted both in and outside disability studies, particularly since the publication of Jasbir Puar's influential 2017 book, *The Right to Maim: Debility, Capacity, Disability*, which places disability and debility into direct conversation.[7] But the term has also been a source of controversy among disability scholars, with some prominent voices in the field asking whether the term "debility" in fact decenters disabled people.[8]

Even scholars (like me) who primarily use the term "disability" have noted for some time the need to think beyond paradigms developed for disability scholarship by (primarily) white scholars working in the global north. Such thinking requires taking seriously the possibility that the scholarship we seek may not, in fact, be about disability—or, at least, not about disability in the forms we have been taught to recognize it or the terms with which we have been taught to describe it. The writings of José Carlos Mariátegui, the disabled Peruvian Marxist philosopher discussed at length in chapter 2 by Paulo Drinot, are not generally considered to be about disability—but how does our understanding of Marxist theory change when we consider that its primary intellectual architect in Latin America was disabled? And how does our understanding of disability change when we examine it through a lens informed by Latin American Marxist philosophy? If the public health effects of an earthquake in colonial Guatemala (like those discussed by Martha Few in chapter 7) do not readily conform to contemporary diagnostic categories for illness, let alone legible disabled identities, can scholarship about the effects of that earthquake nonetheless help us to understand the historical factors that have contributed to the social construction of disability?

As I remember the scholar who asked me whether the writers examined in my dissertation were disabled, I do understand the importance of the question; I would link that question to the slogan "Nothing about us without us." Although it has been used by a range of social justice activists, "Nothing about us without us" is most closely associated with US disability activism and denotes a core tenet of the US disability rights movement. It responds to a fundamental injustice: The fact that dominant cultures, across the Americas and beyond, are often the product of profoundly ableist laws, institutions, belief systems, and aesthetic representations. Because the creation and dissemination of literature, art, archives, scholarship, and policy have historically been much more available to nondisabled people than to disabled people, these entities have often furthered the social and political exclusion of disabled people. In other words, when people who neither experience impairment nor identify as disabled make art, scholarship, and policy about the bodyminds and lives of chronically ill, impaired, aging, or injured people, the objects they produce often cause real damage. At the same time, "Nothing about us without us" poses questions that must be addressed. Who is "us"? How do we know? What are the problems—even potentially the violence—of identifying a woman who experienced *epidémica de la constitución* in the aftermath of the 1773 Guatemala earthquake as disabled when writing about her in the present—and thus including her in the "us" of disability studies? What are the problems of *not* identifying her as such—and thus excluding her from the "us" of disability studies? Over the past 15 years, there has been a flourishing of scholarship—by people like Sony Coráñez Bolton, Mel Y. Chen, Nirmala Erevelles, Eunjung Kim, Jina B. Kim, Therí Alyce Pickens, Sami Schalk, and Cynthia Wu (to name a few)[9]—that puts much-needed pressure on the "us" in "Nothing about us without us," questioning its racial, sexual, and national exclusions. Certainly, *Histories of Disability in Latin America* participates in this work as well, as there remains very little work in the field that centers Latin American perspectives.

But perhaps even more radically, this book inspires us to place the "about" of "Nothing about us without us" under new scrutiny. In their introduction to this volume, Carey and Vrana are scrupulously attentive to their own scholarly formation as historians of Latin America and careful not to claim the objective of offering a major intervention in disability studies: "Even as we recognize that focusing on Latin America decenters North American European perspectives and content that have long dominated disability studies, our primary goal is not to make an internal intervention in disability studies but rather to deploy and incorporate disability studies in Latin American history."[10] I read this statement as an ethical recognition of the "Nothing about us without us" imperative, a gesture of respect for the expertise of trained disability scholars.

At the same time, one of the things I find most invigorating about *Histories of Disability in Latin America* is that most of its contributors were *not* trained as disability scholars. For me, one of the most exciting things about working in disability studies now is the fact that it is seen no longer as a niche field relevant only to those who identify as disabled but instead as a body of knowledge that illuminates larger systems of normativity. And just as I believe, fervently, that Latin American history (a field to which my own work is only adjacent, in terms of both discipline and geopolitical location) stands to benefit greatly from attending to disability scholarship, I also believe that disability studies will gain from more robust knowledge of Latin American history. Without dismissing legitimate concerns about scholars uninterested in disability justice who seek to cash in on the "cultural capital" of disability studies,[11] I am eager for more avenues for conversation across field and discipline. Reading this book, I certainly recognized that some of its contributors brought more knowledge of disability studies to their work than others, but all of the pieces struck me as starting points for ongoing discussion. Furthermore, it is undeniable that I read this book at a moment when the academic enterprise in the United States and around the world is under dire threat from authoritarian regimes aiming precisely to close down the kind of conversation it stages.

Perhaps *Histories of Disability in Latin America* isn't so much a book *about* us as a book *with* us. In a moment when scholarship aimed at forging new intellectual and political alliances among marginalized and oppressed people is under direct threat, we might do well to think about our work in such terms: not "What is this work about?" but "Who is this work with?" More than a decade ago, Kandice Chuh offered a critique of aboutness at a moment when neoliberal multiculturalism dominated higher education curricula and functioned as a means of managing difference within both the university and the larger society; I write at a moment when the very presence of "the studies" (ethnic studies, area studies, gender studies, queer studies, disability studies) is under direct attack and the false inclusion of multiculturalism is replaced by the stark exclusion of white nationalism. Yet I find her critique of aboutness more salient than ever as I think about the future of knowledge created with the aim of contesting power. Chuh writes: "As long as institutionality itself is the horizon of knowledge politics, as was or became for the interdisciplines established in the post–civil rights era, the radicalism that drove that establishment and demanded curricular transformation as part of a wholesale remaking of the social totality could not be sustained. In this light . . . there is an urgency to identifying and elaborating ways of contesting the arrangements of knowledge."[12] If the radicalism at the heart of our fields—Latin American history and disability studies most prominently in this case, but also queer theory, Latinx literature, Marxist philosophy, and so many others—was contained by our institutions long before the rise of the current regime, how do we return to that radicalism? My answer in this moment is to make knowledge *with* one another: across institutions, across disciplines, across fields, as well as across lines of gender, race, nation, (dis)-ability, and class. Our survival, and the survival of radical knowledge, depends on it.

NOTES

1. Kandice Chuh, "It's Not About Anything," *Social Text* 32, no. 4 (Winter 2014): 132.

2. Douglas Baynton, "Disability and the Justification of Inequality in American History," in *The New Disability History: American Perspectives*, ed. Paul K. Longmore and Lauri Umansky (New York University Press 2001), 51.

3. For readers wanting to pursue this line of argumentation further, Jina B. Kim's brief discussion of disability justice and its crucial distinction from disability rights in a recent state-of-the-field essay is the most concise, legible explanation of the limits of disability rights. See Kim, "Disability in an Age of Fascism," *American Quarterly* 72, no. 1 (March 2020): 265–76.

4. Sami Schalk, *Black Disability Politics* (Duke University Press, 2022), 13–14.

5. Julie Livingston, *Debility and the Moral Imagination in Botswana* (Indiana University Press, 2005), 7.

6. Livingston, *Debility and the Moral Imagination in Botswana*, 2.

7. Jasbir K. Puar, *The Right to Maim: Debility, Capacity, Disability* (Duke University Press, 2017).

8. David T. Mitchell and Sharon L. Snyder, "Is the Study of Debility Akin to Disability Studies Without Disability?" *GLQ: A Journal of Lesbian and Gay Studies* 25, no. 4 (October 2019): 663–66.

9. Sony Coráñez Bolton, *Crip Colony: Mestizaje, US Imperialism, and the Queer Politics of Disability in the Philippines* (Duke University Press, 2023); Mel Y. Chen, *Intoxicated: Race, Disability, and Chemical Intimacy Across Empire* (Duke University Press, 2023); Nirmala Erevelles, *Disability and Difference in Global Contexts: Enabling a Transformative Body Politic* (Palgrave Macmillan, 2011); Eunjung Kim, *Curative Violence: Rehabilitating Disability, Gender, and Sexuality in Modern Korea* (Duke University Press, 2017); Jina B. Kim, *Care at the End of the World: Dreaming of Infrastructure in Crip-of-Color Writing* (Duke University Press, 2025); Therí Alyce Pickens, *Black Madness : Mad Blackness* (Duke University Press, 2019); Sami Schalk, *Bodyminds Reimagined: (Dis)Ability, Race, and Gender in Black Women's Speculative Fiction* (Duke University Press, 2018); Cynthia Wu, *Chang and Eng Reconnected: The Original Siamese Twins in American Culture* (Temple University Press, 2012).

10. Carey and Vrana, introduction to this volume, pp. 8–9.

11. Alyson Patsavas, "Disability Studies Gains Cultural Capital? And Now What?," *Feminist Wire*, November 22, 2013, https://thefeministwire.com/2013/11/disabilities-studies-gains-cultural-capital-and-now-what/.

12. Chuh, "It's Not About Anything," 129.

Acknowledgments

First, Ahmed Ragab is a dream editor. His enthusiasm for this project never wavered. We have both sought to be more like Ahmed in our writing and editorial work.

The Johns Hopkins University Center for Black, Brown, and Queer Studies supported our dreams of holding a gathering in summer 2022 to discuss a shared set of readings and workshop chapter drafts. Elizabeth O'Brien offered crucial on-site assistance during that gathering and we remain grateful to her for this labor and Ana María Castillo shared reflections and insights that grounded our work there. A Loyola University Center for the Humanities grant generously funded indexing and photograph permissions, and funds from the UF Research Foundation supported additional photograph permissions.

Phoebe Oathout, Jennifer D'Urso, and Robert Brown at Johns Hopkins University Press ushered us and this project through its final stages. In earlier moments in the project's gestation, outstanding scholars in disability history and disability studies shared with us their excitement and thoughtful critique; we thank you, Stefanie Hunt-Kennedy, Julie Minich, Mike Rembis, and Sara Scalenghe. We also thank the three generous scholars who served as anonymous peer reviewers for our manuscript. Maeve Hill helped us track down, organize, and format obscure citations and sources. Marianne Quijano, Thomas Miller, Charles Davidson, Allen Wells, Matt Mulcahy, Martha Few, and Heather Gonyeau offered helpful comments on the introduction.

Finally, we thank our contributors, many of whom gamely embraced the challenge of writing in new fields or using new archival and oral sources.

Heather Vrana thanks the Stanford Humanities Center for the most precious gift of time and the Fellows of the 2022–23 academic year for important conversations at a critical juncture in this project, especially Isabela Fraga, Elspeth Iralu, Christy Pichichero, Eric Plemons, Judith Rodríguez, and Anna Toledano. Martha Few, Julie Gibbings, Jessica Harland-Jacobs, Kelda Jamison, David Kazanjian, Anne Whiteside, and Sofie Williams deserve much gratitude for engaging in many hours of yapping about the project and about disability history in general. Coediting can be notoriously challenging, but David Carey Jr. kept the book moving forward with so much kindness and enthusiasm that it never felt like a struggle even when we faced difficult things. Finally, thank you to Mary, Jon, and Anna Vrana, my first teachers of the many meanings of disability.

David Carey Jr. thanks Martha Few for the invitation to engage in the manuscript with her Latin American ethnohistory graduate students, who suggested refreshing ways to analyze the material and frame its significance. Undergraduate students in my History of Science, Medicine, and Health course at Loyola similarly expanded my sense of how to maximize the accessibility of the findings and narratives. In a testament to the importance of in-person exchanges, the idea for this volume was hatched when Heather Vrana graciously accepted an invitation to share their research and scholarship at Loyola University in February 2020. I have been enriched by Heather's brilliance and thoughtfulness ever since. As we were in the final stages of preparing the manuscript to submit to the press, I was struck by a box truck while riding my bicycle. The accident and its repercussions—both physical and psychological—reminded me that most of us are at best only temporarily able-bodied and -minded. I am especially grateful to my family, friends, colleagues, and medical professionals—too many to name—who provided support and hope when I needed them most. As always, Sarah, Ava, and Kate continue to inspire my pursuits as they chart their own paths toward integrating intellectual curiosity and social justice.

Contributors

David Carey Jr. holds the Doehler Chair in History at Loyola University Maryland. He received his PhD in Latin American studies at Tulane University and his BA in Political Science at the University of Notre Dame. In addition to writing more than 40 peer-reviewed articles and essays, he is the author of *I Ask for Justice: Maya Women, Dictators, and Crime in Guatemala, 1898–1944* (2013), which was the co-recipient of the 2015 Latin American Studies Association Bryce Wood Book Award. His most recent books are *Health in the Highlands: Indigenous and Scientific Medicine in Guatemala and Ecuador* (2023) and *Oral History in Latin America: Unlocking the Spoken Archive* (2017). He has authored three other books and has edited or coedited three volumes. Among other entities, the Fulbright Program, American Philosophical Society, Wenner-Gren Foundation, and John Simon Guggenheim Foundation have supported his research and scholarship. He also coedited *Untold Truths: Exposing Slavery and Its Legacies at Loyola University Maryland* (2024). He is a coeditor (with Elizabeth O'Brien) of the series Bodies and Ecologies: Histories of Health, Environment, and Medicine in Latin America and the Caribbean with University of Nebraska Press and the editor of the Critical Latin America series with Brill.

Paulo Drinot is Professor of Latin American History at University College London. He is the author of *The Allure of Labor: Workers, Race, and the Making of the Peruvian State* (2011) and *The Sexual Question: A History of Prostitution in Peru, 1850s–1950s* (2020), both also published in Spanish translation, as well as editor or coeditor of several volumes, in English and Spanish, on various aspects of Peruvian and Latin American history. His latest coedited volume (with Alberto Vergara), *Modern Peru: A New History*, was published in late 2025. He has served as coeditor of the *Journal of Latin American Studies* and is a recipient of a Leverhulme Trust Major Research Fellowship. He is currently working on a biography of José Carlos Mariátegui.

Martha Few is Liberal Arts Professor of Latin American History and Gender, Women's, and Sexuality Studies at Pennsylvania State University. Her research concentrates on the histories of Indigenous peoples during

Spanish colonial rule in Guatemala, Central America, and southern Mexico through the lenses of medicine and public health, gender and sexuality, environmental history, and human-animal studies. Her recent books include *For All of Humanity: Mesoamerican and Colonial Medicine in Enlightenment Guatemala* (2015) and (with Adam Warren and Zeb Tortorici) *Baptism Through Incision: The Postmortem Cesarean Operation in the Spanish Empire* (2020). Few was Senior Editor of the *Hispanic American Historical Review* from 2017 to 2022.

JULIE AVRIL MINICH (she/her/hers) is Professor of English and Mexican American and Latina/o Studies at the University of Texas at Austin, where she teaches courses in Latinx literary and cultural studies, gender and sexuality studies, and disability studies. Her scholarly articles are published or forthcoming in a number of journals and anthologies, including *Feminist Formations, GLQ, Modern Fiction Studies*, and the *Journal of Literary and Cultural Disability Studies*. Minich is the author of *Radical Health: Unwellness, Care, and Latinx Expressive Culture* (Duke University Press, 2023) and *Accessible Citizenships: Disability, Nation, and the Cultural Politics of Greater Mexico* (Temple University Press, 2014; winner of the 2013–14 MLA Prize in United States Latina and Latino and Chicana and Chicano Literary and Cultural Studies). She also coedited, with Mel Y. Chen, Alison Kafer, and Eunjung Kim, *Crip Genealogies* (Duke University Press, 2023).

ELIZABETH O'BRIEN is Assistant Professor of History at the University of California, Los Angeles. Her first book is *Surgery and Salvation: The Roots of Reproductive Injustice in Mexico, 1770–1940* (2023). Her research has been published in *The Lancet, Endeavour*, the *Washington Post*, the *Journal of Women's History, Women's History Review*, and *Mexican Studies/Estudios Mexicanos*; has been funded by the National Endowment for the Humanities, National Science Foundation, Fulbright Program, and American Council of Learned Societies/Mellon; and has received prizes from the Latin American Studies Association, Rocky Mountain Council for Latin American Studies, Western Association of Women Historians, History of Science Society's Forum for the History of Human Science, and online publication *Nursing Clio*.

BIANCA PREMO is Distinguished University Professor of Latin American History at Florida International University in Miami. She has published in an array of fields, including the history of childhood, gender, the law, and temporality. Her works on childhood have appeared in the *American Histor-*

ical Review and other journals, and her books include *Children of the Father King: Youth, Authority, and Legal Minority in Lima, 1650–1820* (2005) and the coedited volume *Raising an Empire: Children and Childhood in Early Modern Iberia and Latin America* (2007). Supported by the American Council of Learned Societies, the National Endowment for the Humanities, and a John S. Guggenheim Fellowship, she is currently writing a book on a child mother in twentieth- and twenty-first century Peru and the ethics of history.

HEATHER VRANA is Associate Professor of Modern Latin America in the Department of History at the University of Florida. Vrana is the author of the monograph *This City Belongs to You: A History of Student Activism in Guatemala* (2017) and the anthology *Anti-Colonial Texts from Central American Student Movements, 1929–1983* (2017) and coeditor (with Julie Gibbings) of *Out of the Shadow: Revisiting the Revolution from Post-Peace Guatemala* (2020). Vrana's research on revolutions, student and social movements, disability, and memory has appeared in, among other journals, the *American Historical Review, Hispanic American Historical Review, Radical History Review,* and *Journal of Genocide Research.* Vrana's current research examines the politicization of health before, during, and after El Salvador's civil war, locating disability as a cause for and consequence of the conflict, and an axis around which the guerrilla, government, military, and international actors promoted their interests. This research has been funded by the Consortium for the History of Science, Technology, and Medicine and the Stanford Humanities Center. Vrana is currently the editor for history of the *Latin American Research Review.*

ADAM WARREN is Williams Family Professor of History and Chair of the Department of History at the University of Washington. A specialist in colonial and republican Peru and the history of science, medicine, and disability, he is interested in how medical and scientific research have been used to explain social inequalities and frame projects of population reform and control in the Andes, and how ordinary people have shaped and challenged these practices of knowledge making. He is the author of *Medicine and Politics in Colonial Peru: Population Growth and the Bourbon Reforms* (2010); coauthor (with Martha Few and Zeb Tortorici) of *Baptism Through Incision: The Postmortem Cesarean Operation in the Spanish Empire* (2020); and coeditor (with Julia Rodriguez and Stephen Casper) of *Empire, Colonialism, and the Human Sciences: Troubling Encounters in the Americas and Pacific* (2024). His articles have appeared in the *Bulletin of the History of Medicine* and *História,*

Ciências, Saúde—Manguinhos, among other journals. His ongoing research includes a broader history of the cesarean operation, fetal baptism, and the politics of childbirth in the Spanish Empire and a book project focused on the history of disability and slavery in late colonial Peru and Río de la Plata.

Barbara Weinstein is Silver Professor of History at New York University and a past president of the American Historical Association. She previously taught at Vanderbilt University, Stony Brook University, and the University of Maryland and has been a visiting lecturer at the Hebrew University of Jerusalem, the Universidade Estadual de Campinas, and the École des Hautes Études en Sciences Sociales. Most of her research has explored the social history and political economy of postcolonial Brazil. Her publications include *The Amazon Rubber Boom, 1850–1920* (1983), *For Social Peace in Brazil: Industrialists and the Remaking of the Working Class in São Paulo, 1920–1964* (1996), and *The Color of Modernity: São Paulo and the Making of Race and Nation in Brazil* (2015). She is coeditor, with Ricardo López-Pedreros, of *The Making of the Middle Class: Toward a Transnational History* (2012) and an editor of the Radical Perspectives series for Duke University Press. She has served as senior editor of the *Hispanic American Historical Review* and *International Labor and Working-Class History*. Her research has received support from the John Simon Guggenheim Foundation, the Radcliffe Institute for Advanced Study, the National Endowment for the Humanities, and the Cullman Center for Scholars and Writers of the New York Public Library, where she began the research for her current project, an intellectual biography of Frank Tannenbaum, a pioneering scholar of labor, criminology, the Mexican Revolution, and race relations in the Americas.

K. Eliza Williamson is a medical anthropologist who studies disability, caregiving, and reproduction in Latin America, primarily Brazil. Her current book manuscript is based on a decade of ethnographic research with families affected by Zika in Bahia, in the Brazilian Northeast, and she has also examined the implementation of maternal health policy that aims to "humanize" childbirth in Brazil's public healthcare system. Eliza is currently a Postdoctoral Associate in global health humanities and social medicine at the Duke Global Health Institute at Duke University. Her work has been published in *Cultural Anthropology*, *Medical Anthropology Quarterly*, *Anthropology and Medicine*, *Space and Culture*, and *Interface—Comunicação, Saúde, Educação*, among other journals and edited volumes. Eliza's research has been supported by funding from the Wenner-Gren Foundation and the Fulbright-

Hays program, in addition to other grants and fellowships, and she is a recipient of the Association for Feminist Anthropology dissertation award. She has served on the Disability and Accessibility Committee of the Brazilian Anthropological Association, collaborating with colleagues on public-facing educational materials on anti-ableism, and she is currently a member of the steering committee of the Disability Research Interest Group of the American Anthropological Association.

EMILY XIAO holds a doctor of medicine degree from Johns Hopkins University as well as a bachelor of science, with a major in history, from Yale University. She is currently a Pediatrics Resident in the Baylor College of Medicine. She was awarded the W. Barry Wood Research Award for a podium presentation of her research on the anencephaly cluster in Brownsville, Texas.

Index

Page locators in *italics* indicate figures.

Aase, John (physician), 101

ableism, 8, 87, 88–89n4, 197n4; in archives,
13–17; biorisk, language of, 99; debilitation
produced by, 96; ethnonational stereotypes
reified by, 94; as ideology, 179; systemic,
139, 145, 150n32

abortion, 100–103, 124n35; disability inclusion language co-opted by opponents, 103;
eradication of disability through, 100–101;
and family cap provision, 125n44; flexible
stance for severe abnormalities, 101; "late-
term," 103; respectability linked with, 100.
See also anencephalic births; pregnancy

aboutness, 260

absent presence, 19

Academy of Medicine (Peru), 29

Adler, Miguel, *64*, 80

affective responses to nonnormative bodies,
104–5, 122

African diaspora, x, 2, 9

agency of disabled people, 4, 11, 18, 30, 99

Aguirre, Manuel de (enslaved man), 171–72

Alianza Popular Revolucionaria Americana
(APRA), 61, 71–72

Allende, Salvador, 258n46

Amauta (magazine), 58, 83

Amazon, "scientific colonization" of, 33

Andis, Anne, 115, 117

anencephalic births: abortion decisions,
100–103; activism around, 94, 109–10,
115–17; anthropomorphization of anencephaly, 108; birth defects registry, 18, 94,
115–17; care and kinship in relation to
fetus, 103–6, 117, 122; dehumanizing terms
used, 104–5; environmental factors ignored
in government studies, 108–11; as epidemiologic "mystery," 94; fetal remains, handling of, 103–4; folic acid distribution
campaign, 94, 118–21, 130n152, 130n156;
literature discussion, 95–97; media portrayals of, 93–94, 97, 98, 100–111, 115–16,

121; Mexican-origin mothers blamed for,
94, 97–99, 116, 120; paternalism of health
care providers, 106; simplified public
understanding of, 120; as term, 106. *See
also* border; neural tube defects (NTD);
toxicity

anticolonial politicization of disability,
234–35, 252

Anzaldúa, Gloria, 95

aoccan niyehuati, 1, 9, 261

Archbishopric Archive (Lima, Peru), 153

archives: ableism in, 13–17; accessible presses,
16–17; Ecuador, 181; ethical issues, 14–15,
156; few female-authored sources, 210;
material artifacts, 16; Maya-language
dictionaries and manuscript, 222–23;
medical records, 14–15; oral history, 15;
Peru, 153, 161; sacred and special community knowledge and artifacts, preserva-
tion of, 16; silences in, 156, 181, 195, 207;
violence perpetuated by, 14–16

Arras, John, 100

Asociación de Lisiados de Guerra de El Salvador (ALGES), 253–54

Asociación Salvadoreña de Lisiados y
Discapacitados de Guerra (ASALDIG), 253

Associação Abraço a Microcefalia ("I Embrace
Microcephaly" Association), 134

Associações de Pais e Amigos de Pessoas
Excepcionais (Brazil), 11

Atherton, Martin, 15

Audiencia of Guatemala, 206, 208, 209; *See
also* Protomedicato

Austin American-Statesman, 102

Ávalos y Porras, Manuel, 214, 216–18, 220–22,
227n48

"avidez" (emotional avidity), 42, *43*

Baatz, Christa (Victoria), 249–50

Bahia, Brazil. *See* Zika virus; Zika virus,
children with